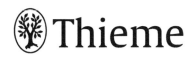

Practical MR Mammography

High-Resolution MRI of the Breast

Uwe Fischer, MD

Professor
Women's Health Care Center
Göttingen, Germany

2nd edition

1347 illustrations

Thieme
Stuttgart · New York

Library of Congress Cataloging-in-Publication Data
Fischer, Uwe, MD.
   [Atlas der MR-Mammographie. English]
   Practical MR mammography : high-resolution MRI of the breast / Uwe Fischer.
—2nd ed.
      p. ; cm.
   This book is an authorized translation of the 2nd German edition published and
copyrighted 2010 by Georg Thieme Verlag, Stuttgart. Title of the German edition:
Atlas der MR-Mammographie. Hochauflösende Mamma-MRT.—T.p. verso.
   Includes bibliographical references and index.
      Translated from German.
   ISBN 978-3-13-132032-2 (hardback : alk. paper)
   I. Title.
   [DNLM: 1. Mammography—methods. 2. Breast Neoplasms—diagnosis. 3. Mag-
netic Resonance Imaging—methods. WP 815]
   618.1'907548--dc23
                        2012002156

Translator: Susanne Luftner-Nagel, MD, Göttingen, Germany

Illustrators: Christiane and Dr. Michael von Solodkoff, Neckargemünd, Germany

1st Chinese edition 2010
1st English edition 2004
1st German edition 2000
2nd German edition 2010

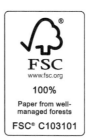

© 2012 Georg Thieme Verlag KG
Rüdigerstraße 14, 70469 Stuttgart, Germany
http://www.thieme.de
Thieme Medical Publishers, Inc., 333 Seventh Avenue,
New York, NY 10001, USA
http://www.thieme.com

Cover design: Thieme Publishing Group
Typesetting by primustype Robert Hurler GmbH, Notzingen, Germany
Printed in the United States of America
by King Printing Co., Inc.
ISBN 978-3-13-132032-2
eISBN 978-3-13-167032-8
                                                123456

Preface

Eight years after the first edition of this book was published, almost nothing is the same as it once was. The idea that publishing the second edition would only entail updating some data and replacing a few MR images has proven to be a great misconception. Breast MRI has experienced dramatic advances during the last 8 years, making it now the most reliable breast examination technique in the early diagnosis of breast cancer. The essential steps that have made this advancement possible pertain predominantly to the increasing capacity of the whole-body magnet, currently making possible high-resolution (HR) MR mammography with a high temporal resolution. In this context, discussions of 2D and 3D techniques are outdated. Another essential cornerstone for the improvement of the MR mammography examination has been the development of open surface coils, which allow access to the breast even after positioning the patient. As a consequence, it is possible to compress both breasts so that movement artifacts can be practically eliminated. The aspect of patient comfort has also increasingly been considered. Additional equipment, such as a head-rest fixture with an integrated inclined mirror, improves patient comfort and results in a further reduction of extraneous disturbances during image generation.

The changes relating to breast MRI in recent years do not involve only the technical and methodical aspects of the examination, however. Breast MRI has become completely established in international breast diagnostic imaging. The American College of Radiology has included a separate chapter pertaining to breast MRI in its latest edition of the BI-RADS Lexicon, specifying terms, lesion characteristics, and lesion categorization used in breast MRI examinations. There are now guidelines that clearly define indications for its performance in the context of early breast cancer detection. In addition, MR mammography stands alongside x-ray (radiographic) mammography and breast ultrasonography as an equally valuable modality in the chapter on breast interventions. The Breast Diagnostics Working Group of the German Radiology Society, for example, has defined the minimum requirements for the performance of diagnostic breast MRI examinations and listed recommendations for the performance of MR-guided interventions.

The significant improvement of spatial resolution in MR mammography has also resulted in greater clinical significance of visualized details in terms of the therapeutic consequences. An extensive intraductal component (EIC) surrounding a proven index tumor, for example, is often visualized only on MRI and has attained an unprecedented importance. In addition, the classical domain of x-ray mammography in the detection of a ductal carcinoma in situ (DCIS) has begun to falter as, here also, the present scientific data show that HR MR mammography is superior to conventional mammography. All these developments raise the legitimate question of whether these improvements must be taken into consideration and eventually lead to a modification of our present-day diagnostic strategies. The superiority of MR mammography in the detection of all malignant tumor forms without radiation exposure and with a similar specificity to that of other breast imaging modalities naturally induces the desire to use it as the primary breast examination for early breast cancer detection, which can be complemented by x-ray mammography and/or breast ultrasonography in individual cases when justified. It is likely that some years will pass before we achieve this state; in the meantime we must perform suitable studies on the efficacy of such strategies.

In this context, other problematic aspects must also be addressed: cost, availability, quality, and expertise.

All of the developments mentioned above have made it necessary to completely rewrite the chapters from technique and methods to terminology and lesion analysis, as well as in terms of quality management. In addition, the images presented in the first edition no longer meet present-day standards for artifact-free, HR MR mammographic images. Thus, all the images in this second edition have been replaced with 512 × 512 matrix images. This book is now an up-to-date work that includes all relevant aspects for the effective performance and analysis of high-quality MR mammography. For a beginner, it is an effective introduction to the basics. On the other hand, it is meant to help with the questions and problems that a "mammophile" breast MRI expert may occasionally encounter.

Uwe Fischer, Göttingen, Germany

Acknowledgments

While the first edition of this book was written during my 9 years working at the University of Göttingen in the field of MR mammography, this second edition reflects not only the innovative changes in the performance and analysis of MR mammography but also my new vantage point modified by the shift of my working field. The current edition includes all the experience I have accumulated during the last 7 years of work at the Women's Health Care Center, Göttingen. In this frame of reference, where individualized and optimal diagnostic strategies are implemented for the early detection of breast cancer, MR mammography has increasingly earned a central role. It has also shown itself to be the most reliable diagnostic method for staging and follow-up after breast cancer.

The diagnostic breast work-up is teamwork. Thus, many co-workers and colleagues have contributed to the success of the second edition of the *Practical MR Mammography*. I would like to mention the most important by name:

From the Women's Health Care Center, Göttingen, are Anja El-Hajab, Doris Hermes, Dr. Dorit von Heyden, Anke Kuechemann, Adelgunde Leicht, Dr. Susanne Luftner-Nagel, Gudrun Meyer, Jeanette Rheinlaender, Jutta Rueschoff, Christina Vujevic, and Dr. Friedemann Baum. For their cooperative and helpful communications I thank the surgeons Dr. Abdallah Abdallah, Professor Werner Audretsch, Dr. Bettina Conrad, Dr. Dieter Kulenkampff, Professor Thorsten Kühn, and Dr. Mahdi Rezai, as well as the breast pathologists Professor Heinz Becker, Professor Gösta Fischer, and especially Dr. Burkhart Sattler. All of the above-mentioned were always available to competently answer questions, give explanations, and provide image material.

Abbreviations

2D	data acquisition in single slices		**IV**	intravenous
3D	data acquisition in volume block		**LCIS**	lobular carcinoma in situ
ACR	American College of Radiology		**MIP**	maximum intensity projection
ADH	atypical ductal hyperplasia		**MLO**	mediolateral oblique (projection)
B-classification	pathological category classification of core biopsy specimens (B1 to B5)		**MPR**	multiplanar reconstruction
			MRE	MR elastography
BCS	breast-conserving surgery		**MRI**	magnetic resonance imaging
BCT	breast-conserving therapy		**MRM**	magnetic resonance mammography
bFGF	basic fibroblast growth factor		**MRS**	MR spectroscopy
BI-RADS	breast imaging, reporting, and data system		**MT**	magnetization transfer
BW	body weight		**Mx**	x-ray (radiographic) mammography
CAD	computer-aided diagnosis/detection		**NMR**	nuclear magnetic resonance
CB	core biopsy		**NOS**	Not Otherwise Specified (= invasive ductal carcinoma)
CC	craniocaudal (projection)			
CCDS	color-coded Doppler sonography		**OIBC**	occult inflammatory breast cancer
CM	contrast medium		**PASH**	pseudoangiomatous stromal hyperplasia
CUP	carcinoma of unknown primary		**REI**	routine examination interval
DCIS	ductal carcinoma in situ		**RF**	radiofrequency
DIN	ductal intraepithelial hyperplasia		**RODEO sequence**	rotating delivery of excitation off-resonance
DTPA	diethylenetriamine pentaacetic acid			
DWI	diffusion-weighted MRI		**ROI**	region of interest
EIC	extensive intraductal component		**SE**	spin echo
FEA	flat epithelial atypia		**SI**	signal intensity
FLASH	an ultrafast GE sequence		**SLNB**	sentinel lymph node biopsy
FNAB	fine-needle aspiration biopsy		**SNR**	signal-to-noise ratio
FNAP	fine-needle aspiration puncture		**STIR**	short-inversion-time inversion recovery
FOV	field of view		**T**	Tesla (field strength)
G	Gauge		**T1w**	T1-weighted
G	pathological grading class		**T2w**	T2-weighted
GCP	good clinical practice		**TE**	time-to-echo, echo time
Gd-DTPA	gadolinium-DTPA		**TIC**	time–signal intensity curve
GE	gradient echo		**TR**	time-to-repetition, repetition time
HPF	high-power field		**TRAM**	transverse rectus abdominis myocutaneous flap technique
HR	high-resolution			
HRT	hormone replacement therapy		**TSE**	turbo-spin-echo
IDC	invasive ductal carcinoma		**US**	ultrasound/ultrasonography
ILC	invasive lobular carcinoma		**VAB**	vacuum-assisted biopsy
IR	inversion recovery		**VEGF**	vascular endothelial growth factor

Contents

1   History of MR Mammography   1

2   Preparing and Informing the Patient   2

3   Technique and Methods   3

Basic Principles of Magnetic Resonance Imaging 3
Surface Coils 4
Time of Examination. 5
Previous Breast Intervention 6
Patient Positioning. 7
Breast Compression 8
Field Strength 9
2 D and 3 D Techniques 10
Parallel Imaging 11
T1-Weighted Sequences (with and without Fat Saturation) . 12
Echo Time 14
T2-Weighted Sequences 16
Temporal Resolution. 17
Spatial Resolution. 18
Slice Orientation 19

Phase-Encoding Gradient 21
Paramagnetic Contrast Materials 23
Image Postprocessing 25
Image Subtraction. 25
Time–Signal Intensity Curve Analysis of
Enhancing Lesions. 25
Maximum Intensity Projection. 27
Multiplanar Reconstruction 27
Computer-Aided Diagnosis / Computer-Aided Detection 28
Examination Protocol 30
Presently Unestablished Breast MRI
Examination Techniques. 31
MR Spectroscopy 31
MR Elastography. 31
Diffusion-Weighted Breast MRI 32

4   Tumor Angiogenesis and Breast MRI   33

5   Diagnostic Criteria   34

Assessment of the T1-Weighted Precontrast Examination . . 34
Assessment of the T2-Weighted Examination 36
Assessment of the Contrast-Enhanced T1-Weighted
Examination. 37
Focus/Foci 37

Mass 37
Nonmasslike Enhancement 40
Dynamic Enhancement Characteristics (Kinetics). 41
Associated Findings. 43
Breast MRI Evaluation Protocols 44

6   Artifacts and Sources of Error   47

Incorrect Positioning 47
Improper Administration of Contrast 49
Motion Artifacts. 50
Documentation and Classification 51
Out-of-Phase Imaging 53
Susceptibility Artifacts 54
Cardiac Flow Artifacts. 55
Surface Coil Artifacts 56

Incorrect Region of Interest (ROI) 57
Insufficient Spatial Resolution. 58
Substandard Subtraction Process (Negative Pixels). 59
Incorrect Pixel Shifting. 59
Inadequate Windowing 60
Ghosting. 61
Inhomogeneous Fat Suppression / Silicone Suppression 62

Contents

7   Normal Findings in Breast MRI   63

Morphology 63
Blood Supply. 63
Parenchyma and Age 64
Parenchymal Asymmetry, Accessory Glandular Tissue 65
Nipple and Retromamillary Region 67

Interindividual Variations 69
Intraindividual Fluctuations 70
Hormone Replacement Therapy 72
Pregnancy and the Lactating Breast 73

8   Benign Changes   75

Fibroadenoma 75
Special Types of Fibroadenomas 79
Adenomas 82
Benign Phyllodes Tumor 87
Lipomas 90
Fibrocystic Breast Condition 91
Adenosis 92
Stromal Fibrosis of the Breast 96
Pseudoangiomatous Stromal Hyperplasia 98
Hemangioma 100
Adenomyoepithelioma 102

Simple Cysts 103
Inflamed Cysts 105
Hemorrhagic Cysts 108
Complicated Cysts 109
Hamartoma of the Breast 112
Acute Nonpuerperal Mastitis 115
Abscess 118
Chronic Nonpuerperal Mastitis 119
Mondor Disease 121
Cutaneous Changes in Breast MRI 123

9   Postoperative/Posttraumatic Changes   125

Fat Necrosis 125
Seroma 128
Hematoma 129
Scar Tissue 130
Changes following Breast-Conserving Therapy plus
Radiotherapy/Mastectomy 133

R1 Resection 136
Recurrence after Breast-Conserving Therapy / Mastectomy /
Breast Reconstruction 137

10   Borderline Lesions   139

Papilloma 139
Radial Scar 145
Lobular Carcinoma in Situ (LCIS) 149

Atypical Ductal Hyperplasia 151
Breast Cysts with Intracystic Proliferation 153

11   Intraductal Carcinomas   155

Classification 155

Study Results 163

12   Malignant Changes   165

Invasive Ductal Carcinoma 165
Invasive Lobular Carcinoma 170
Medullary Carcinoma 175
Mucinous Carcinoma 177
Invasive Papillary Carcinoma 179
Tubular Carcinoma 182
Inflammatory Breast Cancer 184

Paget Disease of the Nipple 186
Malignant Phyllodes Tumor 188
Sarcoma 189
Triple-Negative Breast Cancer 190
Breast Carcinomas during Pregnancy and/or the
Lactational Period 193
Study Results 194

13   Lymph Node Diagnostics   195

14   Autologous and Prosthetic Breast Reconstruction   201

Diagnostic MRI after Autologous Breast Reconstruction. . . . 201
Diagnostic MRI of Breast Prostheses. 203

Normal Findings 205
Complications. 206

15   Breast MRI in Men   213

Gynecomastia 213

Male Breast Cancer 216

16   MRI-Guided Interventions   217

Special Considerations in MRI-Guided Interventions. 217
MRI-Compatible Surface Coils for Breast Interventions 217
Computer-Aided Calculation of Puncture Coordinates 217
Diagnostic MRI-Guided Vacuum-Assisted Biopsy 219
Indications and Objectives 219
Biopsy Equipment 219

Postbiopsy MRI Check That Tissue Samples Are
Representative 222
Therapeutic MRI-Guided Vacuum-Assisted Biopsy 224
MRI-Guided Localization. 225
Indications and Objectives. 225
Localization Equipment. 225

17   Indications for Breast MRI   229

Differentiation between Scar and Local Recurrence after
Breast-Conserving Therapy 229
Carcinoma of Unknown Primary 232
Preoperative Local Staging 235
Tumor Size 235
Extensive Intraductal Component 235
Infiltration of the Pectoral Muscle 235
Multifocality 238
Multicentricity. 238
Synchronous Bilateral Breast Cancer 240

N-Staging 240
Influence of Breast MRI on Therapeutic Strategy 240
Increased Breast Cancer Risk 243
Monitoring during Neoadjuvant Chemotherapy 245
Follow-up after Breast Reconstruction with Prosthesis
Implantation. 247
The Problem Case in Mammography and/or Breast
Ultrasound 247
Early Breast Cancer Detection with Breast MRI. 249

18   Differential Diagnosis and Strategy   251

Solitary Focus 251
Multiple Foci 252
Mass Lesion. 253
Mass Lesion—Differential Diagnosis 253

Nonmasslike Lesion. 255
Nonmasslike Lesion—Differential Diagnosis 256
Architectural Distortion. 259

19   Quality Assurance   261

Minimum Requirements for Breast MRI Examinations 261
Quality Check in Breast MRI 262
Written Report 262
Quality Assurance in Special Cases. 263
Quality Assurance: MRI BI-RADS 3 Findings 263

Quality Assurance after MRI-Guided Vacuum-
Assisted Biopsy. 263
Quality Assurance after MRI-Indicated Open Biopsy
(Surgery) 264

Contents

20   Current Standing, Problems, and Perspectives of Breast MRI   **265**

Current Standing. 265
Value of Breast MRI. 265
Indications for Breast MRI 265
Göttingen Optipack. 265
Problems and Solutions 266

Limitations of Breast MRI 266
Certification. 266
Perspectives 267
Diagnostic and Therapeutic Strategies 267
Early Breast Cancer Diagnostics. 267

21   Further Reading   **269**

Index   **279**

1 History of MR Mammography

In 1973 the development of magnetic resonance imaging (MRI) was triggered by Paul Lauterbur. On the basis of the research of Felix Bloch and Edward Mills Purcell, it was he who made possible the spatial encoding within a static magnetic field, using linear variations of field strength along the spatial coordinates. Today the general advantages of MRI in medical imaging, especially the acquisition of overlap-free multiplanar images with a high contrast range, are well established. It is less well known that the breast was one of the earliest objects of MRI research. Raymond Damadian suggested that it might be possible to differentiate tumors of the breast in 1971. In 1979 Peter Mansfield published the first MR images of breast tumors. However, neither the subsequent in-vitro studies nor the later in-vivo tissue measurements of T1 and T2 relaxation times allowed a reliable differentiation between benign and malignant breast lesions. For this reason, MRI of the breast was initially not widely accepted.

The technical breakthrough of modern MRI of the breast occurred in the mid-1980s, mainly due to the development of fast gradient-echo imaging sequences with small flip angles, dubbed fast low-angle shot (FLASH), by Jens Frahm and Axel Haase of the Max Planck Institute for Biophysical Chemistry in Göttingen, the application of paramagnetic contrast materials, and the use of specialized surface coils. These developments made possible the performance of dynamic contrast-enhanced examinations of the breast with a sufficiently high spatial resolution.

In the following years, MRI of the breast was principally influenced by the research groups of Sylvia Heywang and Wilfried Kaiser. Two schools of thought and much debate resulted. Whereas Kaiser utilized two-dimensional (2D) FLASH sequences and favored a high temporal resolution, Heywang employed three-dimensional (3D) FLASH sequences favoring a higher spatial resolution. The discussion as to which technique yields superior diagnostic results is now of historical interest only. Today's MRI examinations of the breast employ 3D sequences that provide both high temporal as well as high spatial resolution.

Further developments of hardware and software in recent years have made possible the performance of an MR mammography examination with excellent spatial resolution (512×512 matrix) within an adequate time interval. Current studies substantiate that such a high-resolution MR mammography is superior to all other breast imaging modalities in the detection of both invasive and intraductal breast cancer. In addition, we now have specialized instruments available for the performance of MRI-guided biopsies so that it is also possible to histologically verify those lesions seen only on MRI. As a consequence it is foreseeable that the MRI examination of the breast will increasingly be the method of choice for the early detection of breast cancer, the diagnostic work-up of symptomatic women, and the follow-up of women with a history of breast cancer.

2 Preparing and Informing the Patient

Before an examination begins, the patient must remove all ferromagnetic items (jewelry, watch, wallet, etc.). All upper body clothing should be entirely removed and preferably replaced with a bathrobe open to the front.

Contraindications for MR mammography
- Cardiac pacemakers
- Heart valves and surgical clips (in heart or brain) made of MR-incompatible materials
- Heart or brain surgery within the last 2 weeks
- History of adverse reaction to gadolinium in a previous MR examination using contrast (does not apply to MR examinations of prostheses without contrast medium)

There are no acute life-threatening indications for the performance of MRI of the breast. It is, therefore, necessary to avoid any possible injury to the patient that could be caused by performing this examination. In some cases, it may be necessary to do without it.

Obligatory aspects of patient information
- Necessity for contrast medium administration
- Possible contrast medium intolerance
  - risk of minor adverse reactions ~1:5000
  - risk of major adverse reactions ~1:500 000
- Written declaration of consent by patient (informed consent form)

Optional aspects of patient information
- Information about the purpose of the examination
- Information about the length of the examination: ~15 minutes
- Reference to the expected background noise
- The need to remain motionless during the examination to avoid movement artifacts
- Notification of when contrast is administered (temporary feeling of coolness in the arm)

Patient preparation
- Place venous access (18–20 gauge) into the cubital or cephalic vein.
- If possible, avoid using the lower arm veins for contrast medium administration (longer inflow phase).
- Connect extension tubes (1.5 m length, 4 mL volume).
- Allow a short rest period (~5 minutes) before positioning the patient on the MR table
- Place the patient in a comfortable prone position.
- Immobilize the arms alongside the body (e.g., hang them in a loop made from the bathrobe belt, see **Fig. 3.4a**).
- Apply hearing protection (earplugs, MRI-suitable headset with/without music).
- Give the patient a panic bulb to be used in case of claustrophobia, nausea, etc.

Start of examination
- Notify the patient that the examination will begin over a microphone.

3 Technique and Methods

Basic Principles of Magnetic Resonance Imaging

Since Paul Lauterbur published his first reports on magnetic resonance imaging (MRI) 30 years ago, it has developed into the mature and versatile imaging technique of today. The method employs the physical principles of nuclear magnetic resonance (NMR), which have been described by several chemists and physicists including Nobel prize winners Isidor Rabi, Edgar Purcell, Felix Bloch, and Richard Ernst. According to the laws of electromagnetism, the rotating motion of an electrically charged particle induces a localized magnetic field around the particle. Certain nuclei, namely the proton and those possessing an uneven number of protons and neutrons, have an intrinsic angular momentum or spin. For MR imaging, the hydrogen nucleus, or proton, is preferred because of its high concentration in biological tissues (water, fat). In addition to its high abundance, it has the highest magnetic moment of all natural isotopes. In the absence of an external magnetic field, the orientations of the magnetic spins are at random, so that their magnetic dipoles have no net external effect. When hydrogen nuclei are placed in a strong external magnetic field, these atomic nuclei align themselves with the static magnetic field B_0 in one of two orientations (magnetic quantum numbers): parallel, i.e., spin up (low-energy state), or antiparallel, i.e., spin down (high-energy state). Because the energy difference between the two states is small, they are almost equally probable. For protons at 1.5 T, the lower energy state is favored by only 1 additional proton per 100 000 protons. In addition, each proton is spinning around its own axis and experiences a torque when exposed to a magnetic field, similar to a spinning top in the earth's gravitational field. The spin vectors are forced to precess or gyrate at a certain frequency, which is linearly dependent on the magnetic field strength B_0. This precessional frequency ω of the proton's magnetic moments, also called the Larmor frequency, obeys the formula:

$$\omega = \gamma \times B_0$$

The proportionality constant γ is specific for the type of nucleus and is called the gyromagnetic ratio. The joint alignment of the spin vectors in the magnetic field creates the macroscopic magnetic moment or magnetization M. It is this net magnetic moment that is responsible for the induction of the MR signal in the receiver coil.

Excitation and relaxation. A short burst of radiofrequency (RF) excitation at the appropriate material-dependent resonant frequency (42 MHz for protons at 1 T) causes a reorientation of the proton's magnetization vector out of its alignment with the longitudinal axis of the magnetic field; that is, the macroscopic magnetization experiences the torque of the RF field and is forced to rotate about it. The degree of displacement, the flip angle α, is dependent on the amplitude and duration of the excitation pulse and is expressed in angular degrees. After the RF pulse is turned off, the protons resume their original positions of longitudinal alignment with the static magnetic field, i.e., they relax. During this relaxation process, the energy absorbed by the nuclei is emitted as RF radiation, or lost through molecular interactions such as electromagnetic dipole–dipole interactions and thermal dissipation. The emitted electromagnetic signal (MR signal) can be detected as an induced voltage by special receiver coils and translated into an image. The restoration of the magnetization vector to its original orientation is an exponential process described by the increase of magnetization in the longitudinal plane (spin–lattice interaction associated with the T1 relaxation time), and the loss of transverse magnetization (spin–spin interaction associated with the T2 relaxation time). The decay of transverse magnetization is caused by fluctuations of the molecular dipole fields that cause dephasing of the precessing spin vectors. Field inhomogeneities give rise to an additional dephasing of the aligned spins, denoted by adding a star to the relaxation time T2 (T2*). The relaxation times are the times it takes for the RF signal to exponentially rise (T1) or decay (T2) to half its maximum value. Fortunately for the contrast in MR images, T1 and T2 relaxation times are unique for each type of tissue. They can be measured by the receiver coil and are used for image generation.

Spatial encoding. For image generation, the emitted signals or RF echoes must be assigned to a specific location on a three-dimensional matrix. Spatial localization is achieved by applying linear magnetic field gradients in x, y, and z directions in space. Two-dimensional (2D) and three-dimensional (3D) techniques differ in the process of spatial encoding. In the 2D technique, section selection is achieved by simultaneously switching the slice-selection gradient and RF excitation, followed by a phase and frequency encoding in-plane. In the 3D technique, a volume is excited with RF and a second phase encoding is performed orthogonally to the first.

Contrast. The contrast of MR images is influenced by two factors: tissue-specific factors and external factors. Major tissue-specific factors include proton density, and T1 and T2 relaxation times. External factors include hardware and software parameters (e.g., slice thickness, orientation, number of acquisitions), the selected pulse sequence (e.g., spin-echo, gradient-echo, fat saturation), the field strength, and whether or not contrast material is administered.

Pulse sequences. There are numerous different pulse sequences that can be used for acquiring MR images. Some basic aspects of spin-echo (SE) and gradient-echo (GE) sequences, the latter of which is especially important for dynamic MR mammography, are explained in the following text.

In a conventional *SE sequence*, excitation results from a slice-selective 90° RF pulse, which cancels the longitudinal magnetization and converts it into a transverse magnetization. After half the echo time (TE) has passed, it is followed by a 180° RF pulse, which rephases or refocuses the precessing spins to compensate for signal loss due to inhomogeneities in the magnetic field. Hence, a maximum signal emission, the spin echo, will result at the echo time TE. This entire pulse cycle is repeated with a repetition time TR. Depending on the selected echo time and repetition time, the resulting images are T1-, T2- or proton-weighted.

The echo in *GE sequences* is not produced by a 180° RF pulse but by reversing the gradient, causing a refocused RF echo, i.e., gradient-echo. In addition, the initial 90° RF pulse can be substituted by a smaller pulse with a flip angle α < 90°, which does not use the entire longitudinal magnetization. Although this results in a decreased signal intensity compared with that of the SE sequences, image generation and acquisition are much faster.

Due to the greater sensitivity of GE sequences to local field inhomogeneities caused by ferromagnetic substances (e.g., metal clips) and to the susceptibility differences of adjacent tissues (e.g., bone/air, hematoma/normal tissue interfaces), they are more prone to artifacts than SE sequences. The echo time length, however, is also a factor with a major influence on artifact formation. The greater sensitivity of GE sequences to paramagnetic contrast materials is an additional consequence of these factors.

Contrast material. MRI signal production can be modified by the administration of contrast material. Paramagnetic substances are primarily used for this purpose, but superparamagnetic materials are also administered. Both groups of materials have the property of changing the relaxation times of the imaged anatomical structures. The major effect of paramagnetic contrast materials is to shorten the T1 and T2 relaxation times of the tissues. Dynamic MR mammography takes advantage of this shortening effect on the T1 relaxation time, resulting in signal enhancement in the T1-weighted sequences. Superparamagnetic substances, which exert a strong T2 shortening effect, are not utilized in MR mammography.

Surface Coils

To achieve adequate spatial resolution in MR mammography, dedicated surface coils made especially to fit the breast shape must be used. Commercially available devices that allow a simultaneous bilateral examination are designed for the patient lying prone with both breasts hanging freely in the lumen of the breast coil. Although unilateral breast coils have the advantage of a more homogeneous magnetic field, they have the disadvantage of requiring the patient to return for a second examination on another day, and are therefore no longer employed. Currently only bilateral breast coils are used, allowing the simultaneous MR exami-

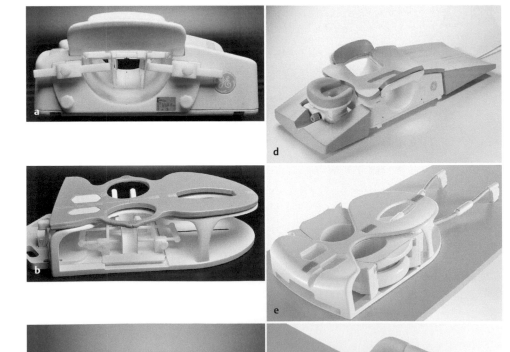

Fig. 3.1 a–f Open breast surface coils from various manufacturers.
a GE HealthCare.
b Noras.
c Invivo.
d GE HealthCare.
e Siemens.
f Philips.

nation of both breasts after a single administration of contrast medium (CM). It is of great advantage for the surface coil to be open to the lateral sides, allowing access to the breast after positioning of the patient. In this way, it is possible to position and immobilize the breasts under visual monitoring (**Fig. 3.1**). It is

also a prerequisite for the performance of MRI-guided interventional procedures.

! Open surface coils are one of the indicative features of high-quality breast MRI equipment.

Time of Examination

The circulation in the female breast is subject to hormonal changes. As expected, CM uptake in the breast also varies with the phase of the menstrual cycle and the endogenous hormonal status. The degree of disturbing signal enhancement is least in the second week of the menstrual cycle, making this the preferred time slot in which to perform breast MRI if the referral indication allows. In spite of the fact that focal contrast-enhancing patterns caused by cyclic fluctuations rarely show a pattern typical for malignancy, MR mammography examination in the first and fourth weeks of the menstrual cycle should be avoided (**Fig. 3.2**). The problem arising from the normally increased parenchymal enhancement pattern seen at an unfavorable phase of the cycle is rather that especially the small and non–mass-enhancing lesions may be masked and more easily missed. In addition to the performance of an early image subtraction, it is therefore recommended to perform an earliest subtraction when MR mammography shows a strong parenchymal enhancement. If

a woman has no menstrual cycle that can be used to asses her hormonal status and give her an appropriate appointment, cyclic breast pain is a reliable criterion for estimating a favorable cycle phase. MR mammography appointments should not be given to coincide with a time when breast pain is strong.

Hormone replacement. There is no restriction on the optimal time for performing MRI of the breast on a postmenopausal woman. However, hormone replacement therapy (HRT) can result in undesirable early contrast enhancement of the parenchyma. Here also, the earliest subtraction should be performed to get the most information out of the examination. In exceptional cases, it may be expedient to repeat the examination 4–6 weeks after discontinuing HRT. In our experience, however, it is not routinely necessary to discontinue HRT before performing an MR mammographic examination.

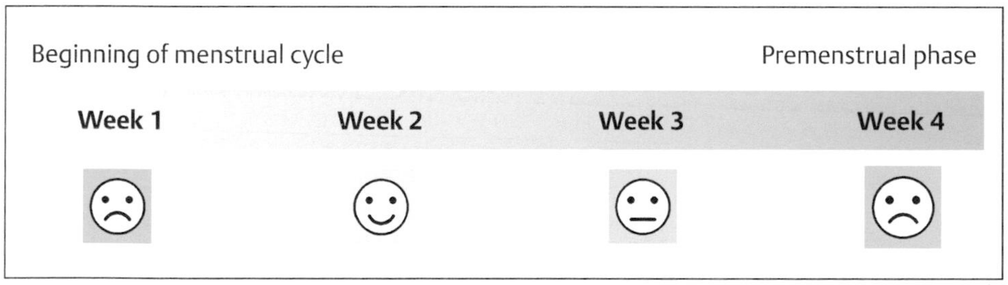

Beginning of menstrual cycle			Premenstrual phase
Week 1	Week 2	Week 3	Week 4
:(	:)	:|	:(

Fig. 3.2 Optimal appointment week for performing MR mammography in terms of the menstrual cycle. The best time to perform a breast MRI examination is during the second week of the menstrual cycle. Less optimal is the third week of the cycle. The least favorable times to perform this examination are during the first and fourth weeks of the cycle.

Previous Breast Intervention

MR mammography may be performed without limitation after both fine-needle biopsy and large-core biopsy of a breast lesion without significant hematoma. Neither of these procedures results in increased contrast enhancement and they do not, therefore, interfere with the interpretation of the examination. After carrying out a vacuum-assisted biopsy one typically finds a relatively large resection cavern with reactive hyperemia at the borders and a central hematoma. Residual tumor (e.g., seen as circumscribed enhancing areas) is occasionally seen under these conditions but is not detected reliably.

> **!** It is always preferable to perform MR mammography before rather than after a breast intervention.

Galactography. If medical and organizational reasons allow it, galactography should not be performed before a planned MR mammography examination because areas of increased enhancement may result in the examined breast segment. If galactography has already been performed, then the differential diagnosis of a segmental contrast enhancement pattern in the examined duct must include reactive hyperemia.

Open biopsy and radiation therapy. To avoid problems in interpreting areas of increased enhancement due to wound healing, MR mammography should not be performed earlier than 6 months after open biopsy. After lumpectomy followed by breast irradiation, this interval is increased to 12 months after completion of radiation therapy (**Fig. 3.3**). However, the degree and duration of changes caused by radiation therapy are subject to significant interindividual differences: they may resolve within a few weeks in some patients, or persist for 1–2 or more years in others.

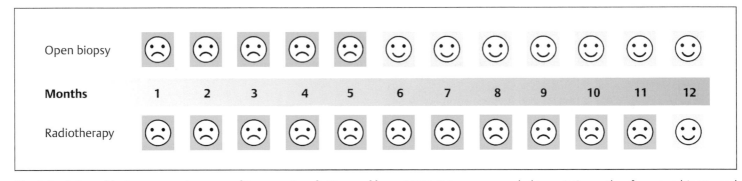

Fig. 3.3   Interval between previous open biopsy or irradiation and breast MRI. It is recommended to wait 6 months after open biopsy, and 12 months after breast irradiation following breast-conserving therapy before performing MRI of the breast.

Patient Positioning

Normally, the patient is examined in a whole-body scanner in the prone position with both arms lying flat against the body. If the patient is wearing a bath robe, the arms can be placed in a loop made from the knotted belt. This has the advantage of allowing the patient to relax the shoulder area (**Fig. 3.4a**), significantly reducing the risk of motion artifacts due to relaxation of the pectoral muscle and adjacent breast tissue during the examination. As an alternative, the arms may be placed above the head. This positioning, however, increases the risk that the breasts are not completely placed inside the breast coil since the cranial portions of the breast are pulled partially out of the coil when the arms are raised. The use of a special head rest, upon which the forehead rests and from which one can look at a picture or postcard through an inclined mirror, has proven useful for relaxing the patient (**Fig. 3.4b–d**). Positioning the head sideways is often found to be uncomfortable and to result in cervical complaints. After sliding the patient into the magnet bore, it is important to be assured that the extension tubing of the venous access is freely accessible.

! Patient comfort is an essential aspect of high-quality MR mammography.

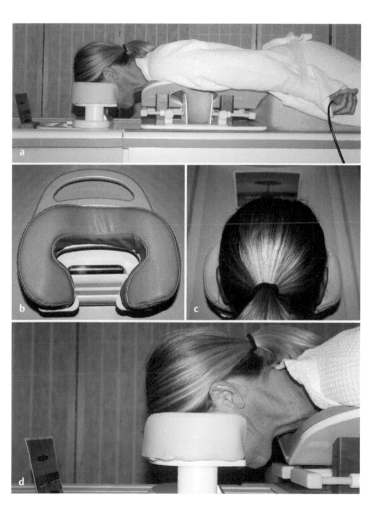

Fig. 3.4a–d Patient positioning for breast MRI.
a Comfortable patient positioning in an open whole-body scanner in the prone position with both arms lying flat against the body, in the bathrobe belt loop.
b Padded head rest with integrated inclined mirror.
c Patient head positioning with view of a picture postcard.
d Lateral view of head positioning.

Breast Compression

Adequate breast compression is necessary to effectively reduce motion artifacts during an MR mammographic examination. This is especially true for the subtraction technique generally used in Europe. Such artifacts are less disturbing in the primary fat saturation technique. There have been numerous endeavors to achieve better compression of the breast inside the coil. Wearing a T-shirt during the examination as well as lateral coil padding have proven to be ineffective, particularly because the breasts are compressed toward the thoracic wall or medially. This is also true for ventral padding of the breast inside the coil with specialized inserts in different sizes. The industry offers a coil-integrated mediolateral compression device. This leads to a maximal spread of breast tissue in the craniocaudal direction, which is undesirable when using the standard axial MRI view. In contrast, it is optimal to use open surface coils with integrated, manually guided compression paddles in the craniocaudal direction (**Fig. 3.5**). Aside from the resulting reduction of motion artifacts, this device decreases the breast thickness in the craniocaudal direction, thereby significantly reducing the slice thickness in the axial MRI view.

! Adequate breast compression is essential for artifact-free MR mammography.

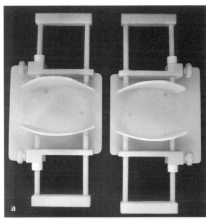

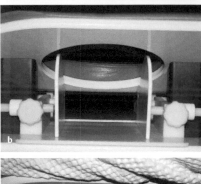
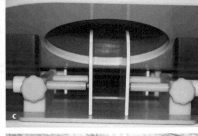

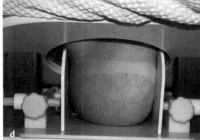
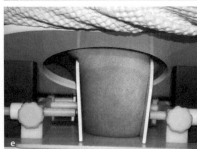

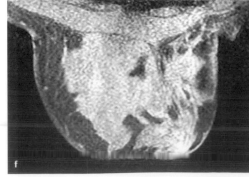
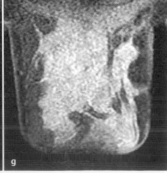

Fig. 3.5a–g   Breast compression in an open breast coil.
a Insertable compression device for bilateral immobilization of the breast in an open surface coil (Noras).
b Device inserted into an open surface coil (open position).
c Device inserted into an open surface coil (closed position).
d Breast positioned in the open surface coil with the compression device open.
e Breast positioned in the open surface coil with applied compression.
f Original image for planning further examination (without compression).
g Original image for planning further examination (with compression).

Field Strength

Presently, systems recommended for the performance of MR mammography with contrast material have a field strength of 1.5 T (1.5 tesla) or more. It is not advisable to use systems with a field strength of 0.5 T or 1.0 T. Preliminary experiences with 3.0 T systems show that these systems are suitable for breast MRI examination and may have a higher sensitivity, though to date it is not statistically significant (**Fig. 3.6**).

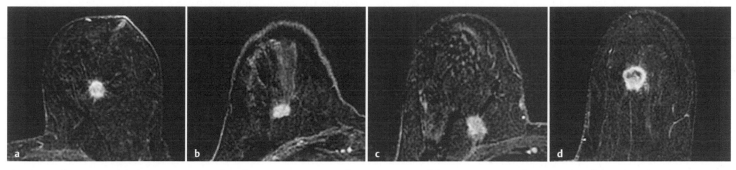

Fig. 3.6 a–d Breast MR images acquired with a 3 T-system. 3D breast images of four carcinomas from MRI performed with a 3 T-system. Representative single subtraction images (images courtesy of Radiology group practice, Bochum, Germany).

2D and 3D Techniques

2D technique. For MR mammography performed using 2D technique, single axial slices are excited (**Fig. 3.7a**). There should be no gaps between these slices, although, for methodological reasons, there is a signal decrease in the peripheral areas of each slice which has no clinical significance. The field of view (FOV) is rectangular and also includes an area within the intrathoracic space. The repetition times (TR) lie in the range of ~200–350 milliseconds, allowing the acquisition of a sufficient number of slices within the TR interval. The ideal flip angle is between 70° and 90°.

3D technique. In 3D technique, the entire breast is excited as a volume (**Fig. 3.7b**). This volume can be divided into so-called partitions, or slices of variable thickness in any desired plane.

3D imaging allows the depiction of thin slices without gaps in a defined slice profile. The selected repetition times are on the order of 10 milliseconds and shorter than those for the 2D technique. The flip angle is typically 25°.

Contrast-enhanced breast MRI. Nowadays both the 2D and 3D techniques may be used without reservation for contrast-enhanced MRI of the breast (**Fig. 3.8**). Both techniques have advantages and disadvantages that do not significantly influence the assessment or predictive value of the breast MRI. The decision on which of these techniques to use depends largely upon the experience of the examiner and it is therefore not advisable to frequently vary the technique used.

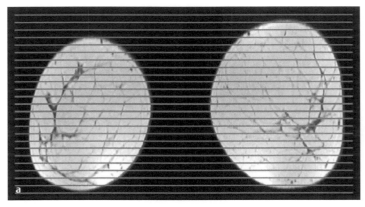
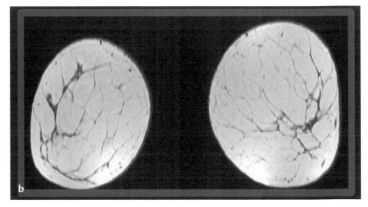

Fig. 3.7 a, b Acquisition of breast MRI images in 2D and 3D techniques.
a Image acquisition of single slices in 2D technique.
b Image acquisition of a volume block in 3D technique.

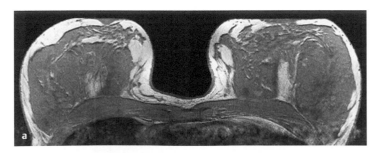
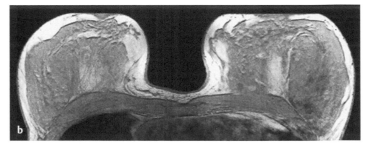

Fig. 3.8 a, b Comparison of breast MRI images in 2D and 3D techniques. No significant difference in image quality is seen.
a Single precontrast T1w slice in 2D technique.
b Single precontrast T1w slice in 3D technique.

Parallel Imaging

The development and implementation of parallel imaging was motivated by the wish to decrease the image acquisition time by reducing the number of phase-encoding steps without decreasing the spatial resolution. Basically, parallel imaging is the acquisition of image data from two or more receiving coils with varying spatial sensitivity. Images are then reconstructed from the complementary data received from each coil element rather than using the time-consuming sequential phase-encoding steps.

Techniques. There are two main groups of parallel imaging algorithms used for image reconstruction: First there is image-based reconstruction after Fourier transformation (SENSE, PILS, and SPACE RIP) by which images with overlapping anatomical coverage obtained from several surface coil elements in phased array are used to form the final image. Second there is k-space-based reconstruction before Fourier transformation (SMASH, AUTO-SMASH, and GRAPPA) in which missing k-space links are calculated by summing k-space data from each coil element and filled in.

! Parallel imaging enables high spatial and temporal resolution in breast MRI.

T1-Weighted Sequences (with and without Fat Saturation)

T1-weighted (T1w) measurements allow the detection of tissue enhancement after administration of an appropriate paramagnetic contrast material. However, the signal-intense fat tissue can significantly reduce the probability of detecting contrast-enhancing lesions in T1w sequences. This makes it essential to suppress or eliminate the fat signal in such studies. There are two basic means of achieving this:

- Subtraction of identical images before and after contrast administration
- Primary generation of fat saturation (FatSat) sequences.

Image subtraction. In Europe, subtraction of corresponding slice images before and after contrast administration has become the established method of choice for eliminating the disturbing fat signal (**Fig. 3.9**). The disadvantage of this method is its susceptibility to motion artifacts.

Primary fat suppression. American groups prefer primary fat saturation sequences (**Fig. 3.10a, b**). This technique was intro-

duced by S. E. Harms as the so-called RODEO sequence (rotating delivery of excitation off-resonance) which combines a frequency-selective saturation of the fat signal with a GE sequence and the so-called magnetization transfer (MT).

Primary fat suppression is achieved by sending a high-frequency impulse at a shift of 220 Hz just before performing the actual measurements. Saturated fat tissue then emits no signal during the examination. It is generally possible to send such a fat-suppressing impulse before any sequence, but doing so prolongs the examination time. One disadvantage of this technique is its high sensitivity to inhomogeneities of the main magnetic field. As a result it is sometimes not possible to achieve homogeneous fat signal suppression. This is particularly true for MR mammography because of the eccentric location of the breasts. In addition, breast parenchyma is signal-intense in the precontrast images when using this protocol, making subsequent image subtraction desirable (**Fig. 3.10c**).

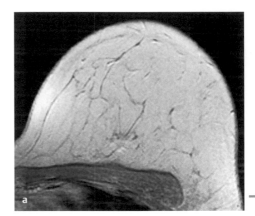 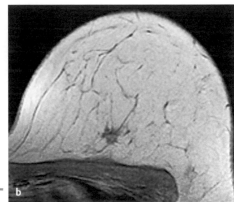 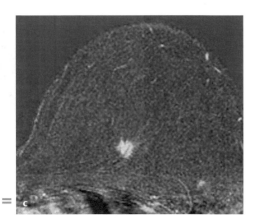

Fig. 3.9a–c   Image subtraction to eliminate disturbing fat signal.
a T1w image 3 minutes after contrast administration (second measurement).
b T1w precontrast image, which is subtracted from the postcontrast image (**a**).

c The resulting subtraction image allows optimal visualization of hypervascularized findings due to suppression of signal from surrounding fatty tissue.

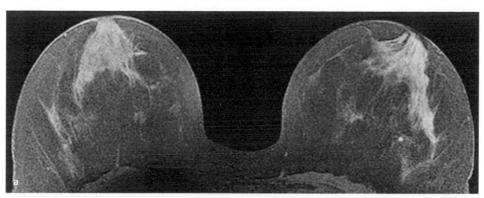

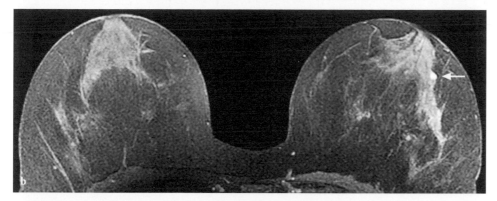

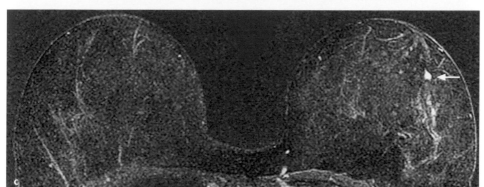

Fig. 3.10 a–c   Frequency-selective saturation of the fat signal in T1w images.

a FatSat T1w precontrast image with suppressed fat signal and signal-intense parenchyma.

b Signal enhancement of a small fibroadenoma (arrow) in the left breast, difficult to distinguish from the signal-intense parenchyma.

c Detection and characterization of this fibroadenoma (arrow) is facilitated by performing a subtraction of the corresponding image slices (image **b**–image **a**).

Echo Time

Protons bound in fat tissue exhibit a different resonance frequency from protons in water (or breast parenchyma). In MRI this is the cause of an effect called chemical shift artifact. Especially for the GE sequences used in MR mammography, the difference in resonance frequency results in a phase difference between the signal of protons in water and that of protons in fat tissue. If this difference is 180°, it is referred to as out-of-phase imaging (synonym: opposed-phase imaging). If this difference is 0°, then fat and water spins are in phase (in-phase imaging). The strength of this effect is dependent upon the magnetic field strength. Out-of-phase imaging results in signal loss at the interfaces between fat- and water-containing tissues. In dynamic breast MRI, this is true at the borders between fat tissue and breast parenchyma. Depending upon the MRI system's magnetic field strength, the echo time (TE) should be selected such that in-phase imaging results and an interfering signal loss at these interfaces is avoided (**Figs. 3.11, 3.12, 3.13**).

> **!** Breast MRI is performed "in-phase" (field strength 1.5 T ≡ TE between 4.2 and 5 milliseconds).

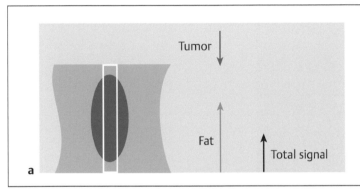 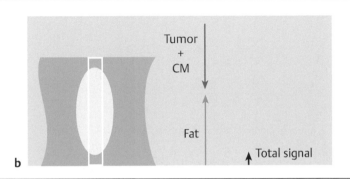

Fig. 3.11 a, b   Out-of-phase (opposed-phase) imaging. Schematic illustrations of pre- and postcontrast images of a voxel containing a tumor (on the left of each illustration).

a In the T1w precontrast image, fat tissue has a high signal intensity and the uncontrasted tumor has an opposing signal. The resulting total signal is low.

b In the T1w postcontrast image fat tissue has the same high signal intensity and the enhancing tumor now has a stronger opposing signal. The resulting total signal is therefore lower still than in the precontrast image.

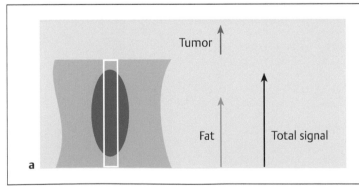 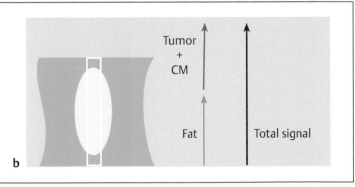

Fig. 3.12 a, b   In-phase imaging. Schematic illustrations of pre- and postcontrast images of a voxel containing a tumor (on the left of each illustration).

a In the T1w precontrast image fat tissue has a high signal intensity and the uncontrasted tumor also has a signal in the same direction. The resulting total signal is high.

b In the T1w postcontrast image fat tissue has the same high signal intensity and the enhancing tumor now has a stronger signal. The resulting total signal is therefore increased in comparison to the signal intensity in the precontrast image.

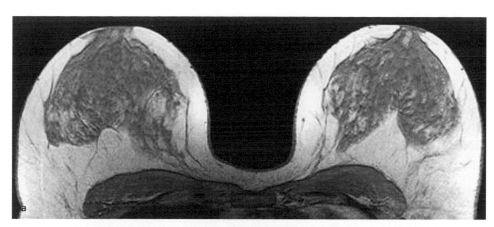

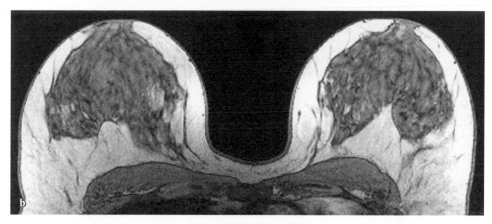

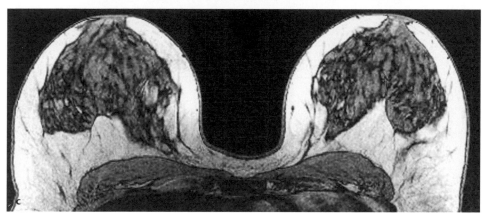

Fig. 3.13a–c   In-phase and out-of-phase imaging in breast MRI. High-resolution breast MRI using a 1.5 T system. Increasing signal loss at the borders between fat tissue and parenchyma when MRI is increasingly out-of-phase.

a Correct performance of breast MRI with an echo time of 4.6 milliseconds (in-phase).

b Echo time of 3.3 milliseconds.

c Inadvisable echo time of 2.1 milliseconds (out-of-phase).

T2-Weighted Sequences

Hydrous or edematous structures emit an intense signal in T2-weighted (T2w) sequences. The most commonly used T2w sequences in MR mammography are SE- or turbo spin-echo (TSE) sequences. Alternatively, inversion recovery (IR) sequences may also be used, with or without simultaneous fat saturation (**Fig. 3.14**). Water-sensitive T2w images are generally acquired before performing contrast enhanced dynamic measurements. It is expedient to plan and perform the T2w measurements with identical slice position and thickness as in the dynamic T1w images because this simplifies their direct comparison.

T2w sequences make it possible to recognize small cysts only a few millimeters in diameter with high sensitivity. In addition, they provide a useful criterion for the characterization of vascularized lesions. Myxoid fibroadenomas, for example, often show a very high CM uptake due to their low degree of fibrosis. In the T2w images, these lesions typically have a very intense signal, occasionally as pronounced as that of cysts. In contrast, carcinomas often show a much lower signal intensity, similar to or lower than that of the normal breast parenchyma. However, a low T2w signal in a questionable finding is not a reliable criterion indicating malignancy. The T2w sequences are also often helpful for the depiction of internal septations, as typically seen in myxoid fibroadenomas. These septations in the T2w images are occasionally more pronounced than in the T1w subtraction images.

! T2w sequences are not suitable for the detection of malignant breast tumors.

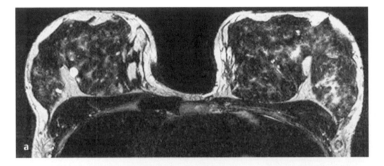
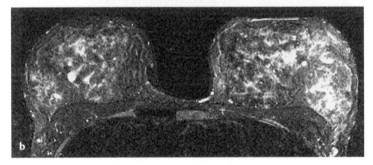
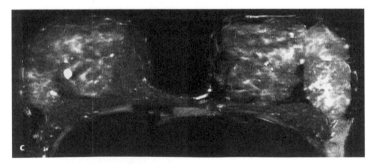

Fig. 3.14a–c   Water-sensitive measurements. Different options for acquiring water-sensitive images of the breast.
a T2w SE sequence without simultaneous suppression of the fat signal (fat saturation).
b T2w SE sequence with simultaneous fat saturation.
c IR sequence with simultaneous fat saturation.

Temporal Resolution

In most cases, hypervascularized tumors of the breast show earlier CM uptake than the normal surrounding parenchyma. This is especially true for invasive carcinomas, which usually reach their signal peak 3 minutes after CM administration. The signal intensity of breast parenchyma, on the other hand, increases continuously during the examination period of 8–10 minutes. The interindividual degree of variation for carcinoma signal intensity is great, however. Some carcinomas may reach their signal maximum in the first minute after CM administration and show a peak with a following washout phenomenon (**Fig. 3.15**). On the other hand, areas within the normal healthy parenchyma may also display an early, intense CM uptake (e.g., adenosis, hormone stimulation) and can result in an early masking of pathological processes (**Fig. 3.16**).

The generally accepted guidelines require that dynamic measurements have a temporal resolution of no more than 2–2.5 minutes per sequence over a period of at least 6 minutes after CM administration. This makes possible the discrimination between pathological processes and the surrounding parenchyma, as well as the acquisition of a sufficiently accurate dynamic curve. Semidynamic measurements (e.g., two measurements after CM administration, sequence length ~5 minutes) are historic and no longer acceptable. Further optimization of the resolution to below 1 minute per sequence or in the range of seconds, however, does not result in greater diagnostic benefit. If the MR system has extra capacity available, it is advisable to use it to increase the spatial resolution rather than the temporal resolution in order to improve the assessment of morphological characteristics.

! The relevant time frame for the detection of lesions in breast MRI encompasses the first 3 minutes after CM administration. Later measurements are used only for the characterization of lesions.

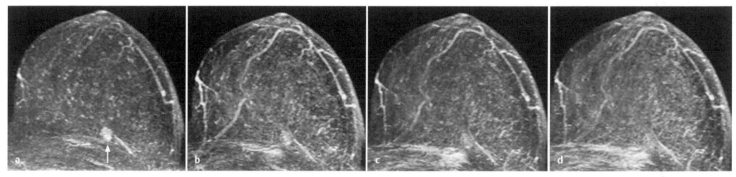

Fig. 3.15a–d Malignant tumor with washout phenomenon. Chronological subtraction images after contrast administration.

a Clear depiction of a small hypervascularized breast carcinoma (arrow) in the earliest subtraction image (first postcontrast image – precontrast image).

b Due to the washout effect in this tumor, a vaguer depiction in the early subtraction image (second postcontrast image – precontrast image).

c Contrast is nearly completely washed out by the third subtraction.

d Tumor enhancement is no longer seen in the fourth subtraction image.

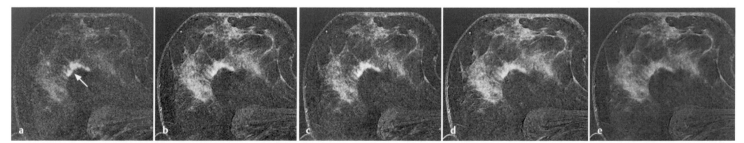

Fig. 3.16a–e Tumor masking effect due to enhancement of normal surrounding breast tissue. Chronological subtraction images after contrast administration.

a Clear depiction of a hypervascularized breast carcinoma (arrow) in the earliest subtraction image (first postcontrast image – precontrast image). Normal parenchyma enhances only slightly at this time.

b–d In the course of time, the carcinoma shows a progressive contrast washout while the surrounding breast tissue shows increasing enhancement.

e In the late phase of the examination (~8 minutes after contrast administration), the carcinoma is masked by the healthy surrounding breast tissue.

Spatial Resolution

The spatial resolution of MR mammography is influenced by various factors and adjustment parameters. In particular these are the matrix, which is dependent upon the chosen FOV, the slice thickness, and the size of the imaged volume.

FOV. Examinations performed with axial orientation have an FOV that is predetermined by the patient's proportions. It is square in shape and generally has an edge length between 300 and 350 mm. Examinations performed with coronal orientation in 3D technique allow the selection of a rectangular FOV, reducing the slice thickness by 50%.

Image volume. For diagnostic purposes, the image volume is defined by the requirement that both breasts must be examined completely. The explicit requirement that craniocaudal compression of the breasts be performed reduces the object thickness significantly.

Matrix. The recommended matrix is at least 256×256 pixels. Ideally, however, a 512×512 pixel matrix (HR-MR mammography) should be used. This matrix should not, however, be the result of interpolation (**Fig. 3.17**).

Slice thickness. The generally accepted slice thickness is 2–4 mm. Ideally, however, breast MRI meeting today's standards should be performed with a single slice thickness of 1.5–2.5 mm to achieve a maximal spatial resolution. This ensures that tumors with a diameter greater than 3–5 mm will be completely imaged in at least one slice (**Fig. 3.18**).

In general, optimizing spatial resolution results in a worsening of temporal resolution. In the past, when MRI systems had a lower capacity, routine examinations had necessarily been a compromise between these two characteristics. Due to technical advances, modern devices and measurement techniques are now available that allow the performance of examinations with very high spatial resolution within the generally recommended time frame.

> ! The potential capacity resources of an MRI system should be used to increase the spatial resolution, and not the temporal resolution. The size of a tumor that can be visualized without a partial volume effect is determined by the slice thickness (diameter = 2 × slice thickness).

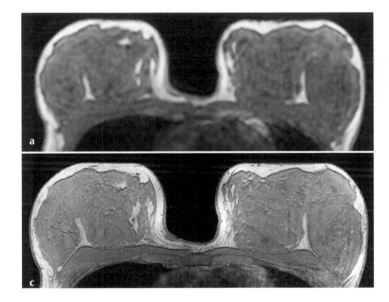

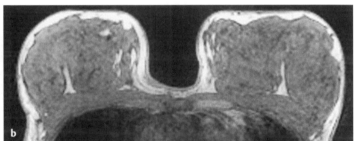

Fig. 3.17 a–c   Comparison of different matrices in breast MRI.
Significant improvement in the visualization of intramammary structures with higher matrices.
a 128 × 128.
b 256 × 256.
c 512 × 512.

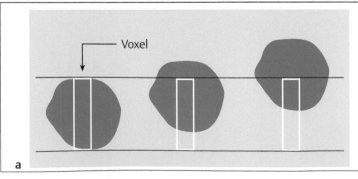
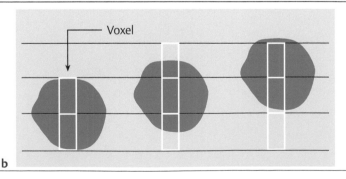

Fig. 3.18 a, b   Relation between slice thickness and tumor size: partial volume effect.
a When the tumor diameter and the slice thickness are equal, partial volume effects may occur if the tumor occupies only part of the voxel in the slice (middle and right lesions).
b When the tumor diameter is at least twice the twice slice thickness, the lesion will always be seen in at least one slice without a partial volume effect.

Slice Orientation

It is, in principle, possible to perform an MRI examination at any orientation. In Europe, contrast-enhanced breast MRI performed to detect or evaluate a breast tumor is generally performed with axial orientation. In the United States, the sagittal slice orientation is generally preferred. The sagittal orientation is recommended for the evaluation of breast prostheses.

Axial view. The main advantage of the axial slice orientation is that it enables a good assessment of breast areas near the chest wall because partial volume effects between breast tissue and the pectoral muscle (i.e., bony thorax) do not produce ambiguous structures (**Fig. 3.19**). In addition, intramammary veins are usually imaged along their course, so they can be recognized as tubular structures and will not be mistaken for round lesions. The main disadvantage of the axial slice orientation is the limited assessment it permits of the parenchymal structures in the axillary region, due to cardiac artifacts caused by the phased encoding gradients.

Coronal View. The coronal slice orientation permits the selection of a rectangular FOV, which allows reduction of the slice thickness and optimization of the spatial resolution (**Fig. 3.20a,b**). In addition, it enables artifact-free imaging of the parenchymal structures in the axillary tail (**Fig. 3.20d**). One disadvantage is that veins are seen in cross section and may be misinterpreted as small, suspicious lesions. For this reason it may be expedient to postprocess images in MIP (maximum intensity projection) technique (**Fig. 3.20c**). The interpretation of breast areas near the chest wall may be hindered by partial volume effects of thoracic structures (**Fig. 3.20e**).

Sagittal view. The sagittal slice orientation in combination with primary fat suppression protocols is very common in American-influenced countries (**Fig. 3.21**). It is explicitly recommended for the evaluation of possible prosthesis complications because it ideally visualizes the cranial aspect of prostheses, the most common weak spot.

! The sagittal view is explicitly recommended for the evaluation of prostheses.

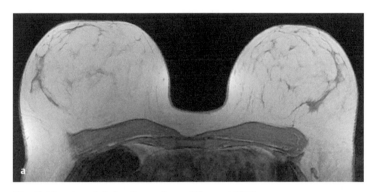 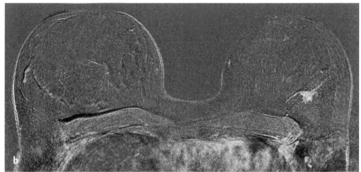

Fig. 3.19a, b   Axial orientation of breast MRI.
a T1w precontrast (single slice) with complete depiction of both breasts, including pre- and parapectoral aspects.

b Corresponding single slice subtraction image after intravenous CM administration.

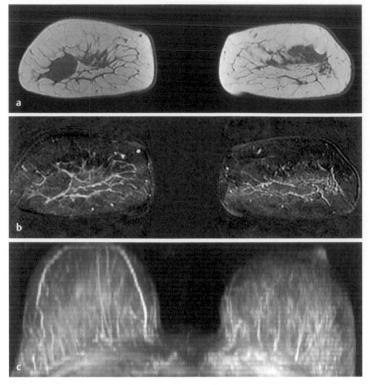

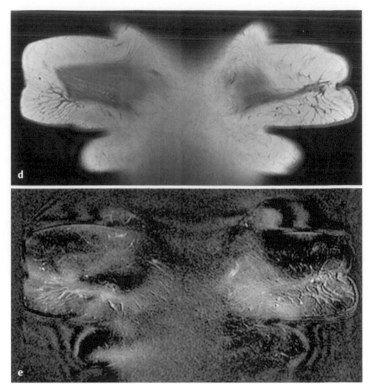

Fig. 3.20a–e   Coronal orientation of breast MRI.
a T1w precontrast examination in coronal orientation with 50% reduced FOV.
b Subtraction image after CM administration with depiction of subcutaneous veins in cross section.
c Axial reconstruction of the data.
d Coronal precontrast slice of the breast aspect near the thoracic wall.
e Coronal subtraction slice image near the thoracic wall.

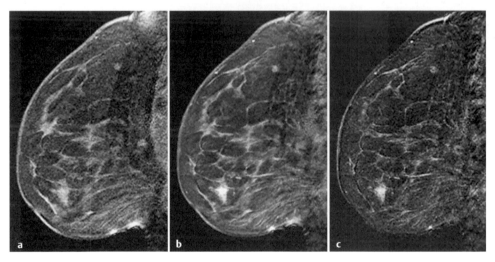

Fig. 3.21a–c   Sagittal orientation of breast MRI.
a T1w fat-saturated, precontrast examination in sagittal orientation.
b T1w fat-saturated examination 3 minutes after CM administration.
c Subtraction image.

Phase-Encoding Gradient

The spatial localization of a signal in three-dimensional space is achieved in MRI by encoding the slice position, the frequency, and the phase shift. For the axial view commonly used in Europe, the phase-encoding gradient is typically positioned in the mediolateral direction. This, however, occasionally results in an impairment of the evaluation of the axillary breast aspects, which is usually stronger on the left side (heart) than on the right (**Fig. 3.22a**). This problem can be solved by modifying the examination protocol to feature alternation of the direction of the phase-encoding gradient ("swapping") (**Fig. 3.22b**). Because of the decreasing importance of signal dynamics in HR-MR mammography, this examination protocol modification offers an alternative to, and will likely lead to a change of, the established examination protocol. In this context, the following two variations seem feasible.

Sandwich protocol. (**Fig. 3.23**). This involves a supplementary examination with phase-encoding gradient swapped to the ventrodorsal direction before and after the established dynamic examination (mediolaterally aligned phase-encoding gradient). The

advantage of this protocol is that it is still possible to perform an analysis of the time–signal intensity curve. The disadvantage is that the images with improved visualization of the axillary breast aspects are not available until 6–8 minutes after CM administration. If a contrast-enhancing lesion is found here at this late phase, a repeat breast MRI examination with a primary ventrodorsal phase-encoding gradient is the logical consequence.

Zebra protocol. (**Fig. 3.24**). This protocol involves swapping the phase-encoding gradient after each measurement. The advantage of this protocol is that the images with improved, artifact-free visualization of the axillary breast aspects are available very quickly after CM administration. If a contrast-enhancing lesion is found here, however, it is not possible to perform an analysis of the time–signal intensity curve with high temporal resolution.

! The sandwich and zebra protocols are examination protocols in which additional scans with a perpendicular phase-encoding gradient direction are performed.

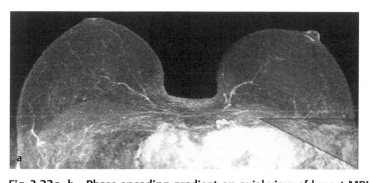
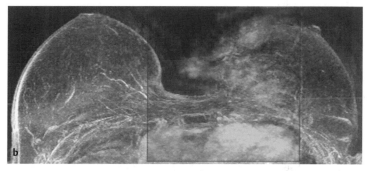

Fig. 3.22a, b Phase-encoding gradient on axial view of breast MRI. Established protocol.

a MIP of contrast-enhanced breast MRI in axial view with mediolateral direction of the phase-encoding gradient. A typical cardiac motion artifact overlays the axillary tail of both breasts (triangle), on the left more than on the right.

b A possible solution to this problem can be achieved by swapping the phase-encoding direction by 90° to the ventrodorsal direction. Now the depiction of the axillary structures is free of artifact, but the cardiac motion artifact overlays the medial aspect of both breasts (square), on the left more than on the right.

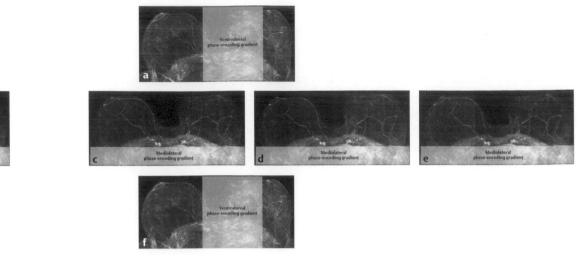

Fig. 3.23a–f Sandwich protocol. Established dynamic axial breast MRI examination with mediolateral phase-encoding gradient direction (middle row: **b** precontrast, **c–e** postcontrast). Additional scans with phase-encoding gradient swapped to the ventrodorsal direction before the precontrast scan (**a**) and after the last postcontrast scan (**f**). This provides the option to perform an earliest and an early subtraction with the mediolateral phase-encoding gradient direction, and a very late subtraction of the images with the ventrodorsal phase-encoding gradient direction. In addition it is possible to perform a kinetic curve analysis with a high temporal resolution.

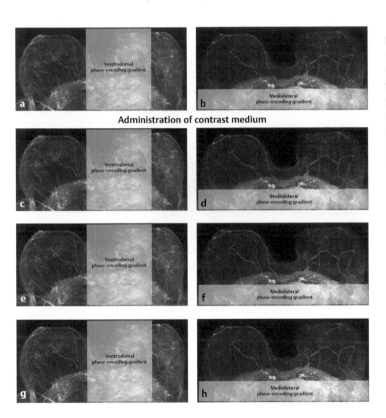

Fig. 3.24 Zebra protocol (a–h). Dynamic axial breast MRI examination with alternating ventrodorsal (left column) and mediolateral (right column) phase-encoding gradient direction. Each scan is performed once before contrast administration (**a** and **b**). Postcontrast scans are performed by turns. This provides the option to perform an earliest subtraction of scans with the ventrodorsal phase-encoding gradient direction and an early subtraction of scans with the mediolateral phase-encoding gradient direction. It is not possible to perform a kinetic curve analysis with a high temporal resolution.

Paramagnetic Contrast Materials

The distinguishing characteristic of all paramagnetic substances is that they have at least one unpaired electron. This electron has a magnetic moment that is ~1000 times stronger than that of a proton and it is this characteristic that effects a shortening of the T1 and T2 relaxation times. Thus paramagnetic substances cause an increased signal intensity in the T1w sequences, which are used in dynamic MR mammography. Intravenous administration of an extracellular paramagnetic CM provides a means for imaging the perfusion in the breast. Repetitive measurements after CM administration can provide information about the time course of CM uptake and washout.

Gd-DTPA. The greatest experience with contrast material in MR mammography is with gadolinium-DTPA (Gd-DTPA). Its chemical structure comprises a Gd ion with a triple positive charge combined with a DTPA derivative, forming a very stable complex (effective stability constant $K_{eff} = 10^{18.3}$ at pH 7.4). Gd-DTPA is also extremely stable under physiological conditions.

Dosage. The recommended contrast dosage for dynamic MR mammography (1.5 T) is 0.1 mmol Gd-DTPA/kg body weight, independent of the technique used. There are no studies showing any potential advantage in using a higher or lower CM dosage. It is important to consider, however, that the threshold value for the evaluation of contrast-enhancing lesions is dose-dependent and must be adapted accordingly (**Fig. 3.25**). There are user observa-

tions that speak for the practicability of using contrast materials with a higher concentration (**Fig. 3.26**).

Mode of administration. Contrast medium should be administered mechanically through a previously placed cubital venous access, at a rate of 2–3 mL/s. Use of a venous access in the lower arm and hand veins should be avoided. Immediately after CM administration, 20 mL or more of 0.9% NaCl should be administered to flush out any residual contrast.

Elimination. Gadolinium-DTPA is eliminated rapidly and completely by renal excretion without tubular reabsorption. The half-time of Gd-DTPA in blood is ~90 minutes. More than 91% of the administered dose is eliminated after 24 hours.

Tolerance and adverse effects. Gadolinium-DTPA is very well tolerated by most patients. On present data, Gd-DTPA is estimated to have an adverse reaction rate under 2%, of which 80% are minor reactions. These minor adverse reactions include nausea, vomiting, allergy-like skin and mucous membrane reactions, and local sensations of pain or warmth. It is necessary to inform the patient of these possibilities and to obtain a signed consent form before beginning the examination. Emergency measures to be taken in case of a major adverse reaction are the same as those for adverse reactions to radiographic CM.

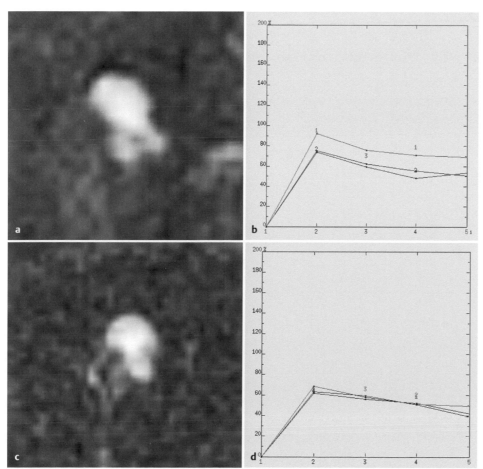

Fig. 3.25 a–d Intraindividual comparison of breast MRI with different doses of contrast medium. Breast tumor shows identical contrast and morphology in breast MRI after administration of a full CM dose (a) and half the dose (c). The initial enhancement is higher when the full dose is administered. The kinetic curves show identical characteristics with regard to the postinitial washout phenomenon (**b, d**).
a CM dose: 0.1 mmol Gd-DTPA/kg body weight.
b Initial signal increase of 95%.
c CM dose: 0.05 mmol Gd-DTPA/kg body weight.
d Initial signal increase of 70%.

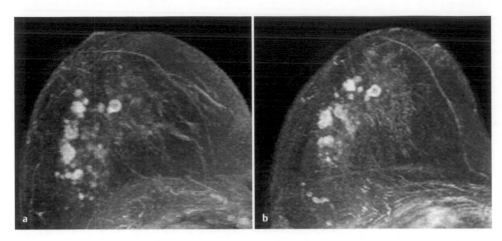

Fig. 3.26a, b Intraindividual comparison of breast MRIs with different concentrations of contrast medium. Multicentric breast tumor shows identical contrast and morphology in breast MRI after administration of contrast medium in different concentrations.
a Breast MRI with 0.1 mmol Gd-DTPA/kg body weight (Magnevist, 0.5 mol/L).
b Breast MRI with 0.1 mmol gadobutrol/kg body weight (Gadovist, 1 mol/L).

Gd-DTPA in pregnancy. The absolute safety of Gd-DTPA administration in pregnancy has not yet been proven. Dynamic MR mammography should therefore not be performed on pregnant women.

Gd-DTPA during lactation. Approximately 0.011% of CM administered intravenously is eliminated in the breast milk of lactating women. About 2% of this is absorbed by the gastrointestinal tract of a breast-fed child. Calculations show that the plasma concentration of Gd-DTPA in a child weighing 3 kg is 1/1000 of the mother's plasma concentration. It is generally recommended, however, that breast feeding be interrupted for 24 hours after CM administration.

Gd-DTPA and renal Insufficiency. Administration of a CM based on Gd-DTPA can lead to the development of nephrogenic systemic fibrosis in patients with renal insufficiency. This risk is especially high for patients with acute or chronic renal insufficiency and a glomerular filtration rate < 30 mL/min/1.73 m^2, as well as for patients with acute renal failure associated with a hepatorenal syndrome or after receiving a liver transplant.

Image Postprocessing

The great number of images acquired in dynamic MR mammography makes postprocessing necessary. This serves to improve the detection, characterization, and presentation of enhancing lesions.

Image Subtraction

Early and earliest image subtraction. The subtraction of precontrast from postcontrast images with identical slice position is performed to eliminate the intense fat signal and improve the detection of hypervascularized lesions. Normally, the precontrast image series is subtracted from the second series after CM administration (early subtraction) on a pixel-by-pixel basis (**Fig. 3.27**). If the breast parenchyma shows strong enhancement at this time, a complementary subtraction of the precontrast image series from the first postcontrast image series (earliest subtraction) should be performed (**Figs. 3.28g, 3.29**).

The subtraction of precontrast images from later postcontrast images has not proven useful because these images provide no additional diagnostic information (**Fig. 3.28i–k**) and the increasing enhancement of healthy breast tissue can lead to a masking of suspicious lesions.

! Early and earliest image subtractions are useful for the detection of suspicious lesions. Subtraction images from later postcontrast image series do not provide additional information.

Time–Signal Intensity Curve Analysis of Enhancing Lesions

The analysis of time–signal intensity curves (TICs) measured within representative areas of enhancing lesions allows further differentiation with respect to the probability of malignancy. A region of interest (ROI) should be selected such that it includes the greatest possible portion of the maximally enhancing area while disregarding less vascularized tumor areas (e.g., central necrotic portions). The size of the ROI should be between two and five pixels. The placement of three ROIs per lesion is recommended (**Fig. 3.30**). The numerical results of the TIC measurements should be expressed in terms of a percentage increase over the initial values (**Fig. 3.31**).

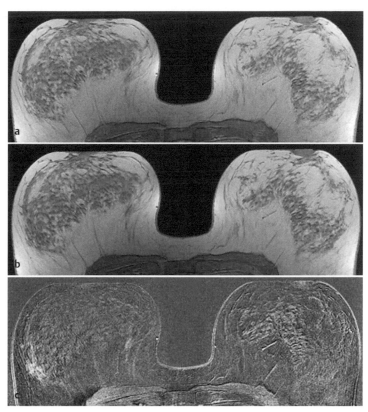

Fig. 3.27 a–c Early subtraction in contrast-enhanced breast MRI.
a Second postcontrast image.
b Corresponding precontrast image.
c Subtraction image = second postcontrast image – precontrast image.

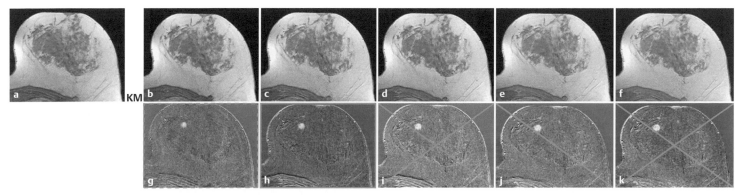

Fig. 3.28 a–k Early, earliest, and later subtractions in contrast-enhanced breast MRI. T1w precontrast image and the corresponding five consecutive postcontrast images of the left breast (upper row, **a–f**). The earliest subtraction image (**g**, first postcontrast image – precontrast image) and the early subtraction image (**h**, second postcontrast image – precontrast image) are useful for the detection of enhancing findings. Later subtraction images are of no additional help in detecting suspicious findings (crossed out images **i–k**).

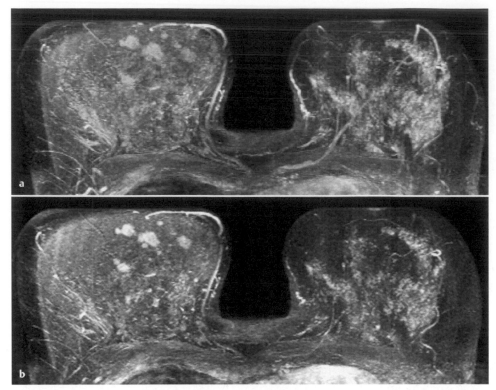

Fig. 3.29 a, b   **Early and supplementary earliest subtraction in contrast-enhanced breast MRI with strong parenchymal enhancement.** Multicentric breast cancer in the right breast.
a MIP of early subtraction images (second postcontrast image – precontrast image).
b MIP of earliest subtraction images (first postcontrast image – precontrast image) with improved visualization of breast tumors.

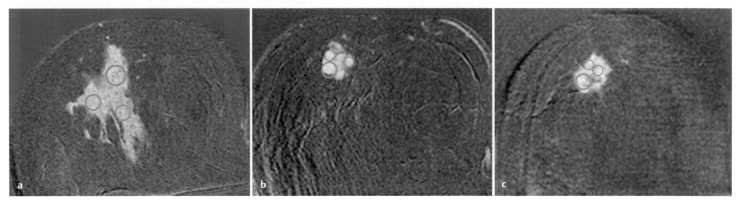

Fig. 3.30 a–c   Correct positioning of ROIs in three different tumors. Correct placement of three ROIs in each tumor for the kinetic curve analysis.
a Tumor with homogeneous enhancement.   **c** Tumor with ring enhancement.
b Tumor with inhomogeneous enhancement.

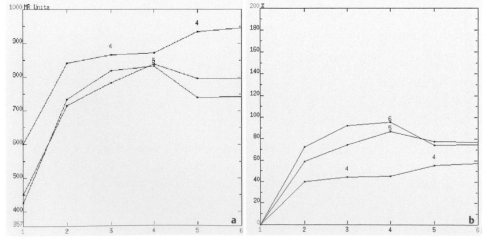

Fig. 3.31 a, b   Numerical and percentage increase presentation of kinetic curves. Multicentric breast cancer in right breast.
a Numerical signal intensity presentation on the *y*-axis of the kinetic curve (not recommended).
b Signal intensity increase on the *y*-axis of the kinetic curve as percentage increase relative to baseline signal intensity value (recommended).

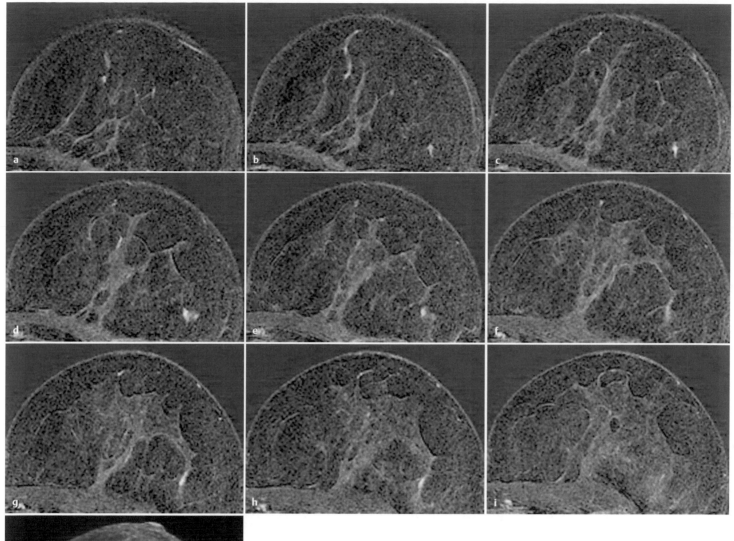

Fig. 3.32a–j MIP presentation of a linear-dendritic enhancing lesion
a–i Focal punctiform enhancement in continuous axial slices.
j A linear-dendritic enhancement pattern (arrow) is more easily recognized in the MIP.

Maximum Intensity Projection

The maximum intensity projection (MIP) technique yields a three-dimensional comprehensive view of both breasts. Based on postprocessed subtraction images in which only image pixels having at least a certain signal intensity are taken into account (threshold value algorithm), the representation of image information gives the impression of a transparent breast that can be viewed from different angles. This form of imaging allows a simpler spatial orientation and is especially suitable for the presentation of suspicious findings. In addition, it can be helpful for depicting the extent and dimensions of the tumor, especially for nonmass lesions (**Fig. 3.32**). Normally, the MIP technique does not provide additional diagnostically relevant information.

! Because the MIP technique allows a simple spatial orientation, it is especially suited for the presentation of breast findings. Generally, however, it does not provide additional diagnostically relevant information.

Multiplanar Reconstruction

Multiplanar reconstruction (MPR) images allow three-dimensional views of partial volumes within the breast. These are also based on postprocessed subtraction images. In special cases, these may help clarify the topographic relationship between a suspicious lesion and defined anatomical structures (e.g., mamillary region). The MPR technique is rarely used in MR mammography. Like MIP, this technique does not normally provide additional diagnostically relevant information.

Computer-Aided Diagnosis / Computer-Aided Detection

Both terms are in use and are abbreviated as CAD.

Automated image postprocessing. Various models for computer aided analysis of dynamic MR examinations of the breast have been published. These range from color-coded parameter images, automatically defined ROIs, and cine sequences with repeat rates of 1–2 seconds, to the employment of pharmacokinetic models (**Figs. 3.33, 3.34**). Newer versions of CAD systems evaluate not only the dynamic aspects (TICs) of a finding but also morphological criteria. To date, however, there are no large-scale studies defining the value of these postprocessing and analysis modalities.

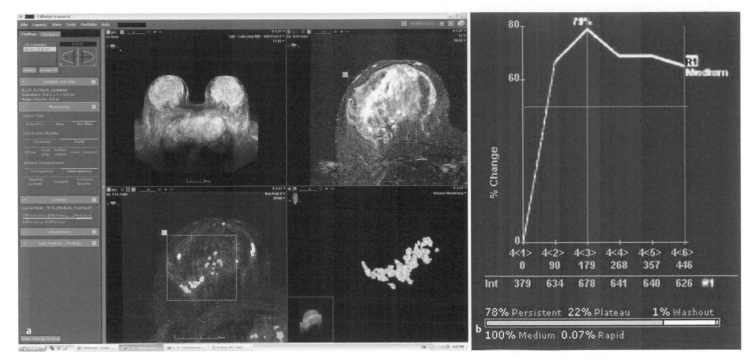

Fig. 3.33a, b Lesion analysis with a CAD system. Example of computer-aided analysis in contrast-enhanced breast MRI (CADstream, Confirma Co., WA, USA).

a Color-coded labeling of findings with enhancement above a defined threshold. Computer presentation of the surface 3D reconstruction.

b Representative kinetic curve.

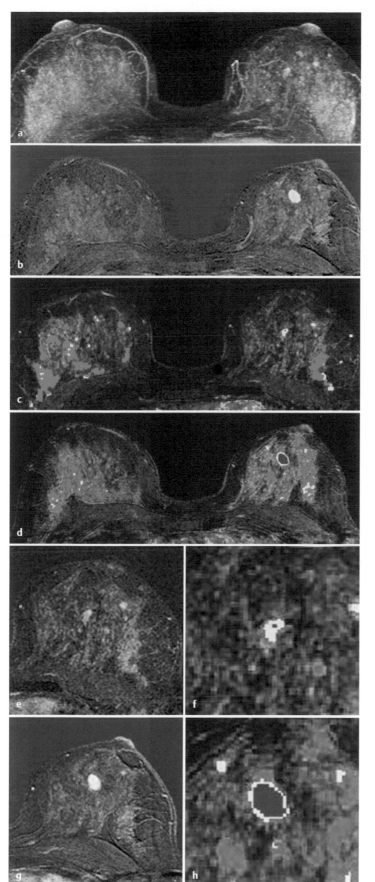

Fig. 3.34a–h CAD labeling of an early breast cancer.

a Breast MRI in a symptom-free patient with extremely dense breast tissue (ACR IV) and no ultrasound finding. Diffuse bilateral breast tissue enhancement (MRI density III). Several foci, more numerous in the left breast. No abnormality was detected (MRI-BIRADS 1 for both breasts).

b Breast MRI of same patient 2 years later. Similarly increased bilateral enhancement of breast parenchyma. No pathological finding in the right breast. A new hypervascularized, oval lesion with a diameter of 8 mm in the central aspect of the left breast.

c Retrospective analysis of first breast MRI (**a**) using a newly acquired CAD system shows extensive areas of hypervascularization in the peripheral aspects of both breasts (blue and yellow labeling indicate postinitial increase and plateau, respectively). In the central aspect of the left breast, identification of a circumscribed, hypervascularized area with postinitial plateau (yellow). Two red pixels within this area indicate a small region with a postinitial washout phenomenon.

d The lesion found in the breast MRI 2 years later (**b**) is retrospectively shown to correspond to the area described in (**c**). It is now larger in size and displays a prominent red labeling of the central tumor portion.

e Single slice subtraction of the microcarcinoma in (**a**).

f Corresponding CAD analysis with red labeling of the carcinoma.

g Single slice subtraction of the larger carcinoma 2 years later (**b**).

h Clear red labeling of the carcinoma in the corresponding CAD analysis.

Histology: IDC 12 mm, pT1c, pN0, G2.

Examination Protocol

MRI examinations typically feature numerous parameters that can be adjusted in various ways. As an example, the examination protocol used for contrast-enhanced, high-resolution breast MRI at the Women's Health Care Center, Göttingen is presented in **Table 3.1**.

Table 3.1 Protocol for breast MRI at the Women's Health Care Center, Göttingen in 2010

Field strength	1.5 T
Surface coil	Bilateral, open
Breast fixation	Craniocaudal compression paddle
Orientation	Axial
Technique	3D
Phase-encoding gradient	Alternating (zebra protocol)
Sequences	T1w GE sequence, T2w sequence (SE, TSE, IR)
Dynamic examination	1 precontrast, 5 postcontrast series
Paramagnetic contrast material	0.1 mol/kg BW
Contrast administration	IV, cubital vein, mechanically (flow 3 mL/s), postinjection of 20 mL saline solution
Spatial resolution	2.5 mm per slice
Temporal resolution	87 second sequence
FOV	300–350 mm
Matrix	512 × 512
Time-to-repetition, TR	8.4 ms
Time-to-echo, TE	4.1 ms
Flip angle, α	10°

Presently Unestablished Breast MRI Examination Techniques

Further MR examination techniques have been and are constantly being evaluated for their worth in the assessment of conspicuous lesions. A few of these are MR spectroscopy (MRS), MR elastography (MRE), and diffusion weighted MRI (DWI). The significance of these methods is not yet well defined.

MR Spectroscopy

MR spectroscopy (MRS) is based on the interactions between molecules and electromagnetic fields. It allows the evaluation of molecular characteristics such as the bonding strength, as well as the identification of atomic nuclei and their concentrations within the selected measurement volumes. The observed spectra of molecules, however, differ from those of atomic nuclei by having many more, usually overlapping spectral lines ("bands"). In the diagnostic evaluation of breast tumors, the choline peak is of special interest because choline-containing compounds can be found in high concentrations in malignant tumors, and only rarely in normal breast tissue or benign breast lesions. Factors such as

the placement and size of an MRS voxel, affecting the associated partial volume proportion of neighboring or endotumoral necrosis, parenchyma and/or fat, result in large variations in sensitivity and pose an unresolved problem (**Fig. 3.35**).

MR Elastography

The goal of MR elastography (MRE) is to present the viscoelastic properties (shear stiffness) and derived parameters such as anisotropy and elasticity tensor of examined breast tissue in a visual form. Benign and malignant tumors, which have different elastic properties, can therefore be more easily differentiated. To perform this examination, a breast surface coil with an integrated oscillator that generates acoustic shear waves via contact plates (e.g., 60 Hz) is required. The measured wave pattern is then translated into a corresponding color pattern that allows the analysis of the shear stiffness of suspicious lesions in the single MRI slice images (**Fig. 3.36**).

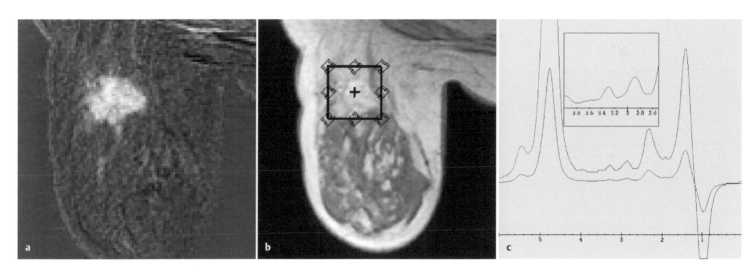

Fig. 3.35a–c   MR spectroscopy of large breast carcinoma.
a Subtraction image.

b Placement of the measurement voxel for spectroscopy.
c Resulting spectrogram.

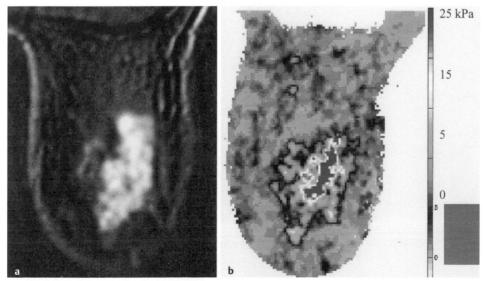

Fig. 3.36a, b   MR elastography of large breast carcinoma. (Image courtesy of Professor Joern Lorenzen, Zentrum für Radiologie und Endoskopie, Klinik und Poliklinik für Diagnostische und Interventionelle Radiologie, Universitaetsklinikum Hamburg-Eppendorf.)
a Subtraction image of invasive breast carcinoma.
b MR elastography with color coding of shear stiffness.

Diffusion-Weighted Breast MRI

Diffusion-weighted MR imaging (DWI) is a technique that provides image contrast that is dependent on the molecular motion of water between tissue compartments. The technique is primarily used for examinations of the brain because the diffusion of water molecules is characteristically altered in many brain diseases. It is also the case for breast tissue that the diffusion rate of water molecules is restricted, depending upon the type and extent of the pathological changes at the cellular level. Thus the aim of diffusion-weighted breast MRI is to provide adjunct information for improving the differentiation of benign and malignant breast lesions (**Fig. 3.37**).

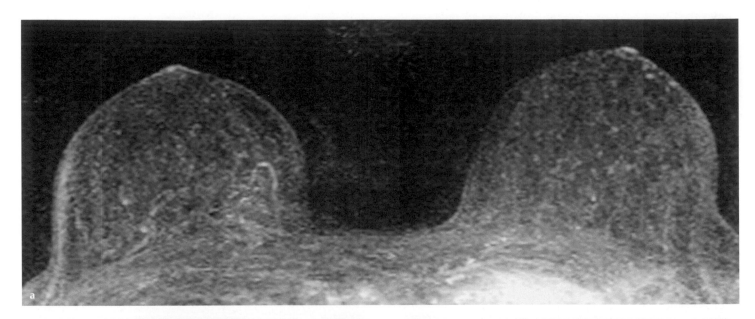

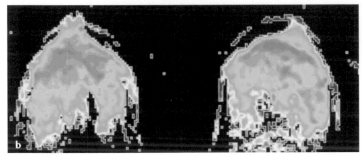
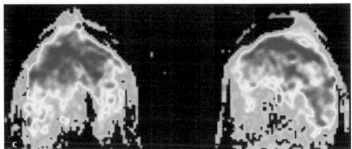

Fig. 3.37 a–c   Diffusion-weighted breast MRI. Normal findings.
a   MIP of subtraction MR images.
b, c   Corresponding diffusion-weighted images.

4 Tumor Angiogenesis and Breast MRI

Nutritional supply to the tumor. The nutritional requirements of malignant breast tumors, which almost always originate within the milk duct system, are initially acquired by diffusion. With increasing size, the growth of solid tumors is dependent upon an increasing network of capillaries to supply it with oxygen and other essential nutrients (tumor-induced angiogenesis, or tumor angiogenesis). Impressive animal experiments have shown that malignant tumors up to a diameter of 1–2 mm are supplied with nutrients via diffusion. From a tumor diameter of 2–3 mm, the formation of a sufficient capillary network is essential for further tumor growth because the nutrient requirements can no longer be adequately met by diffusion over such distances.

Angiogenic growth factors. The growth of new, tumor-associated blood vessels is a complex physiological process. Endothelial cells, which can be in a dormant state for months or years and are necessary for the development of new blood vessel walls, are activated in angiogenesis by various growth factors such as the basic fibroblast growth factor (bFGF) and the vascular endothelial growth factor (VEGF). In addition, numerous other growth factors have been identified. During angiogenesis, angiogenic growth factors activate endothelial cells in preexisting blood vessels to release enzymes that degrade the basement membrane (lysis) and allow endothelial cells to escape. New capillaries develop by the proliferation and migration of these endothelial cells into the surrounding matrix as small sprouts. These newly formed capillaries have a discontinuous basement membrane with an elevated permeability and an increased loss of plasma proteins. The further development of capillaries to arterioles and arteries, as well as to venules and veins, constitutes the completion of the angiogenic process triggered by angiogenic growth factors and determined by the activation of certain biological messenger substances.

! Tumor angiogenesis in breast carcinomas requires the activation, proliferation, and migration of dormant endothelial cells by angiogenic growth factors.

Increased perfusion. In breast MRI, increased enhancement in the first-pass images after IV administration of an appropriate paramagnetic contrast material is used to detect malignant breast tumors and to differentiate them from benign breast lesions. The increased tumor perfusion depicted by MRI has its root in the angiogenic changes associated with breast cancer. These include higher vessel density in the tumor matrix, increased vessel permeability, and the formation of carcinoma-associated arteriovenous shunts. Both the early tumor contrast enhancement and the typical contrast washout only minutes thereafter are thus the visible consequences of these angiogenic processes.

5 Diagnostic Criteria

As in other areas of imaging-based diagnostics, the evaluation of a breast MRI examination entails both the detection and also the characterization of suspicious lesions. High-quality MRI technique and methodology are necessary to depict hypervascularized changes reliably and free of artifacts, and are prerequisites for the detection of relevant breast lesions. Once detected, hypervascularized findings must be substantiated and characterized according to morphological and dynamic contrast criteria. Here, the personal expertise of the examiner is of great importance.

Assessment of the T1-Weighted Precontrast Examination

In certain constellations, the T1w precontrast examination can provide important additional information that sometimes permits a better interpretation of MRI findings. Especially notable are architectural distortions, peritumoral structural changes, fatty inclusions within ambiguous lesions, and therapy-induced and/or artificial changes (**Table 5.1** and **Fig. 5.1**). However, the reliable detection of breast cancer and adequate differentiation between benign and malignant tumors cannot be achieved without the intravenous administration of contrast.

! In T1w precontrast images, structures with a high signal intensity correspond to fat, protein, or blood.

Table 5.1 Typical findings in MRI

Substance	Signal in T1w	Signal in T2w	Examples
Water	Intermediate	High	Cyst
Oil, fat	High	Intermediate	Oil cyst, lipoma, fat in lymph node hilus
Blood, fresh	Low	Low	Fresh hematoma
Blood, old	High (ring form)	High	Subacute hematoma
Calcification	Low	Low	Fibroadenoma, fat necrosis
Metal fragments	Extinguished	Extinguished	Foreign body
Metal residues	Extinguished	Extinguished	Postoperative site

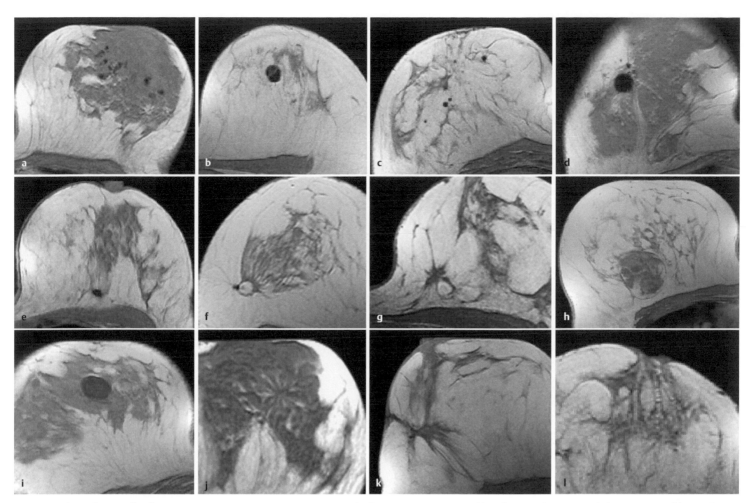

Fig. 5.1 a–l   Relevant findings in T1w precontrast images. Even before contrast material has been administered, important additional information is sometimes obtained from the T1w precontrast image.

a Spotty signal-free areas (diffuse, intramammary macrocalcifications).

b Endotumoral signal-free region (macrocalcification within a regressive fibroadenoma).

c Punctate, round signal extinction (susceptibility artifacts due to electrocautery during surgery).

d Large round signal extinction (susceptibility artifacts due to broken needle tip).

e Small oval signal extinction (susceptibility artifact due to clip marking).

f Round lesion with high signal intensity surrounded by signal-free zone (calcified oil cyst).

g Lesion with high signal intensity after vacuum biopsy (blood in resection cavity).

h Encapsulated space-occupying lesion with inhomogeneous internal signal intensity (hamartoma).

i Smooth-bordered, homogeneous lesion with low signal intensity (e. g., cyst, fibroadenoma).

j Architectural distortion within breast parenchyma (e.g., radial scar, tubular carcinoma).

k Hypointense architectural distortion showing retraction of surrounding tissue (postoperative scar).

l Increased signal intensity within retromamillary ducts (lactation phase).

Assessment of the T2-Weighted Examination

In T2w imaging, water has a very high signal intensity. The supplementary evaluation of these images allows a better assessment of hypervascularized lesions (**Fig. 5.2**). In addition, internal septations, which are a characteristic feature of myxoid fibroadenomas, are often best visualized in the T2w images.

> *!* Internal septations are characteristic features of myxoid fibroadenomas and are frequently best visualized in the T2w images.

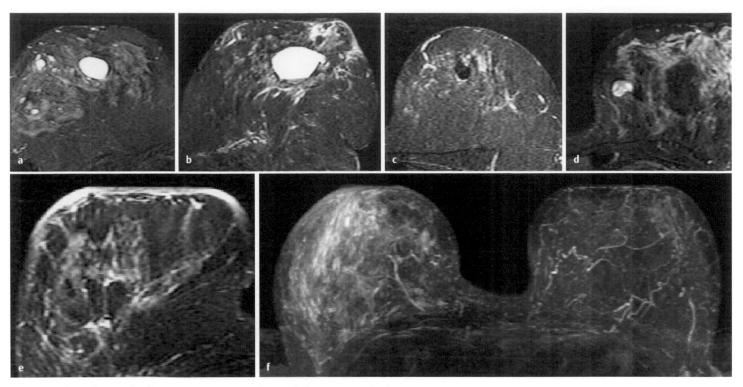

Fig. 5.2 a–f   Relevant findings in T2w images (IR with fat suppression).

a Oval, smooth-bordered lesion with very high signal intensity (cyst).
b Lesion with very high signal intensity and parietal areas with lower signal intensity (seroma).
c Hypointense round lesion (fibrous fibroadenoma).
d Hypointense septations within hyperintense lesion (myxoid fibroadenoma).

e Global skin thickening with high signal intensity (after breast radiotherapy).
f Asymmetric, diffuse increase of signal intensity in the right breast (after radiotherapy of the right breast).

Assessment of the Contrast-Enhanced T1-Weighted Examination

The assessment of hypervascularized structures in breast MRI is generally performed using the early subtraction slice images. If the breast parenchyma shows strong enhancement in this phase of the examination, the supplementary assessment of the earliest subtraction images may be more useful. In accordance with the ACR BI-RADS–MRI Lexicon, three types of lesions can be differentiated:

- Focus/foci
- Mass
- Nonmasslike enhancement

The following description of each type of enhancing lesion includes illustrative image examples.

Focus/Foci

A focus is a tiny spot of unspecific enhancement whose morphology cannot be characterized further due to its small size, and which has no corresponding structure on the T1w precontrast image (**Fig. 5.3**). Foci are multiple, tiny, circumscribable enhancing areas (**Fig. 5.4**). Typically, a focus is smaller than 5 mm in diameter.

Mass

A mass is a three-dimensional, space-occupying lesion that either displaces or has some other influence on the surrounding tissues.

> **!** The morphological criteria of a mass are its shape, margin, and enhancement pattern.

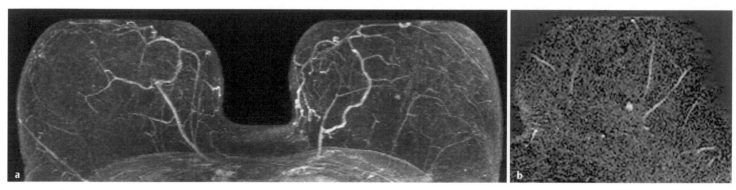

Fig. 5.3a, b   Focus.
a MIP of subtraction images shows a solitary, hypervascularized lesion with a diameter of 3 mm (focus) in the central aspect of the left breast.

b The same focus in a subtraction slice image.

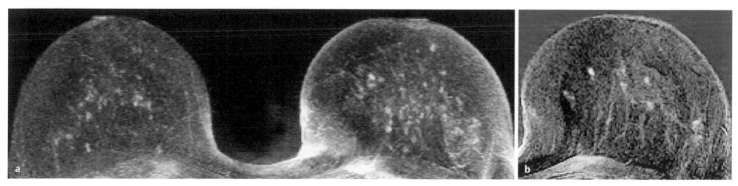

Fig. 5.4a, b   Foci.
a MIP of subtraction images shows multiple, finely speckled hypervascularized areas with a maximum diameter of 4 mm (foci) in both breasts.

b Representative subtraction slice image.

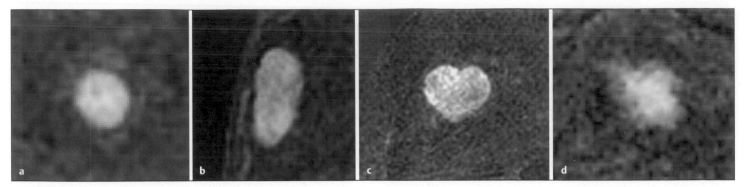

Fig. 5.5a–d   Shapes of hypervascularized mass lesions.
a Round.
b Oval.
c Lobulated.
d Irregular.

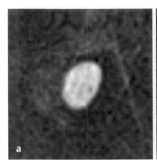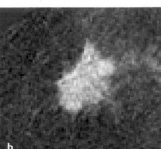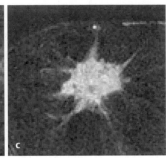

Fig. 5.6a–c   Margins of hypervascularized mass lesions.
a Well-circumscribed/smooth.
b Irregular.
c Spiculated.

Shape

The shape of a contrast-enhancing region in the subtraction image describes its spatial form. A round, oval, or lobulated shape usually designates a benign lesion, whereas a lesion with an irregular shape has a greater probability of malignancy (**Fig. 5.5**).

Shape of Contrast-Enhancing Lesion
• Round
• Oval
• Lobulated
• Irregular

Margins

The margins of a contrast enhancing region in the subtraction image describe its outer contours. Smooth, well-defined margins usually designate a benign lesion. Irregular margins or spiculations extending into the parenchyma designate a greater probability, but are not proof of malignancy (**Fig. 5.6**).

Margins of Contrast-Enhancing Lesions
• Well-defined, smooth
• Irregular
• Spiculated

Enhancement Pattern

The contrast enhancement pattern describes the spatial distribution of contrast within the contrast-enhancing lesion (internal enhancement).

Internal Patterns of Contrast-Enhancing Mass Lesions
• Homogeneous
• Heterogeneous
• Peripheral enhancement (rim sign)*
• Dark internal septations
• Enhancing internal septations
• Central enhancement

Rim-enhancement (*) designates a stronger contrast uptake in the tumor periphery than in the tumor center (signal loss in tumor center = necrosis; signal attenuation in tumor center = tumor fibrosis). The term "rim-enhancement" must be distinguished from the term "wall-enhancement" which is used to designate peripheral enhancement associated with inflamed cysts or abscesses.

Homogeneous, inhomogeneous, rim-enhancement. A homogeneous internal contrast enhancement pattern in a mass lesion is usually indicative of a benign proliferating process. An inhomogeneous internal contrast enhancement pattern is considered unspecific. Because a carcinoma has its biologically active zone in the tumor periphery, however, a rim-enhancement pattern can correspond to an increased perfusion of these areas relative to the tumor center and must be considered suspicious for malignancy.

Septations, central enhancement. Internal, hypovascularized septations are a reliable criterion for myxoid fibroadenomas. Great caution is recommended, however, because wide septations in the center of a fibroadenoma are occasionally very difficult to differentiate from a rim-enhancement associated with carcinomas. Hypervascularized internal septations, on the other hand, are an indication of an increased proliferation rate and must

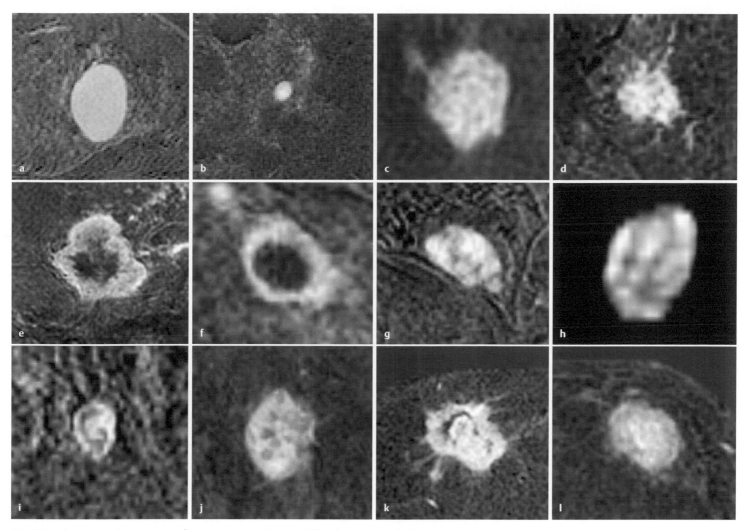

Fig. 5.7 a–l   Internal contrast enhancement patterns within hypervascularized mass lesions.

a, b Homogeneous.
c, d Heterogeneous.
e   Rim-enhancement (thick rim).
f   Rim-enhancement (thin rim).

g, h Dark internal septations (not enhancing).
i, j Enhancing internal septations.
k, l Central enhancement.

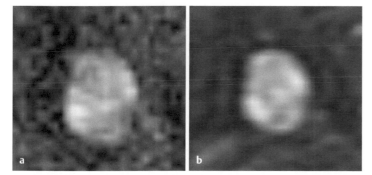

Fig. 5.8 a, b   Dark versus enhancing internal septations. Intraindividual comparison of a mass lesion in subtraction and corresponding IR T2 w, fat-saturated images. In the subtraction image there appear to be enhancing internal septations. In contrast, the corresponding IR T2 w, fat-saturated image gives the impression that the septations are dark (not corresponding to the enhancing areas in **a**).
a Subtraction image.
b IR T2 w, fat-saturated image.

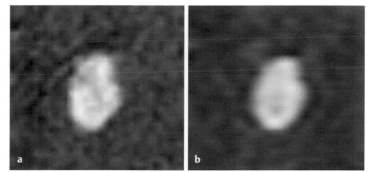

Fig. 5.9 a, b   Dark internal septations versus rim-enhancement. Intraindividual comparison of a mass lesion in subtraction and corresponding IR T2 w, fat-saturated images. In the subtraction image there appear to be dark internal septations. The corresponding IR T2 w, fat-saturated image gives the impression that the tumor rim has a high water content.
a Subtraction image.
b IR T2 w, fat-saturated image.

always prompt one to include malignancy in the differential diagnosis. This is also true when a central region with increased vascularization is seen within a mass lesion (**Fig. 5.7**).

! A rim-enhancement must always be considered suspicious for malignancy.
However, not all rim-enhancements are carcinomas.

Limitations. Note that the clear differentiation of internal mass features (e.g., septation versus rim sign) can sometimes be very difficult. In some cases, the T1 w and T2 w images do not yield corresponding findings (**Figs. 5.8, 5.9**).

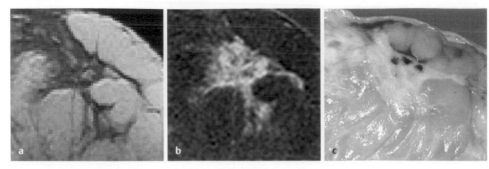

Fig. 5.10a–c Nonmasslike lesion in breast MRI. A nonmasslike lesion respects the boundaries of the surrounding intramammary fat tissue. Only parenchymal structures are infiltrated.

a T1w precontrast image shows parenchymal/tumor structures with intermediary signal intensity. Fat tissue has a high signal intensity.

b Corresponding subtraction image shows strong contrast enhancement of tumor and no enhancement in surrounding fat tissue.

c Macroscopic histology specimen shows carcinoma in areas corresponding to enhancing structures and healthy fat tissue in nonenhancing areas.

Histology: invasive lobular breast carcinoma.

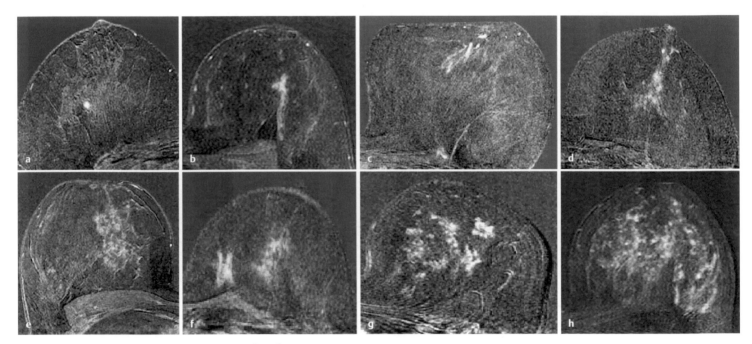

Fig. 5.11a–h Nonmasslike enhancement: distribution.

a Focal area.

b Linear.

c Ductal.

d Segmental.

e Regional (solitary).

f Multiple regions (two).

g Multiple regions.

h Diffuse.

Nonmasslike Enhancement

A nonmasslike enhancement is neither a mass nor a focus, and typically respects the surrounding intramammary fatty tissue boundaries. There is normally no increase in volume, and no displacement of or influence on adjacent structures (**Fig. 5.10**).

! The differential diagnosis of nonmasslike enhancing lesions must always include intraductal proliferative lesions, radial scars, and invasive lobular breast carcinomas.
The analysis of these lesions includes characterization of enhancement distribution, internal characteristics, and symmetry.

Enhancement Distribution

The distribution of a nonmasslike enhancement is a description of the enhancing area in the subtraction image. The terminology used to describe these areas is very much like that used for the distribution of microcalcifications in x-ray mammography. Ductal and segmental distribution are especially indicative of intraductal proliferation, i.e., a potentially malignant lesion (**Fig. 5.11**).

Nonmasslike Enhancement Distribution
- Focal (spread over < 25% of a breast quadrant)
- Linear
- Ductal (linear branching along a milk duct)
- Segmental (triangular with peak toward nipple)
- Regional (solitary and multiple)
- Diffuse

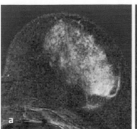 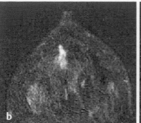 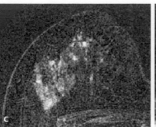 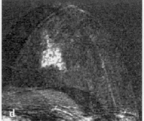 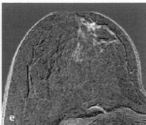

Fig. 5.12a–e   Nonmasslike enhancement: internal characteristics.

a Homogeneous.

b Inhomogeneous.

c Stippled/punctate.

d Clumped.

e Reticular/dendritic.

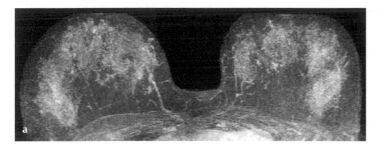 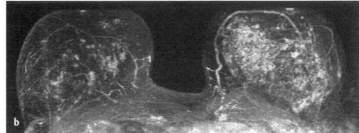

Fig. 5.13a, b   Symmetric versus asymmetric nonmasslike enhancement. MIP of subtraction images.

a Symmetric bilateral enhancement.

b Asymmetric enhancement of left breast.

Internal Enhancement Characteristics/Pattern

The internal enhancement pattern of a nonmasslike lesion describes the internal contrast distribution within the enhancing area in the subtraction image. Clumped, blotchy enhancing areas are especially suspicious for ductal carcinoma in situ (DCIS), while small, stippled enhancing areas, especially when not distributed along a milk duct, are usually a physiological finding. Ultimately, however, neither pattern alone allows the reliable classification of a nonmasslike lesion as malignant or benign (**Fig. 5.12**).

> Nonmasslike Internal Enhancement Pattern
> • Homogeneous
> • Inhomogeneous
> • Stippled/punctate (multiple, scattered, punctate foci 1–2 mm in size)
> • Clumped (aggregate of enhancing masses or foci, occasionally confluent)
> • Reticular/dendritic

Symmetry

The symmetry of nonmasslike enhancing areas requires the comparison of enhancement within both breasts. This can be done by comparing enhancement distribution in the subtraction image (**Fig. 5.13**). It is more informative, however, to compare the distribution of breast parenchyma in the T1w precontrast images first. If there is an asymmetry of parenchymal distribution in these images, then it can be expected that there will be asymmetric parenchymal enhancement. The term asymmetry should therefore only be used when asymmetric enhancement is present in symmetrically distributed parenchymal structures (**Fig. 5.14**).

> Symmetry
> • Symmetric
> • Asymmetric

Dynamic Enhancement Characteristics (Kinetics)

Time–signal intensity curves generated by kinetic techniques describe the signal intensity changes occurring in a contrast-enhancing region (ROI) within the breast with respect to time. These so-called TICs are especially useful and should be evaluated when dealing with mass lesions where the appropriate placement of ROIs is reliable. When evaluating foci, the small size of the individual contrast-enhancing areas does not always allow a suitable ROI placement. From experience, signal analysis within nonmasslike lesions is usually impracticable. Because the enhancing areas are very fine and inhomogeneous, the acquired TICs show an unspecific course due to inclusion of lipomatous areas.

When evaluating a TIC one distinguishes between the initial phase (1–3 minutes after CM administration) and the postinitial phase (3–8 minutes after CM administration).

> Enhancement Dynamics in Breast MRI
> • Initial phase (1–3 minutes after CM administration)
> • Postinitial phase (3–8 minutes after CM administration)

Initial Signal Increase

The initial signal increase is the maximum signal intensity increase (in %) within the first 3 minutes after CM administration based on the signal intensity in the precontrast image (**Fig. 5.15**).

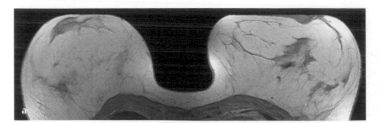

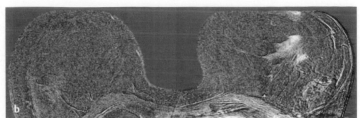

Fig. 5.14a, b   Asymmetric nonmasslike enhancement.
a T1w precontrast image.
b Subtraction image shows no contrast enhancement in the right

breast and conspicuous contrast enhancement in the parenchyma of the left breast.

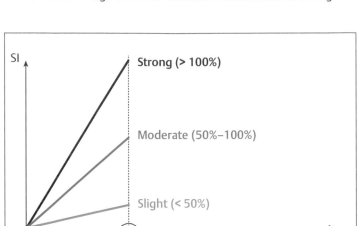

Fig. 5.15   Initial signal increase. The initial signal increase is the maximum signal intensity increase within the first 3 minutes after contrast administration, expressed as a percentage of the precontrast signal intensity. SI = signal intensity.

It is calculated using the formula:

$$\text{Initial signal increase [\%]} = \frac{\text{Signal post CM} - \text{Signal pre CM}}{\text{Signal pre CM}} \times 100$$

Initial Signal Increase (1–3 minutes after CM)
- Slow: less than 50% increase in signal intensity compared with precontrast
- Medium: between 50% and 100% increase in signal intensity compared with precontrast
- Rapid: over 100% increase in signal intensity compared with precontrast

The initial signal intensity increase is dependent upon the system's field strength, the concentration and volume of administered contrast material, and the measurement sequence among other factors. The applied threshold values must therefore be adjusted and defined according to the system and settings used.

❗ The peak of contrast enhancement within breast carcinomas is usually ~3 minutes after IV contrast administration.

Postinitial Signal Course

The postinitial signal course is described by the development of the signal intensity curve between the signal intensity peak within the first 3 minutes after contrast administration and the

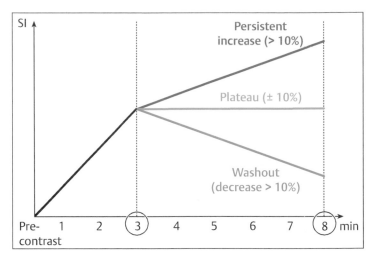

Fig. 5.16   Postinitial signal course. The reference point at which the postinitial signal intensity course begins is the maximum signal intensity within the first two measurements after contrast administration. SI = signal intensity.

8th minute after contrast administration (**Fig. 5.16**). The signal intensity value after the 8th minute is put in relation to the maximum value in the initial signal increase phase. The calculation is made with the formula:

$$\text{Postinitial signal course [\%]} = \frac{\text{Signal 8th min} - \text{Signal}_{\text{MAX}} \text{ 1st–3rd min}}{\text{Signal}_{\text{MAX}} \text{ 1st–3rd min}} \times 100$$

Postinitial Signal Course (3–8 minutes after CM)
- Persistent increase: continuous signal increase to at least 10% over peak signal intensity
- Plateau: constant signal intensity (± 10%)
- Washout: signal decrease to at least 10% under peak signal intensity

❗ The postinitial washout phenomenon of malignant tumors is a consequence of the increased permeability of tumor blood vessels and the presence of tumor-associated AV-shunts.

Kinetic pattern. The distribution pattern of contrast with respect to time has lost much of its past significance due to the increasing and overriding importance of morphological criteria. In the past centrifugal kinetics (*blooming* = mass size increase over time as an indication of benignity) and centripetal kinetics (*iris diaphragm phenomenon* = early initial rim-enhancement, filling in toward the tumor center) were differentiated. Findings displaying the latter phenomenon, however, are already suspicious for malignancy due to the rim sign seen in the early subtraction image.

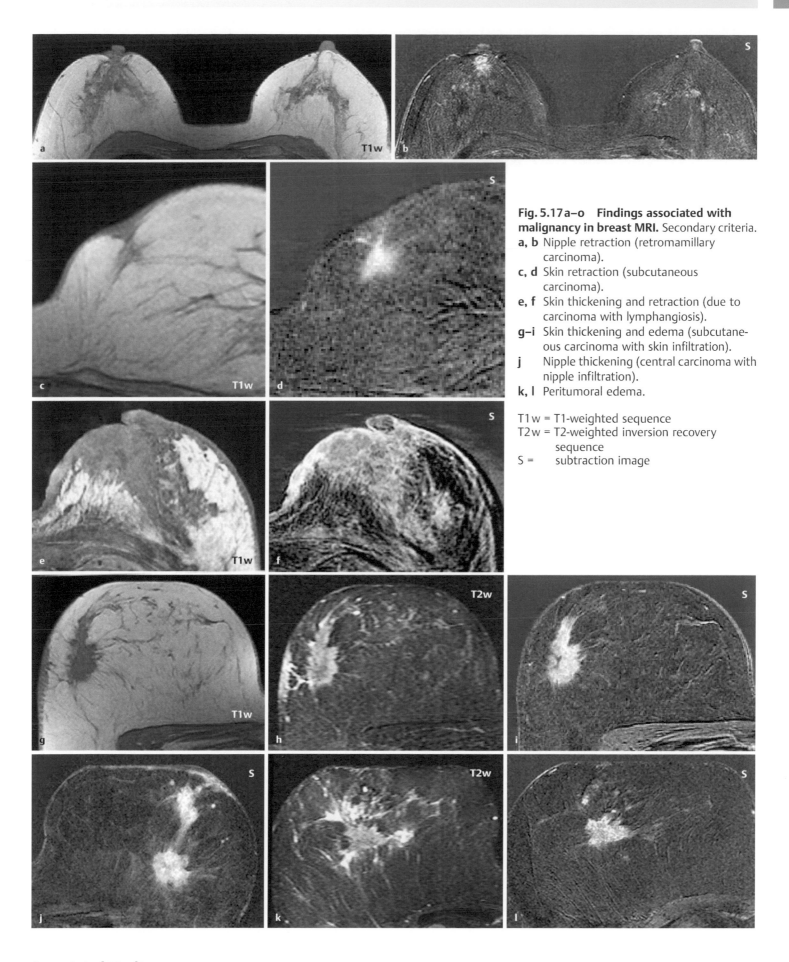

Fig. 5.17a–o Findings associated with malignancy in breast MRI. Secondary criteria.
a, b Nipple retraction (retromamillary carcinoma).
c, d Skin retraction (subcutaneous carcinoma).
e, f Skin thickening and retraction (due to carcinoma with lymphangiosis).
g–i Skin thickening and edema (subcutaneous carcinoma with skin infiltration).
j Nipple thickening (central carcinoma with nipple infiltration).
k, l Peritumoral edema.

T1w = T1-weighted sequence
T2w = T2-weighted inversion recovery
sequence
S = subtraction image

Associated Findings

Associated findings are those breast changes that are often, but not always, found to occur alongside malignant breast lesions. They often support the diagnosis, and sometimes provide additional therapy-relevant information (**Fig. 5.17**).

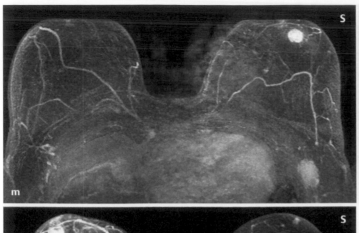

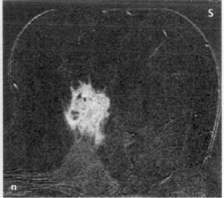

Fig. 5.17 (Continued)
m Lymphadenopathy.
n Infiltration of pectoral muscle.
o Dilated veins.

T1w = T1-weighted sequence
T2w = T2-weighted inversion recovery
      sequence
S =   subtraction image

Table 5.2 Comparison of unifactorial and multifactorial breast MRI evaluation protocols. High sensitivity for all protocols. Lower specificity for protocols using only one criterion for evaluation. Significant improvement of specificity using multiple evaluation criteria

Protocol	Sensitivity	Specificity	Accuracy
Unifactorial			
Threshold SI > 90%	96%	31%	78%
Threshold SI > 500	98%	27%	86%
Multifactorial			
3 Criteria[a]	94%	64%	82%
4 Criteria[b]	98%	59%	87%
5 Criteria[c]	96%	78%	88%

[a] Shape, initial signal increase, postinitial signal course.
[b] Shape, margin definition, initial signal increase, postinitial signal course.
[c] Shape, margin definition, internal CM distribution, initial signal increase, postinitial signal course

Breast MRI Evaluation Protocols

Unifactorial evaluation protocols. Unifactorial evaluation protocols that take only one threshold parameter into consideration (e.g., signal increase > 100% in the 1st minute after CM administration) have a sensitivity equivalent to that of multifactorial evaluation protocols but significantly lower specificity. Today such protocols have only historical value. There is wide consensus that several criteria must be taken into account when evaluating a breast finding to take full advantage of the information that MRI can provide (**Table 5.2**).

Multifactorial evaluation protocols. Multifactorial evaluation protocols typically take several morphological and dynamic criteria into account. Currently the morphological evaluation of a lesion applies to its shape and margins. The dynamic evaluation involves the analysis of contrast distribution and TICs. It should be noted here that with the increasing improvement of spatial resolution in breast MRI, morphological criteria continue to gain importance and time–signal intensity analysis is falling into the background.

! Multifactorial evaluation protocols primarily increase the specificity of breast MRI.

Göttingen Score

The so-called Göttingen score is an established multifactorial evaluation protocol that has proven especially useful for the characterization of hypervascularized mass lesions. The evaluated criteria are shape, margins, internal contrast distribution, and initial and postinitial contrast signal course. The respective findings are given a value, with the more suspicious findings receiving a higher value. After taking all criteria into account, findings with a total score under 3 points generally correspond to benign lesions. Total scores over 3 are more suspicious for malignancy (**Fig. 5.18**).

Figures 5.19, 5.20, 5.21 provide examples for the implementation of the Göttingen score in the evaluation of mass lesions.

Additional criteria. To modify and improve this protocol, attempts are continually being made to integrate further criteria into the overall evaluation process of lesions. Especially promising are the criteria pertaining to the water content of lesions and internal dark septations (both indicating a somewhat greater probability of benignity).

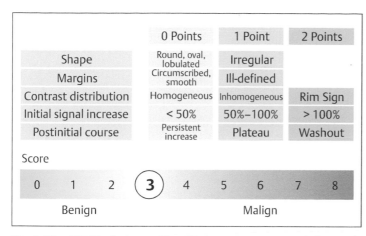

	0 Points	1 Point	2 Points
Shape	Round, oval, lobulated	Irregular	
Margins	Circumscribed, smooth	Ill-defined	
Contrast distribution	Homogeneous	Inhomogeneous	Rim Sign
Initial signal increase	< 50%	50%–100%	> 100%
Postinitial course	Persistent increase	Plateau	Washout

Score

0	1	2	**③**	4	5	6	7	8

Benign   Malign

Fig. 5.18 Göttingen score. The Göttingen score is a multifactorial evaluation protocol in which each of five defined criteria per lesion receives 0 to 2 points. Rim-enhancement, strong initial enhancement, and postinitial washout are the strongest criteria indicating malignancy (each receives 2 points). A total score of 0 to 8 points per lesion is possible.

Findings that achieve a total Göttingen score of 1 or 2 points are benign and can be classified in the MRI BI-RADS categories 1 and 2. Findings achieving a total Göttingen score of 4 or more points have an increasing probability of being malignant and are classified in the MRI BI-RADS categories 4 (4 and 5 points) and 5 (6 to 8 points). Findings with a Göttingen score of 3 points are placed in the MRI BI-RADS category 3.

❗ The Göttingen score is primarily useful for the evaluation of hypervascularized mass lesions.

ACR BI-RADS–MRI

The American College of Radiology first included breast MRI in the 4th edition of its ACR BI-RADS Lexicon in 2003. This provided standardized terminology and characterization criteria for breast MRI findings in analogy to the terms used for mammography evaluation.

After breast MRI lesions are analyzed and described, they must be categorized according to their probability of being malignant (**Table 5.3**). The categories used are the MRI BI-RADS assessment categories 0, 1, 2, 3, 4, 5, and 6. The MRI BI-RADS category 4 can be subdivided into 4A, 4B, and 4C.

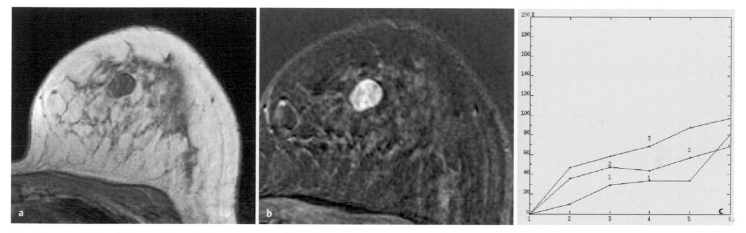

Fig. 5.19a–c Mass lesion with a Göttingen score of 2. Shape is oval (0 points), margins are smooth (0 points), internal contrast distribution is heterogeneous (1 point), initial signal increase has a maximum of 60% (1 point), postinitial course is a persistent increase (0 points). Total Göttingen score = 2. MRI BI-RADS 2.

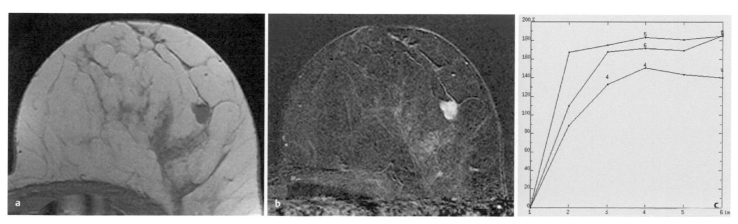

Fig. 5.20a–c Mass lesion with a Göttingen score of 4. Shape is lobulated (0 points), margins are smooth (0 points), internal contrast distribution is heterogeneous (1 point), initial signal increase has a maximum of 160% (2 points), postinitial course is a plateau (1 point). Total Göttingen score = 4. MRI BI-RADS 4.

Table 5.3   MRI BI-RADS and risk of malignancy

MRI BI-RADS	Description	Risk of malignancy
1	Negative	0.00%
2	Benign finding(s)	0.00%
3	Probably benign finding	<2%
4[a]	Suspicious abnormality	2%
5	Highly suggestive of malignancy	>90%

[a] May be classified further into categories BI-RADS 4A (2%–30%), BI-RADS 4B (31%–60%), and BI-RADS 4C (61%–90%)

Table 5.4   Assignment of MRI BI-RADS category depending upon the Göttingen score

MRI total points (Göttingen score)	MRI BI-RADS
0,1	MRI BI-RADS 1
2	MRI BI-RADS 2
3	MRI BI-RADS 3
4,5	MRI BI-RADS 4
6,7,8	MRI BI-RADS 5

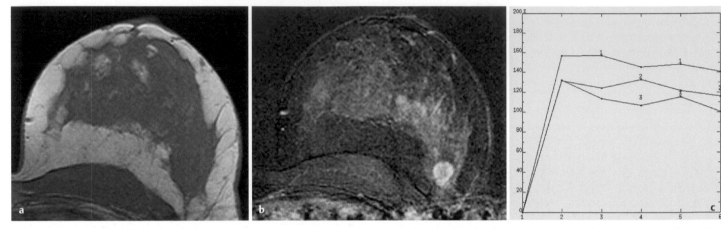

Fig. 5.21 a–c   Mass lesion with a Göttingen score of 7. Shape is round (0 points), margins are ill-defined (1 point), internal contrast distribution is a ring-enhancement (2 points), initial signal increase has a maximum of 160% (2 points), postinitial course is a washout (2 points). Total Göttingen score = 7. MRI BI-RADS 5.

BI-RADS 0. This category is used for findings that cannot be evaluated conclusively and require additional imaging. For breast MRI findings, this category is rarely used because MRI is usually the last step in the diagnostic cascade.

BI-RADS 6. Findings are placed in this category when percutaneous biopsy (large-core biopsy, vacuum-assisted biopsy) has revealed a lesion with malignant histology (intraductal, invasive). This categorization persists until definitive therapy (usually surgical removal) has been initiated.

Göttingen Score and MRI BI-RADS assessment categories. The ACR BI-RADS Lexicon does not elaborate on when to apply which assessment category for a breast MRI finding. The Göttingen scoring system provides a basis upon which an assessment category can be assigned to a MRI finding according to the total score such finding has received (**Table 5.4**).

> In general, clinical, radiological, and ultrasonographic findings must be taken into account to fully characterize ambiguous breast lesions and to decide on the further course of action.

6 Artifacts and Sources of Error

Incorrect Positioning

The patient to be examined is typically placed in the prone position. Ideally, the breasts are examined in a hanging position in an open breast coil. It is important to take care that all areas of the breast hang freely and completely in the coil lumen and not outside its sensitive volume. The complete imaging of the breast within the breast coil lumen can be verified before beginning dynamic measurements. The T2w sequence performed before the dynamic examination is well suited for this purpose and can easily be repeated if inadequate positioning must be corrected (**Figs. 6.1, 6.2, 6.3**).

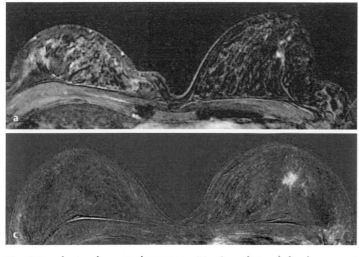 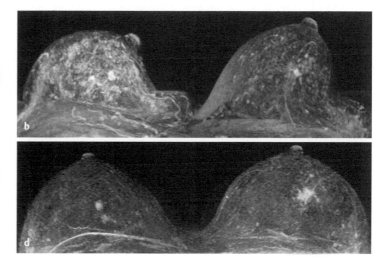

Fig. 6.1 a–d Inadequate breast positioning—lateral displacement.
a Subtraction slice image. Incorrect positioning of the breast inside the surface coil with bulging of breast tissue on the left side of both breasts.
b MIP of subtraction images (external examination).

c Repeat examination with correct positioning of the breasts and better depiction of several fibroadenomas in the right breast, and a radial scar in the left breast.
d MIP of subtraction images.

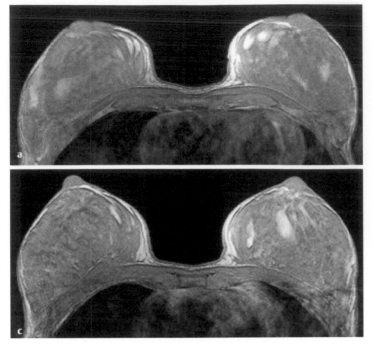

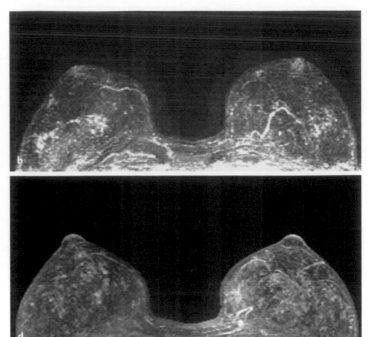

Fig. 6.2a–d   Inadequate breast positioning – nipple.

a T1w precontrast slice image. Incorrect positioning of the nipple (not imaged hanging free and in ventral position).

b MIP of subtraction images with false impression of retromamillary enhancement.

c Repeat examination with correct positioning of the nipples.

d MIP of subtraction images now shows nipples in profile.

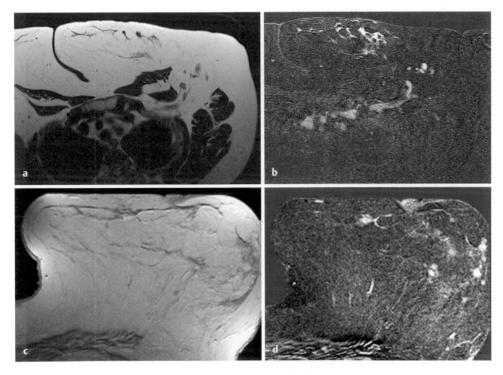

Fig. 6.3a–d   Inadequate breast positioning—use of body coil in supine body position.

a External breast MRI examination performed using a body coil in supine position because of large breast size (T1w image).

b Corresponding subtraction image with unusual depiction of thoracic and mammary structures.

c Repeat examination with correct positioning of the breasts using a dedicated open breast coil.

d Corresponding subtraction image with familiar depiction of mammary structures.

Improper Administration of Contrast

Perivenous injection of contrast medium. The perivenous injection of contrast medium (CM) can remain undetected if only the precontrast and subtraction images are evaluated. Subtraction images, in particular, will simulate normal findings in this case. Occasionally, white ribbonlike zones due to motion artifacts can be mistaken for contrasting veins (**Fig. 6.4**). To ensure the correct intravasal administration of contrast, therefore, it is necessary to detect a definite enhancement in typical reference points (e.g., intramammary veins, internal mammary arteries, **Fig. 6.5**). If the complete contrast dose has been injected perivenously, the breast MRI examination can be repeated as soon as the source of error has been rectified.

!

● Typical reference points to check for correct contrast material administration (**Fig. 6.5**):
● Internal mammary arteries
● Nipples
● Intramammary veins

Inadequate NaCl flushing. The failure to inject a sufficient volume of normal saline after contrast administration results in ~4 mL of contrast material not being administered because it remains in the extension tubing. This leads to a significant underdosage of CM. For a woman with a body weight of 70 kg and a desired dosage of 0.1 mmol Gd-DTPA/kg body weight, this volume results in a 30% reduction of the effective dose. Since this has an effect on the signal enhancement, it may result in misinterpretation of the results. These examinations should be repeated after an interval of at least 12 hours.

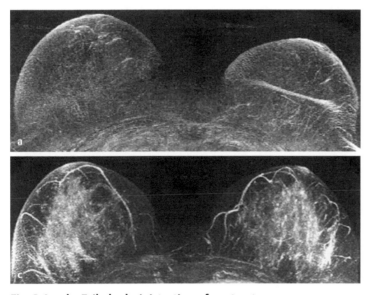
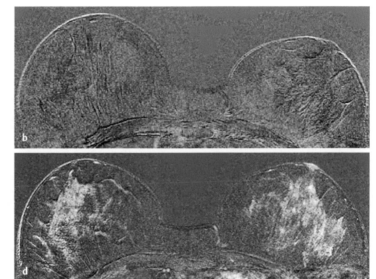

Fig. 6.4a–d   Failed administration of contrast.
a MIP of subtraction images.
b Representative subtraction slice image shows slight motion artifacts without definite indications of correct contrast administration.
c Repeat examination after reconnection of IV tubing (MIP image).
d Representative subtraction slice image of repeat examination.

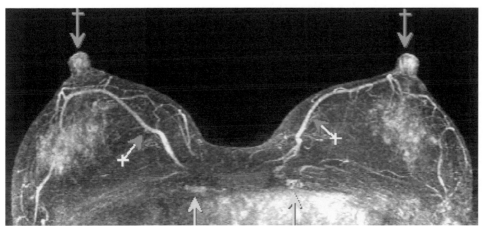

Fig. 6.5   Reference points for verification of correct contrast administration.
● Contrasted internal mammary arteries (yellow arrows).
● Nipple enhancement (green arrows).
● Contrasted intramammary veins (blue arrows).

Motion Artifacts

Motion artifacts seen in MR mammography have two major causes. One is the transmission of heart pulsations, which predominantly affects the left breast of slender patients. The other main cause is movement by the patient during the examination (**Figs. 6.6, 6.7**). Performing breast MRI with an open breast coil and a special compression device to assure adequate breast compression (see Chapter 3) reduces the degree of motion artifacts significantly (**Fig. 6.8**).

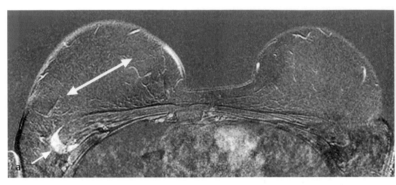 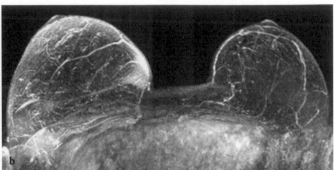

Fig. 6.6 a, b   Motion artifacts due to relaxation of pectoral muscle during dynamic examination.

a Subtraction image. Motion due to relaxation of pectoral muscle results in an artifact band at the lateral end of the right pectoral muscle (arrow), as well as white and black motion artifacts at respectively the medial and lateral skin boundaries (double-headed arrow).

b MIP.

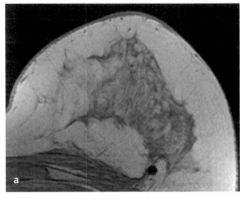 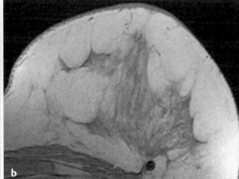 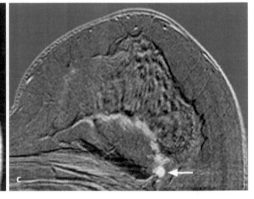

Fig. 6.7 a–c   Motion artifact mimicking masslike abnormality.

a T1w precontrast image. Clip artifact near pectoral muscle.
b T1w postcontrast image. Movement of the pectoral muscle results in a relative displacement of the clip.

c Subtraction image. Ribbonlike zones with signal loss (black) or signal summation (white) result from movement. False-positive "mass" results from displacement of the clip artifact (arrow) in image subtraction.

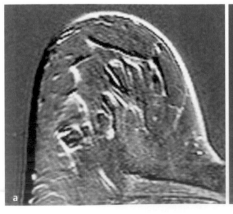 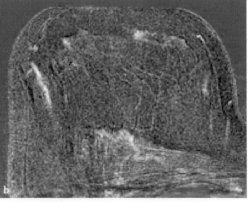

Fig. 6.8 a, b   Motion artifact due to not using breast compression device.

a Subtraction image with unacceptable motion artifacts (MRI artifact level III). External examination was performed without using an appropriate breast compression device. Interpretation yielded a nonmasslike lesion.

b Repeat examination with adequate breast compression (MRI artifact level I). Normal findings.

Subtraction images. The quality of subtraction images is especially sensitive to motion artifacts during the dynamic measurements. The effect is generally seen as the presence of black-and-white ribbonlike zones lacking image information. Such artifacts are occasionally seen to a lesser degree in the peripheral areas of the affected breast. They also occur within the breast parenchyma, however, and are most often seen near the pectoral muscle due to thoracic breathing movements (**Fig. 6.7a**).

> **!** The MIP presentation is the most reliable image to check for motion artifacts. Executed with excellent quality, it can be used to rule out artifacts caused by breast movements (**Fig. 6.9**).

False-negative and false-positive findings. Even minor motion artifacts can mask relevant breast findings. In particular the presence of a nonmasslike lesion can then easily be missed (**Fig. 6.10**). On the other hand, motion artifacts can produce areas that look like a lesion but are not (a false-positive, **Fig. 6.11**).

Documentation and Classification

The degree of motion artifacts should be assessed and documented in the written report of each breast MRI examination. This helps indicate how informative this specific examination is and the relative possibility that a pathological lesion could be missed. In this context, a 4-level classification system equivalent

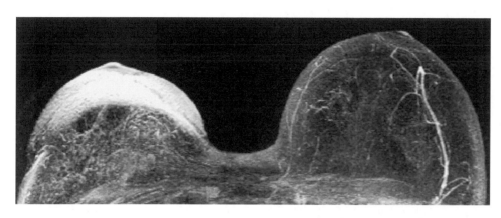

Fig. 6.9 "Snow-peak" effect—motion artifacts in MIP presentation of subtraction images. The MIP is the most reliable image for assessing motion artifacts: The right breast shows a "snow-peak" effect due to significant movement of the breast in the ventrodorsal direction during the early dynamic phase. Optimal, artifact-free presentation of the left breast.

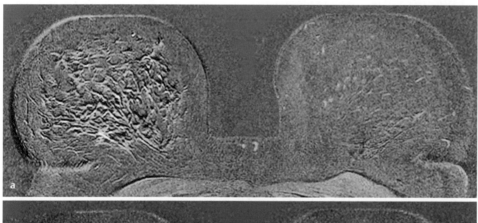
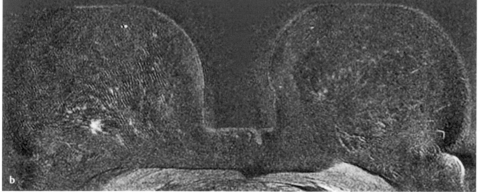

Fig. 6.10a, b Masking of DCIS by motion artifacts.
a Subtraction slice image with linear, ribbon-like motion artifacts in the right breast (MRI artifact level II). Ideal imaging of the left breast. No obvious abnormalities in either breast.
b Repeat examination with fewer motion artifacts (MRI artifact level I). Detection of now obvious, nonmasslike lesion in the central aspect of the right breast.

Histology: DCIS.

to the x-ray mammograpy ACR breast composition patterns has proven itself useful (**Table 6.1**). Breast MRI examinations with no motion artifacts (MRI artifact level I) consequently have optimal sensitivity for the detection of breast cancer. Breast MRI examinations with an unacceptable level of motion artifacts (MRI artifact level IV), on the other hand, are not suitable for the early detection of breast cancer (**Fig. 6.12**).

! The excellent sensitivity of breast MRI in the detection of DCIS can only be achieved when imaging is of optimal quality without (motion) artifacts.

Corrective measures. Interfering motion artifacts can be largely eliminated by using appropriate equipment (open breast coil, compression device) and informing the patient of what is to be expected before the examination begins. If motion artifacts occur in the subtraction images despite these precautions, then a careful

Table 6.1 Classification of artifact levels in breast MRI

MRI artifact level	Degree of intra-mammary artifacts	Pathologic findings that may easily be missed
I	None	None
II	1–2 mm	DCIS
III	2–4 mm	pT1a, pT1b
IV	>4 mm	pT1c and larger

inspection of each slice image in its dynamic course is recommended. The evaluation of images with identical slice position in the so-called cine mode is useful for this purpose since motion artifacts are less disturbing when one is viewing the corresponding images in rapid succession. If the presence of motion artifacts is extreme (MRI artifact level IV, or when appropriate III), the examination must be repeated at a later time.

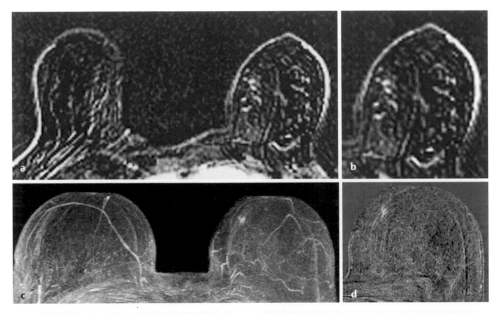

Fig. 6.11a–d Motion artifact resulting in false tumorlike abnormality.
a Subtraction image with inadequate examination technique. External examination yielded an "enhancing area" in the medial aspect of the left breast interpreted as an intraductal lesion.
b Partial magnification of **a**.
c Repeat examination (MIP) with adequate compression and high image quality. Detection of now obvious, dendritic nonmasslike lesion in the medial aspect of the left breast which does not, however, correspond to that seen in **a**.
d Subtraction slice image of **c**.

Histology: DCIS.

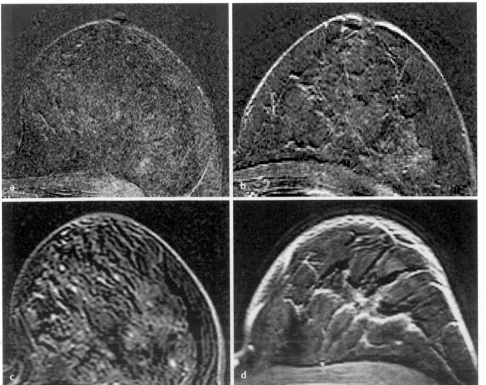

Fig. 6.12a–d Classification system for motion artifacts in breast MRI (MRI artifact levels I–IV).
a No motion artifacts. Optimal image quality. MRI artifact level I.
b Intramammary motion artifacts with maximal width of 2 mm. MRI artifact level II.
c Intramammary motion artifacts with maximal width of 4 mm. MRI artifact level III.
d Intramammary motion artifacts with maximal width >4 mm. Examination is insufficient. MRI artifact level IV.

Out-of-Phase Imaging

Depending upon the magnetic field strength of the system used, the echo time (TE) should be selected such that in-phase, and not opposed-phase (out-of-phase) imaging results. If the echo time is incorrect, then an interfering signal loss at the interface between fat and water containing tissues occurs (**Fig. 6.13**). In severe cases, such signal loss can mask fine linear pathological findings (**Fig. 6.14**).

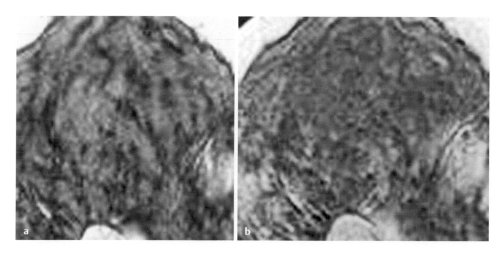

Fig. 6.13a, b Interfering artifacts caused by out-of-phase imaging.
a Subtraction image with signal loss at the borderlines between fat and parenchyma due to inappropriate echo time (opposed-phase imaging).
b Elimination of these artifacts by selection of correct echo time (in-phase imaging).

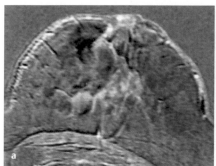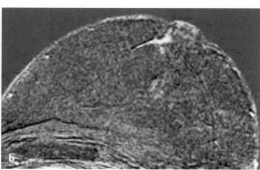

Fig. 6.14a, b Masking of linear enhancement caused by out-of-phase imaging.
a Subtraction image with significant signal loss at the borderlines between fat and parenchyma (external examination).
b Repeat breast MRI examination with correct echo time and reduction of motion artifacts. Now a linear enhancement in the retromammillary area can be clearly detected.

Histology: DCIS.

Susceptibility Artifacts

Susceptibility artifacts in the breast occur when ferromagnetic foreign material lies within the breast or close to the thoracic wall. These artifacts are most commonly seen after surgery, where use of an electrocautery leaves fine metal residues in the tissue, causing typically round signal loss artifacts up to 10 mm in diameter in the MR image. The artifacts are so characteristic that previous surgery can be assumed even without access to the patient's history (**Fig. 6.15a**).

Other intramammary causes of susceptibility artifacts include broken needle parts after surgery (**Fig. 6.15b, c**), port systems (**Fig. 6.16**), metal plates of prosthesis expanders (**Fig. 6.17a**), and metal clips used to mark the tumor bed after breast-conserving therapy. Examples of extramammary causes are sternal wire cerclages after thoracic surgery (**Fig. 6.17b**).

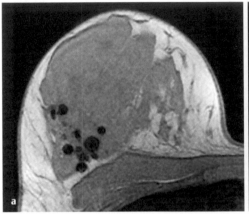 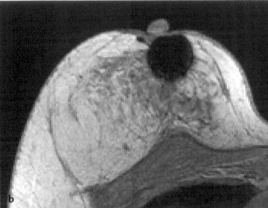 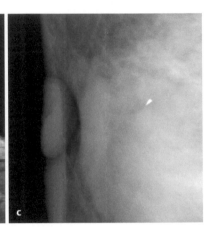

Fig. 6.15a–c   Susceptibility artifacts.
a Extensive region with round areas of signal loss after intraoperative hemostasis using an electrocautery (T1w precontrast image).
b Signal loss of 1 cm diameter in the retromamillary region.

c Mammography reveals small needle fragment as the cause of the susceptibility artifact in **b**.

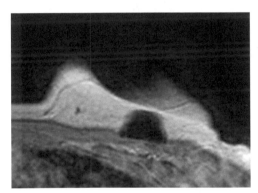 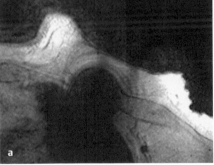 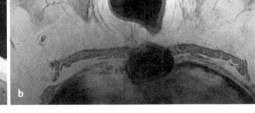

Fig. 6.16   Susceptibility artifact due to port system. Signal loss due to a port system implanted in the prepectoral region does not cause diagnostic problems.

Fig. 6.17a, b   Susceptibility artifact due to a prosthesis expander and sternal wire cerclage.
a *Expander.* Signal loss due to an implanted expander in preparation for prosthesis implantation may cause interference with the diagnostic evaluation of the MRI examination.
b *Wire cerclage after thoracotomy.* Signal loss near the sternum does not cause diagnostic problems.

Cardiac Flow Artifacts

Cardiac flow artifacts are seen as an interfering, overlapping band of artifacts in the direction of the phase-encoding gradient. For an MRI examination performed with transversal imaging of the breasts, the mediolateral phase-encoding gradient should be selected so that the direction of the cardiac artifact band crosses the image through the thorax, dorsally of the breasts. Parenchymal structures may be incompletely imaged (i.e., obscured), however, when these are localized in the lateral areas of the breast and/or in the axillary tail (**Fig. 6.18**). This problem is often encountered in patients with breast implants. Implants often reach far laterally, limiting the evaluation of the lateral areas of the implant and the surrounding parenchyma. In our experience, performing examinations with a modified protocol, including swapping the phase- and frequency-encoding gradients, is advantageous in such cases (see Chapter 3 p. 21).

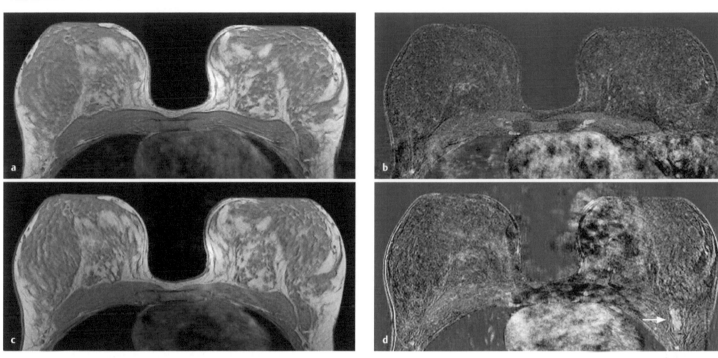

Fig. 6.18a–d Masking of lesion due to mediolateral cardiac flow artifacts.

a Transversal T1w precontrast image with phase-encoding gradient in mediolateral direction.

b Transversal subtraction slice image. Limited evaluation of axillary structures due to cardiac flow artifacts.

c Same examination with ventrodorsal phase-encoding gradient. Artifacts no longer superimpose on axillary structures (T1w precontrast image).

d Hypervascularized breast cancer tumor can now be easily detected in the axillary tail of the left breast (arrow).

Surface Coil Artifacts

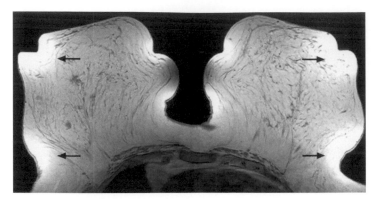

Fig. 6.19 **Coil artifacts.** Increased signal intensity in the marginal areas of both breasts near the coil windings (arrows). The internal breast structure is not assessable in these areas.

Dedicated breast coils available from most medical suppliers have the transmitting and receiving coils arranged as circular elements that partially or completely surround the breasts in the coronary orientation. An increased signal occurs at the level of the coil windings, so that the breast areas localized nearest to the coil show a higher signal intensity. Normally, these effects are seen in the subcutaneous fat tissue and do not interfere with image interpretation. In breasts with an extremely high proportion of parenchyma to fat tissue and a thin subcutaneous layer of fat, misinterpretation of findings in the marginal parenchymal areas is possible (**Fig. 6.19**). In cases with questionable findings, these areas should be further evaluated using an adapted window setting. As a rule, the sufficiency and homogeneity of signal intensity in both breasts should always be assessed (**Figs. 6.20, 6.21**).

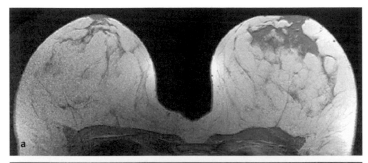
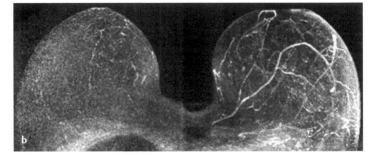
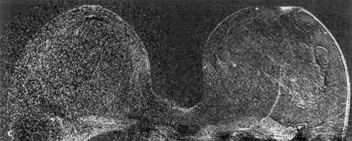

Fig. 6.20a–c **Insufficient signal yield due to a defective right breast coil.** Insufficient signal yield is already obvious in the T1w precontrast image, but more pronounced in the subtraction image. The problem source is a defective right breast coil.
a T1w precontrast image.
b MIP.
c Subtraction slice image.

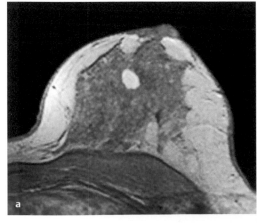
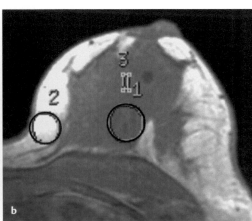
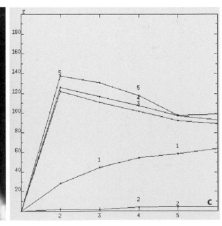

Fig. 6.21a–c **Quality assurance test of transmitter and receiver coils.**
a T1w postcontrast image reveals hypervascularized retromamillary tumor.
b Positioning of measurement regions within the tumor (3) (three ROIs) representative healthy breast tissue (1), and representative fat tissue (2).
c During dynamic measurements, fat tissue has a constant signal intensity without significant enhancement as verification of the system's operation (curve 2). Continuous slow enhancement of parenchyma (curve 1). Typical contrast dynamics within carcinoma (curves 3–5).

Incorrect Region of Interest (ROI)

The evaluation of the signal changes after IV contrast administration is performed in so-called regions of interest (ROIs). These measurement regions must be placed so that they include areas of maximal enhancement within a hypervascularized lesion and yet do not enclose less strongly enhancing areas, so as not to misrepresent the signal curve characteristics. This is especially important for lesions with a ring-enhancement pattern. Here the ROI must be placed in the peripheral, strongly enhancing region of the lesion and not in the central, less vascularized necrotic or fibrotic areas (**Fig. 6.22**). The recommended ROI size is between 2 and 5 pixels. In addition, it is sometimes necessary and prudent to perform several measurements using ROIs in different enhancing areas within the same lesion. The signal curve with the most suspicious course should then be used for assessment of the lesion.

! The most suspicious signal–time curve derived from a lesion is the most significant.

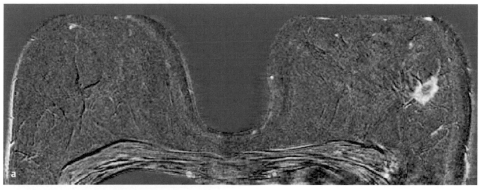

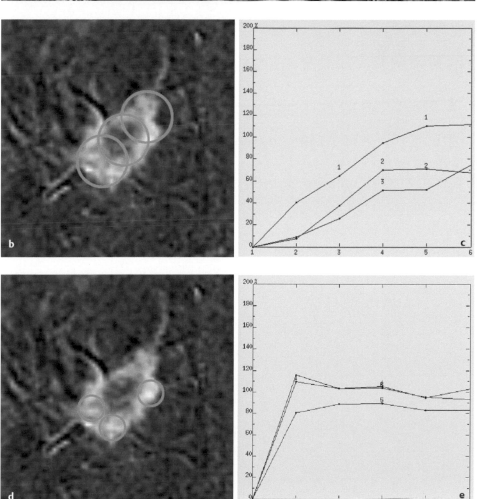

Fig. 6.22 a–e Placement of an ROI.
a Breast carcinoma with ring enhancement in the left breast (subtraction image).
b Incorrect positioning of several ROIs that include necrotic, nonenhancing tumor areas.
c Signal–time curves corresponding to ROIs in **b**.
d Correction by using smaller ROIs placed in tumor areas with maximal enhancement.
e Signal–time curves corresponding to ROIs in **d** show a typical course suspicious for malignancy.

Insufficient Spatial Resolution

Breast MRI can only deliver excellent results when the technical and methodical prerequisites for excellent quality of image acquisition and assessment are fulfilled. High spatial resolution in all three imaging planes without interpolation is one of the major requirements. High-resolution (HR) breast MRI is defined as hav- ing a large acquisition matrix (512 × 512) and a thin slice thickness (2–3 mm). Breast MRI examinations with a lesser spatial resolution have a significantly reduced diagnostic value (**Fig. 6.23**). Breast MRI examinations with a matrix under 256 × 256 are below the minimum recommended standards (**Fig. 6.24**).

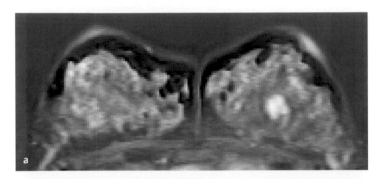

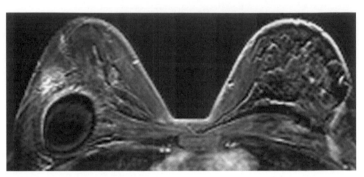

Fig. 6.24   Insufficient spatial resolution. External breast MRI examination performed with a 256 × 218 matrix. Insufficient image quality.

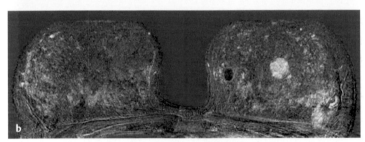

Fig. 6.23 a, b   Insufficient spatial resolution.
a Breast MRI with insufficient spatial resolution and inadequate subtraction technique. Internal characteristics of a suspicious hypervascularized lesion in the left breast cannot be adequately assessed (external examination).
b Repeat examination with large matrix (512 × 512). Internal characteristics of left lesion, as well as other structures are now discernible.

Substandard Subtraction Process (Negative Pixels)

Signal fluctuations during the pre- and postcontrast dynamic MR measurements can result in negative pixel values in the subtraction images of identical slice images. These pixels are coded black in the subtraction image. If this affects large areas, black "holes" are seen, in which no further differentiation of grayscale values is possible (**Fig. 6.25**). This problem is easily alleviated if the manufacturers producing image subtraction software include a constant in the subtraction calculation process that eliminates the occurrence of negative pixels. The resulting images must, however, be windowed to a different level.

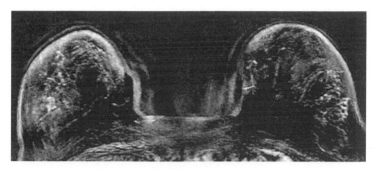

Fig. 6.25 Insufficient spatial resolution. "Black holes" in image subtraction due to negative pixels. Extensive areas are black and cannot be adequately assessed (external examination).

Incorrect Pixel Shifting

Postprocessing software for the correction of motion artifacts, so-called pixel shifting, is now available. Caution: Images postprocessed with such a program look pleasing and seem to be of higher quality. However, the correction algorithm cannot differentiate between undesirable motion artifacts and the sometimes similar-looking pathological findings (**Fig. 6.26**).

> **Goal:** Avoid the creation of image artifacts instead of "eliminating" them by postprocessing.

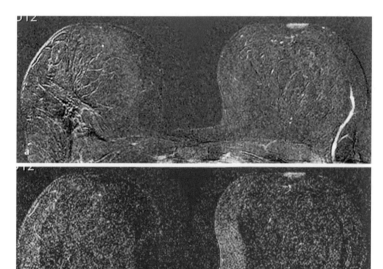

Fig. 6.26a, b Pixel shifting postprocessing.
a Subtraction image with slight motion artifacts in the right breast. Signal-intense vein in the lateral aspect of the left breast.
b After pixel shifting correction there are no more visible artifacts. Note, however, that the vein in the left breast has also been "corrected" and is no longer visible.

Inadequate Windowing

As is true for all digital imaging modalities, breast MRI should take advantage of the spectrum of possible grayscale values available to best detect and visualize pathological breast findings. In this context, monitor assessment of digital images is advantageous (**Figs. 6.27, 6.28**).

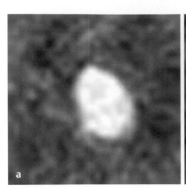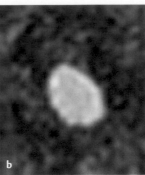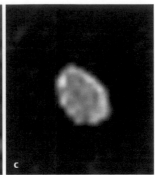

Fig. 6.27 a–c   Adequate windowing of breast MRI with mass lesion showing rim-enhancement. Examples of different window settings for a breast carcinoma. Visualization of the rim-enhancement improves with increasing contrast.
a Low-contrast window setting.
b High-contrast window setting.
c Very high-contrast window setting.

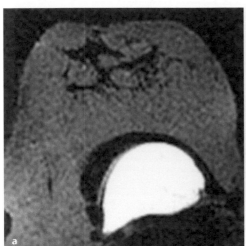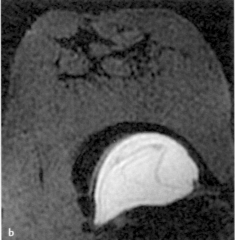

Fig. 6.28 a, b   Adequate windowing of silicone implants in breast MRI. Examples of different window settings.
a High-contrast window setting.
b Lower-contrast window setting. Visualization of the ruptured shell is made possible.

Ghosting

Artifacts that appear as repetitive stripes or contours of the original image in the phase-encoding direction are usually caused by movements and often make the acquired images inadequate for high-quality image assessment (**Figs. 6.29, 6.30**). The appearance of such "ghosts" can be avoided by using appropriate equipment such as an open breast coil and a dedicated compression device.

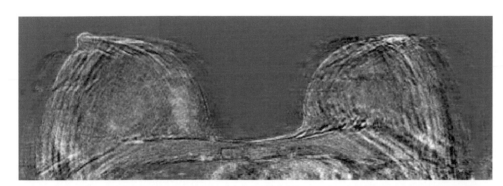

Fig. 6.29 Ghosting. Motion artifacts with significant reduction of the examination's diagnostic value (external examination).

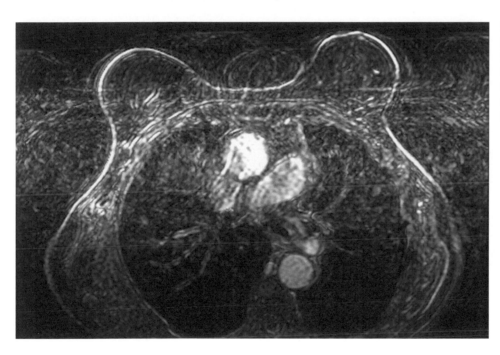

Fig. 6.30 Ghosting. Extreme example of insufficient examination quality with several deficiencies. Motion artifacts with ghosting are also visible in the direction opposed to the phase-encoding direction. There is significant reduction of the examination's diagnostic value (external examination).

Inhomogeneous Fat Suppression / Silicone Suppression

The high signal intensity of certain tissues is sometimes undesirable and can interfere with the interpretation of MR images. In such cases, frequency-selective excitation techniques can be used to suppress the signal of these substances. If suppression is not performed, or is performed inadequately, bothersome phenomena result that can interfere with image assessment (**Figs. 6.31, 6.32**).

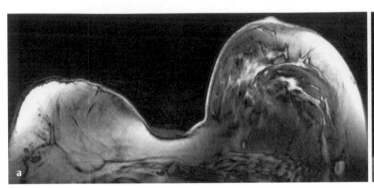
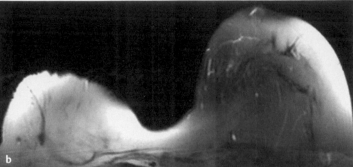

Fig. 6.31 a, b   Insufficient frequency selective fat suppression. Inhomogeneous suppression of intense fat signal, interfering especially with assessment of the left breast.
a T1w image.   **b** T2w image.

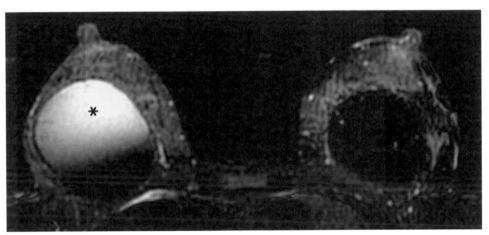

Fig. 6.32   Insufficient frequency-selective suppression of silicon signal. Inhomogeneous signal suppression, especially in the ventral portions of the right silicone implant (*).

7 Normal Findings in Breast MRI

Morphology

The adult female breast is composed of three different tissue components: skin, subcutaneous tissue, and breast tissue (parenchyma and stroma).

Skin. The skin is thin and contains hair follicles, sebaceous glands, and exocrine sweat glands. The *mammary papilla*, or *nipple*, contains sebaceous and exocrine sweat glands as well as abundant sensory nerve endings, but no hair follicles. The skin around the nipple constitutes the *areola* and is pigmented. Near its periphery there are elevations, *Morgagni's tubercles*, formed by the openings of the ducts of *Montgomery's glands*. These are large sebaceous glands of an intermediate type between sweat and mammary glands.

Parenchyma. The parenchyma is divided into 15–20 cone-shaped lobes (*lobi glandulae mammariae*), whose collecting ducts in-crease in diameter to form the subareolar lactiferous sinuses (*ductus lactiferi colligentes*). Between 5 and 10 major collecting milk ducts open at the nipple. Each lobe is itself made up of 20–40 lobules (*lobuli glandulae mammariae*) that consist of 10–100 alveoli or tubulosaccular secretory units (*acini*).

Stroma. The stroma of the breast contains strongly varying amounts of fat, connective tissue, blood vessels, nerves and lymphatics. Stromal tissue forms a mantle around the epithelial tissue of the lobes and along the peripheral ducts. Interlobular connective tissue surrounds the lobules and the central ducts. Fibrous bands called *Cooper's suspensory ligaments* connect the fascial tissue enveloping the breast with the deep pectoral fascia covering the major pectoral and anterior serratus muscles, and support the breast.

Blood Supply

Approximately 60% of the arterial blood supply to the breast, mostly to the medial quadrants and central portions, is provided by the perforating branches of the internal thoracic artery. Approximately 30% of arterial blood flow, chiefly to the upper outer quadrant, is supplied by the lateral mammary branches of the lateral thoracic artery. Branches of the thoracoacromial, 3rd–5th intercostal, subscapular, and thoracodorsal arteries may also contribute to the arterial blood supply to a smaller extent. The fact that the blood supply to different areas of the breast derives from different arteries is of no importance in dynamic MR mammography.

Parenchyma and Age

Morphological aspects of the female breast undergo fundamental changes that depend upon age. Parenchymal changes occurring during pregnancy and the peripartum period will not be discussed here since they are not relevant for MR mammography. Breast enlargement and development of the mammary ducts begins a few years before the menarche. Development of the lobuli, however, does not begin until one to two years after the menarche and continues through the 35th year of life. At this time the physiological process of breast involution with regressive lobular changes begins. **Figure 7.1** shows T1-weighted precontrast images as examples of the different development stages. Interindividual variability is very great, however.

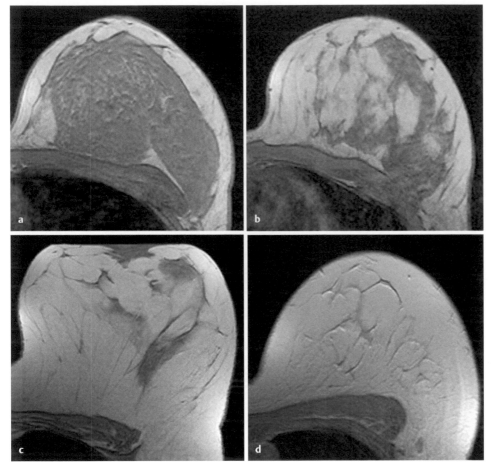

Fig. 7.1 a–d Typical T1w precontrast images in women of different age groups.
a A 20-year-old woman.
b A 40-year-old woman.
c A 60-year-old woman.
d An 80-year-old woman.

Parenchymal Asymmetry, Accessory Glandular Tissue

The following forms of asymmetry can be differentiated when comparing the breasts with each other:

- Size asymmetry
- Parenchymal asymmetry
- Focal asymmetry
- Enhancement asymmetry

Size asymmetry. When size asymmetry is present, inspection of the breasts reveals a visible difference in the volume of the right and left breast. Size asymmetries are frequent findings, the left breast more often being the larger of the two (**Fig. 7.2**). When no palpable mass is present, and mammography shows no characteristics suggestive of malignancy, such an asymmetry is of no clinical significance.

Parenchymal asymmetry. A parenchymal asymmetry is defined as being a clinically unremarkable difference in the proportion of parenchyma within the same-sized breasts (**Fig. 7.3**). This kind of asymmetry also has no clinical significance if there are no additional criteria suggesting malignancy (e.g., regional or diffuse enhancement).

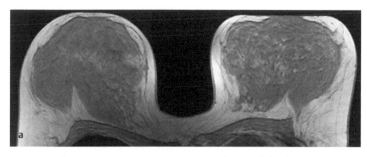
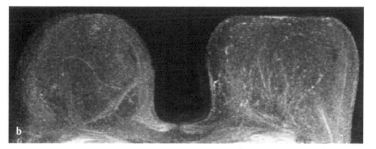

Fig. 7.2a, b   Size asymmetry. Greater volume of the left breast is visible on breast MRI. Because the left breast reaches the base of the breast surface coil, it is flattened ventrally. In contrast, the right breast hangs freely in the breast coil.
a T1w precontrast image.   **b** Symmetric enhancement in the MIP.

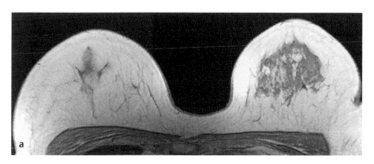
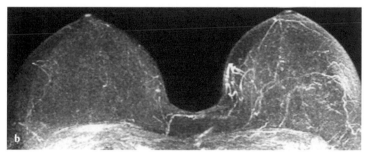

Fig. 7.3a, b   Parenchymal asymmetry.
a T1w precontrast image reveals that there is more parenchyma in the left breast than in the right breast.

b In spite of the parenchymal asymmetry, neither breast shows increased enhancement in the subtraction MIP.

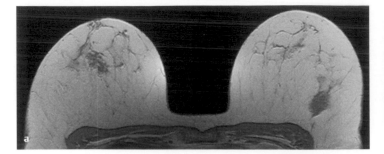

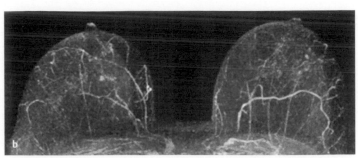

Fig. 7.4a, b   Focal asymmetry.

a T1w precontrast image reveals a regional, nonadipose area in the lateral aspect of the left breast without a mirror-image area in the right breast.

b No increased enhancement is seen in this area after contrast administration (MIP). This is a reliable indication that a harmless focal asymmetry is present.

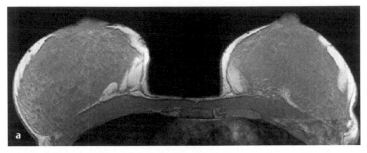

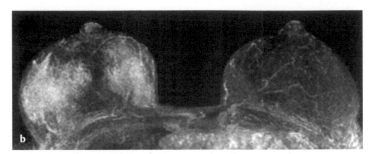

Fig. 7.5a, b   Enhancement asymmetry.

a T1w precontrast image reveals symmetric, dense breast parenchyma.

b The subtraction MIP shows diffuse enhancement of most of the parenchyma in the right breast, and no enhancement in the left breast. The follow-up examination 6 months later showed unremarkable symmetrical enhancement.

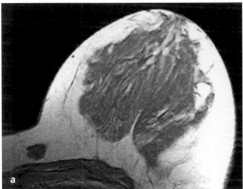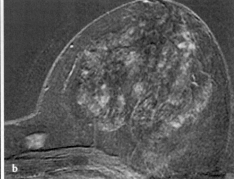

Fig. 7.6a, b   Accessory glandular breast tissue.

a T1w precontrast image reveals a localized area of nonadipose tissue medial to the main body of breast parenchyma.

b In the subtraction image this area shows hypervascularization similar to that of the main body of breast parenchyma. Histological verification of normal breast tissue by large core biopsy.

Focal asymmetry. A focal asymmetry is characterized by a regional, nonadipose area of tissue that does not have a mirror-image area in the contralateral breast (**Fig. 7.4**). This can be a normal finding. When other criteria suggestive of malignancy are present, however, this can also conform to a malignant lesion.

Enhancement asymmetry. An asymmetric, diffuse enhancement of parenchymal structures is designated an enhancement asymmetry (**Fig. 7.5**). Such findings may be physiological. Often, however, these have another underlying cause (e.g. after radiation therapy, inflammation, tumor), so that further diagnostic workup is usually indicated.

Accessory glandular breast tissue. Breast tissue in an atypical location that does not have immediate contact with the main body of breast parenchyma is designated accessory glandular tissue. Typically it is located in the axillary tail of one or both breasts and has a similar morphological structure to the main body parenchyma. Rarely, accessory glandular tissue can be found in the medial aspects of the breast (**Fig. 7.6**). The risk of malignancy in these areas is no greater than that in the main body of breast parenchyma.

Nipple and Retromamillary Region

Physiological enhancement. The nipple has a higher physiological CM uptake than the surrounding skin and breast parenchyma. This increased enhancement is typically seen as a line at the ventral surface of the nipple (**Fig. 7.7a**) or around the circumference of the nipple (**Fig. 7.7b**), or as diffuse enhancement of the nipple–areolar complex (**Fig. 7.7c**). The corresponding signal intensity curve usually shows a rapid initial signal increase (> 100% over baseline values) and a persistent postinitial increase or postinitial plateau.

Atypical perimamillary enhancement. Atypical enhancement in the immediate retromamillary region can be suggestive of an intraductal process (papilloma, DCIS, inflammation) and should therefore be histologically verified or followed up (**Fig. 7.8a, b**). A focal enhancement in the areolar region can be indicative of an inflamed Montgomery gland (**Fig. 7.8c**). Such findings are usually associated with clinical changes and are therefore easy to assess.

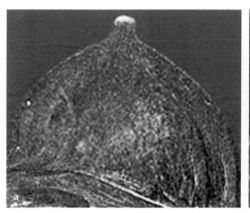 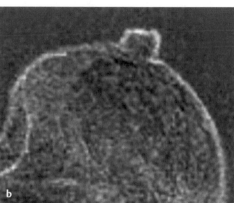 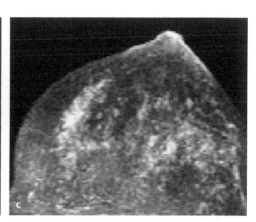

Fig. 7.7a–c Nipple enhancement patterns. Physiological enhancement of the nipple on breast MRI (subtraction images).
a Line of enhancement at the ventral surface of the nipple.
b Enhancement of the nipple circumference.
c Diffuse enhancement of the nipple–areolar complex.

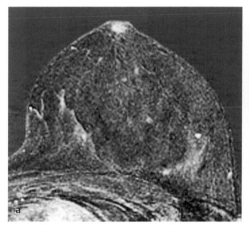 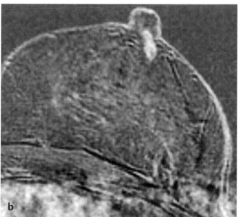 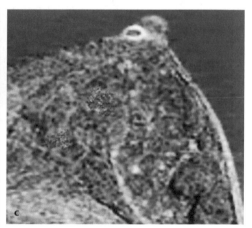

Fig. 7.8a–c Enhancement of the nipple and areola. Subtraction images.
a Focal enhancement within the nipple. Follow-up over many years showed constant findings.
b Linear enhancement in the nipple. Histopathology revealed an intraductal papilloma.
c Focal enhancement at the areola edge. Clinical examination revealed inflammation of a Montgomery gland.

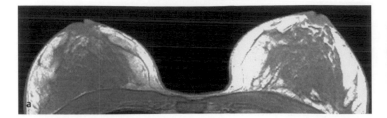

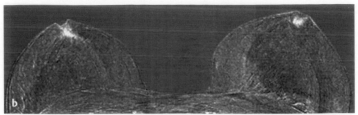

Fig. 7.9 a, b   Atypical enhancement position of bilateral creviced nipples.
a T1w precontrast image reveals bilateral creviced nipples (clinically unchanged over years).
b The subtraction image shows physiological enhancement of the nipples in the retromamillary regions in both breasts.

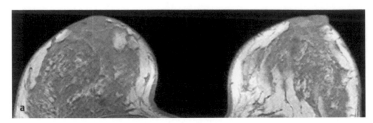

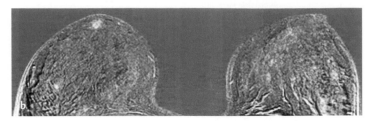

Fig. 7.10 a, b   Atypical enhancement position of a unilateral inverted nipple.
a T1w precontrast image reveals unilateral thickening of the areolar region on the right side. The nipple is not seen in profile.
b The subtraction image reveals an asymmetric focal enhancement of the right inverted nipple (clinically unchanged over years).

Nipple form variants. Unilateral and bilateral creviced (**Fig. 7.9**) and inverted nipples (**Fig. 7.10**) can sometimes cause conspicuous enhancement in the mamillary and retromamillary areas. Such findings should not be misinterpreted if one considers the personal history and clinical status.

Unilateral enhancement. In contrast to the findings described above, a unilateral enhancement in the mamillary region without evidence of a nipple form variant is a finding that requires further diagnostic work-up (clinical examination, mammography, ultrasonography). The differential diagnosis includes inflammatory changes, Paget disease, DCIS, and papillomas.

Interindividual Variations

There are strong interindividual differences in the level and distribution of contrast uptake in the female breast and it is not possible to make a prospective estimation of the expected parenchymal enhancement after contrast administration. Palpation findings, parenchymal pattern in mammography, or echogenicity in ultrasonography do not allow a selection of those patients whose breast parenchyma will display an intense and/or complex contrast enhancement pattern (**Figs. 7.11, 7.12, 7.13**). Our own experience indicates that even examinations providing information about the vascularization (color-coded duplex sonography, contrast-enhanced color-coded duplex sonography) show no significant correlation to the contrast enhancement in MR mammography. Just as the overall breast composition in mammography influences the

possibility of missing a breast cancer in this examination, it is important to note that the informative value of a breast MRI is dependent upon the early parenchymal enhancement pattern. Therefore, in analogy to the breast composition patterns reported in mammography, four MRI density patterns are differentiated to indicate the relative possibility that a lesion could be hidden by the normal tissues in the MRI examination (**Fig. 7.13 a–d**). In contrast to the relatively large proportion of women with high-density parenchyma on mammography, however, the number of women with a high MRI density is very low (**Fig. 7.13 e**).

> **!** Parenchymal density on mammography does not correlate with the breast MRI density.

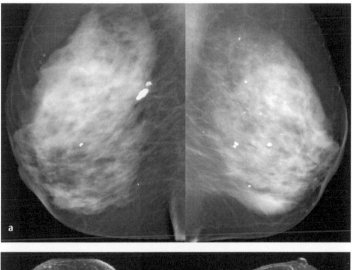
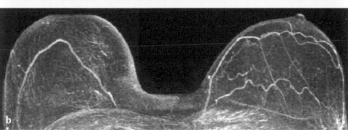

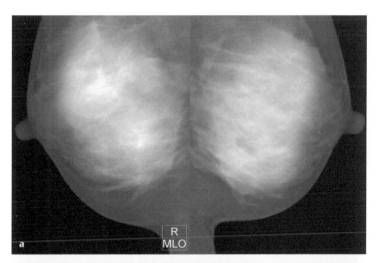

Fig. 7.11 a, b Comparison of mammographic density and breast MRI density.
a Mammography in MLO-projection. Breast tissue of ACR density IV (extremely dense breast tissue).
b Breast tissue is transparent in the early subtraction MIP of the woman in **a** (MRI density I).

Fig. 7.12 a, b Comparison of mammographic density and breast MRI density.
a Mammography in MLO-projection. Breast tissue of ACR density IV (extremely dense breast tissue).
b The early subtraction MIP of the woman in **a** shows strong early enhancement of normal breast parenchyma, limiting the diagnostic value of the examination (MRI density IV).

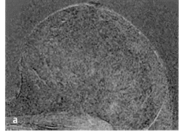
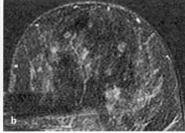
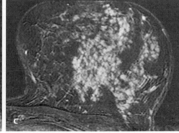
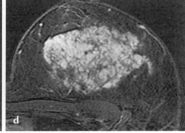

Fig. 7.13 a–e MRI density and the influence on the diagnostic value of the examinations. Parenchymal enhancement in early subtraction image.
a MRI density I: no parenchymal enhancement. Very high diagnostic value.
b MRI density II: focal areas of enhancement, not confluent. Slightly limited diagnostic value.
c MRI density III: confluent focal areas of enhancement. Limited diagnostic value.
d MRI density IV: confluent diffuse parenchymal enhancement. Very limited diagnostic value.

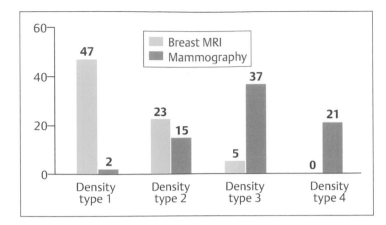

Fig. 7.13 e   (continued)
e **Relative frequency of density types in mammography and enhancement patterns in MRI (MRI density).** Distribution of density types in a group of women who underwent both mammography and breast MRI ("screening" examinations). A large proportion (> 50%) of women have a high mammographic density (III or IV). In contrast, only 5% of women have a rapid parenchymal enhancement pattern (MRI density III or IV). In other words, a large proportion of women (70%) have a transparent parenchymal enhancement pattern (MRI density I or II). In contrast, less than 20% of women have a low mammographic density (ACR I or II). MRI, Mx

Intraindividual Fluctuations

Systematic longitudinal and cross-sectional studies show that parenchymal contrast uptake is subject to intraindividual fluctuations. As expected, this is especially true for younger, premenopausal women. Studies confirm that the intensity and pattern of early parenchymal enhancement is subject not only to fluctuations from week to week but also from month to month. Parenchymal enhancement in breast MRI is least pronounced during the second and third weeks of the menstrual cycle and usually strongest during the premenstrual fourth week and the postmenstrual first week (**Fig. 7.14**). Occasionally, however, very pronounced fluctuations of parenchymal enhancement intensity can also be seen in postmenopausal women (**Fig. 7.15**).

> **!** Parenchymal density on mammography does not correlate with the early parenchymal enhancement pattern seen in breast MRI (MRI density).

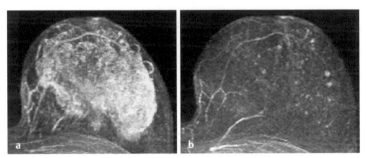

Fig. 7.14 a, b   **Intraindividual fluctuations of parenchymal contrast enhancement depending on the week of the menstrual cycle.**
a Early subtraction MIP of the left breast. Examination in the fourth week of the menstrual cycle. Diffuse enhancement of the entire body of breast parenchyma.
b Early subtraction MIP of examination performed in the second week of the menstrual cycle.

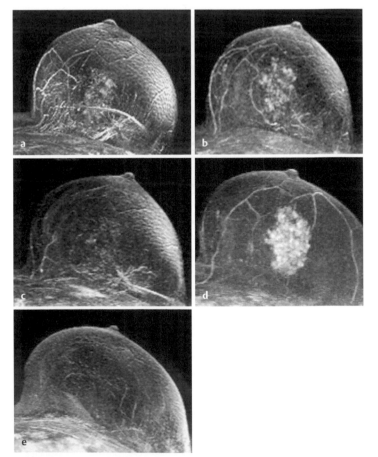

Fig. 7.15 a–e   **Intraindividual fluctuations of contrast enhancement in an area of adenosis.** Yearly breast MRI examinations show pronounced fluctuations in an area of histologically verified adenosis in the left breast of a postmenopausal woman.

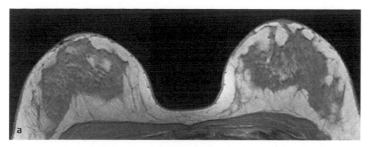

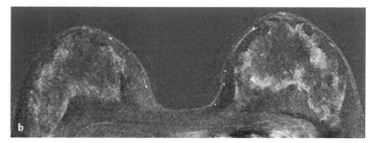

Fig. 7.16a, b   Hormonal influence on contrast enhancement in peripheral aspects of the breast.
a A premenopausal woman with symmetric parenchyma (T1w pre-contrast image).
b Enhancement of peripheral parenchymal areas (subtraction image).

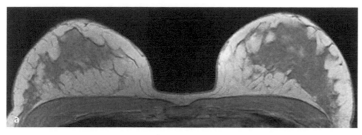

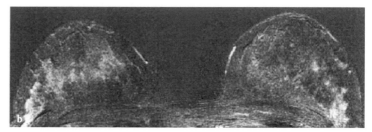

Fig. 7.17a, b   Hormonal influence on contrast enhancement in lateral aspects of the breast.
a A premenopausal woman with symmetric parenchyma (T1w pre-contrast image).
b Enhancement of lateral parenchymal areas in both breasts (subtraction image).

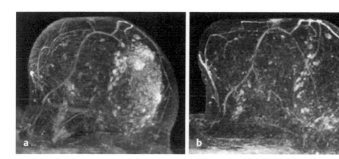

Fig. 7.18a, b   Intraindividual fluctuations of nodular contrast enhancement.
a Early subtraction MIP of the left breast. Examination in the fourth week of the menstrual cycle. Segmental enhancement of lateral parenchymal areas with a masslike lesion.
b Early subtraction MIP of examination performed at the end of the first week of the menstrual cycle shows significant reduction of parenchymal and masslike enhancement.

Patterns. Hormonally induced increases in postcontrast signal intensity can be seen as regionally enhancing areas, typically in the peripheral (**Fig. 7.16**) and/or in the lateral aspects of the breast (**Fig. 7.17**). On the other hand, focal and/or masslike enhancement can also occur and may need to be differentiated from a malignant lesion (**Fig. 7.18**). The signal intensity curves of most hormonally induced enhancing lesions generally show typical characteristics of benign findings; thus a reliable differentiation between benign and malignant lesions is usually possible. In addition, most of these lesions have a high relative water content, also indicating a benign finding.

Hormone Replacement Therapy

Hormones influence the morphology, function, and vascularization of breast parenchyma. As is to be expected, hormone replacement therapy also affects signal behavior in dynamic breast MRI. The influence of hormonal stimulation on breast parenchyma can cause a regionally increased (**Fig. 7.19**) or blotchy enhancement pattern (**Fig. 7.20**). Interindividual and intraindividual studies have shown that hormone replacement therapy in postmenopausal women results in increased parenchymal signal enhancement. Enhancement is significantly higher than that of women in a control group without hormone replacement therapy, and is comparable to that of premenopausal women.

In women taking hormones, hypervascularized mass lesions may be seen that occasionally cause differential diagnostic problems (**Fig. 7.21**). Hormonal changes are reversible 4–8 weeks after discontinuation of hormone replacement, so that this interval should be observed when a repeat examination is planned to rule out malignancy. The hormonal influence on parenchymal enhancement appears to be dependent upon the hormones being taken. Medications containing progestogens seem to have a greater influence than estrogen-containing medications.

Our experience indicates that it is not generally necessary to discontinue HRT before performing a breast MRI examination. Although increased parenchymal enhancement due to hormonal stimulation may be disturbing, it rarely causes findings that are suspicious for malignancy, especially when using a multimodal evaluation protocol.

! It is not generally necessary to discontinue HRT before performing a breast MRI examination.

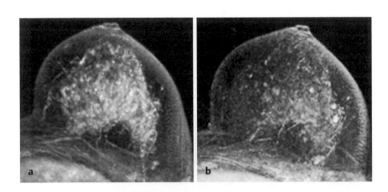

Fig. 7.19a, b Diffuse enhancement due to hormone replacement therapy.
a Early subtraction MIP of the left breast shows rapid and strong enhancement of the entire parenchyma in a woman taking hormones.
b After discontinuation of HRT, early subtraction MIP shows significant reduction of parenchymal enhancement.

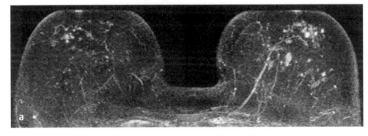

Fig. 7.20a, b Nodular enhancement due to hormone replacement therapy.
a Early subtraction MIP shows several focal and masslike enhancing areas (left greater than right) in a woman taking hormones.
b After discontinuation of HRT, early subtraction MIP shows significantly fewer enhancing areas.

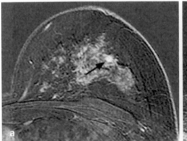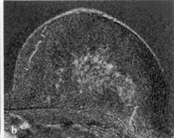

Fig. 7.21a, b Pseudolesion due to hormone replacement therapy.
a Early subtraction image indicates a mass lesion with rim-enhancement (arrow) in a woman taking hormones.
b After discontinuation of HRT, the early subtraction image shows almost complete remission of masslike findings.

Pregnancy and the Lactating Breast

During pregnancy and the following lactation period, the female breast is subject to strong hormonal stimulation. As a result, the parenchyma of the breast shows a pronounced increase of CM uptake in dynamic breast MRI. This has been demonstrated in examinations performed on nursing women (**Figs. 7.22**, **7.23**).

Indications. The use of MRI for examining the breasts of pregnant women is limited and is practically obsolete since the administration of paramagnetic CM is not approved for these women. When an early pregnancy cannot definitely be ruled out, breast MRI should be avoided. The diagnostic indications for breast MRI are never acutely life-threatening, so when pregnancy is a possibility, either a pregnancy test must be performed or the examination date delayed for a few weeks.

During the lactational period, a breast MRI examination may be advisable as part of the pretherapeutic local staging of a proven carcinoma since other diagnostic methods are usually significantly more limited in their diagnostic value. In spite of the expected maximal parenchymal enhancement, breast MRI can often provide important additional information (e.g. tumor extent).

> **!** The performance of a breast MRI examination during the lactational period is sometimes indicated and can provide relevant diagnostic information (e.g., pretherapeutic local staging).

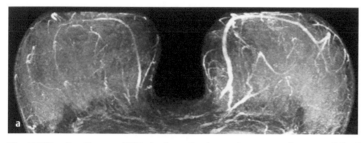
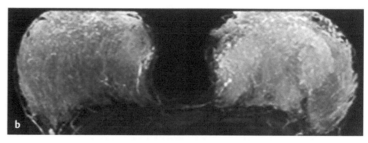

Fig. 7.22a, b   Breast MRI during the lactation period. Normal findings.
a Early subtraction MIP shows maximal enhancement of the entire parenchymal body.
b The corresponding T2w MIP shows the extreme water content of the parenchyma in both breasts.

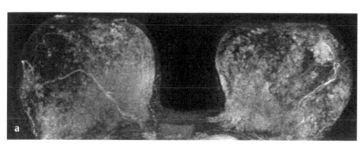
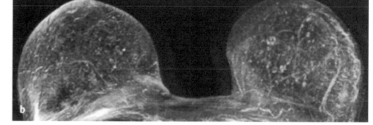

Fig. 7.23a, b   Comparison of breast MRI during the lactation period and years later. Normal findings.
a Early subtraction MIP shows maximal enhancement of the entire parenchymal body.
b Early subtraction MIP of an examination performed several years later shows normalization of parenchymal enhancement.

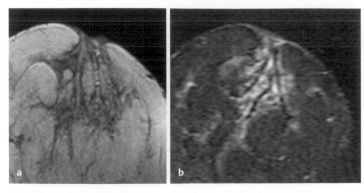

Fig. 7.24a, b   Dilated mammary ducts and galactostasis.
a T1w precontrast single-slice image shows dilated milk ducts with intraductal fat-containing fluid (intense signal) in the retromammillary region.
b The corresponding IR T2w image with suppression of fat signal within milk ducts is a sign of galactostasis.

Specific changes during the lactational period. During the lactational period, dilatation of the mammary ducts is a normal finding. These changes can be seen especially in the T1w precontrast and the water-sensitive T2w images of a breast MRI (**Fig. 7.24**). Galactocele (**Fig. 7.25**) and galactophoritis (**Fig. 7.26**) should also be considered here as they are typically encountered during the lactational period. Although it is not usually difficult to distinguish these findings from malignant tumors, it is important to be familiar with the typical image characteristics of these changes on breast MRI.

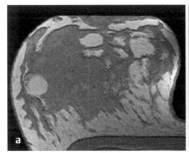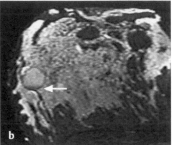

Fig. 7.25a, b   Galactocele.
a T1w precontrast single-slice image shows round mass with protein/fat-containing inclusion.
b Fat-suppressed IR T2w image shows slight reduction of signal intensity in the fat-containing portion of the internal fluid (arrow).

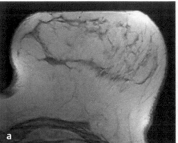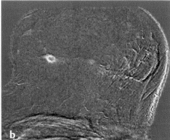

Fig. 7.26a, b   Galactophoritis.
a T1w precontrast single-slice image shows a circumscribed round duct ectasia.
b An early subtraction image shows circumscribed wall enhancement of an inflamed milk duct.

8 Benign Changes

Fibroadenoma

Fibroadenomas are mixed fibroepithelial tumors. Depending on the endotumoral distribution of the stromal and epithelial components, they are classified as **intracanalicular** and **pericanalicular fibroadenomas**. This differentiation is of no clinical importance. In younger women, fibroadenomas typically show a high proportion of epithelial tissue (**myxoid fibroadenomas**). With increasing age, and especially in postmenopausal women, the fibrotic component of these tumors increases and predominates. In this phase, progressive hyalinization and calcification takes place (**fibrotic fibroadenomas**).

! If there is any doubt concerning histology, a percutaneous biopsy is indicated to verify a fibroadenoma. This is preferably performed under ultrasound guidance.

Fibroadenoma: General information

Incidence:	The most common benign breast tumor (~10% of all women).
Age peak:	All ages. Peak between 20 and 50 years.
Risk of malignant transformation:	No increased risk.
Multifocality:	10%–15%.

Findings

Clinical:	Small fibroadenomas are clinically occult.
	Larger tumors are well-circumscribed, movable, painless nodules.
Mammography:	Small fibroadenomas and ones that are within dense parenchymal areas are often mammographically occult.
	Larger tumors appear well-circumscribed, homogeneously dense, oval or lobulated (typically no more than 3 lobuli).
	Occasional halo sign.
	Fibrotic fibroadenomas may display endotumoral dumbbell-shaped and/or popcorn macrocalcifications.
	Note: In the beginning stages of calcification, fibroadenoma-associated calcifications may appear as suspicious clustered, pleomorphic microcalcifications.
Ultrasonography:	Small fibroadenomas within lipomatous breast tissue may be sonographically occult.
	Larger tumors appear smooth-bordered, oval or lobulated, with homogeneous internal echotexture.
	The longitudinal axis is parallel to the skin. The surrounding architecture is undisturbed. Depending upon their water content, they display a moderate to strong posterior acoustic enhancement and possibly a lateral posterior acoustic shadowing.
	Fibrotic fibroadenomas with endotumoral calcifications may display acoustic extinction posterior to macrocalcifications.
	Lesion compressibility is slight to good, depending upon histological composition.

Myxoid fibroadenomas are the most common benign solid tumors in young women. With increasing age, the water content of these tumors decreases, and the fibrotic component increases.

MR Mammography: Fibroadenoma

T1-Weighted Sequence (Precontrast)

Small fibroadenomas located within the parenchyma are not usually visible in the precontrast examination. Larger tumors are oval or lobulated lesions with well-circumscribed borders (**Fig. 8.2b**). Myxoid fibroadenomas have a higher water content than the surrounding parenchyma and are therefore usually hypointense (**Fig. 8.1c**). With progressing fibrosis, however, they gradually become isointense (**Figs. 8.5c, 8.6b**). Fibroadenomas located within fatty tissue are more easily detected (**Figs. 8.7c, 8.8c**). Dystrophic macrocalcifications cause endotumoral signal extinction. In rare cases, a lipomatous peripheral border may be present (MR equivalent of halo sign) (**Fig. 8.3c**).

T2-Weighted Sequence

The signal intensity of a fibroadenoma in the water-sensitive T2w series is also dependent upon its histological composition.

Myxoid fibroadenomas. Myxoid and predominantly myxoid fibroadenomas are tumors with a high internal water content. Because of this, they typically have a high signal intensity in the T2w images (**Figs. 8.1b, d, 8.3b, d**), sometimes making the differentiation from a cyst difficult (**Fig. 8.5b**). The previously described internal septations are sometimes more easily seen in the T2w images than in the subtraction images (**Fig. 8.2c**).

Fibrotic (hyalinized) fibroadenomas. Fibrotic fibroadenomas are tumors with a low internal water content that usually have intermediate (**Fig. 8.6c**) or absent signal (**Fig. 8.8b, d**) in the T2w images. Partially fibrotic fibroadenomas only show a higher signal intensity in the less fibrotic areas within the tumor (**Fig. 8.7b, d**).

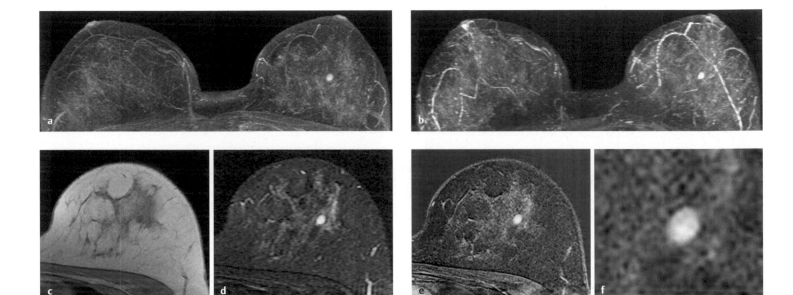

Fig. 8.1 a–g   Myxoid fibroadenoma.
a Subtraction MIP: solitary oval, well-circumscribed mass lesion in the left breast.
b T2w MIP: high signal intensity (water content).
c T1w precontrast slice image: well-circumscribed, oval, hypointense lesion.
d IR T2w slice image: high water content.
e Early subtraction slice image: homogeneous hypervascularization.
f Zoomed subtraction image.
g Time–signal intensity curve (TIC): moderate initial enhancement (just under 100%) and postinitial plateau.

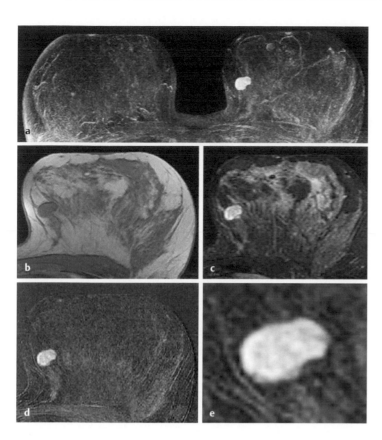

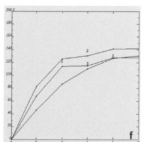

Fig. 8.2a–f Myxoid fibroadenoma with internal septations.
a Subtraction MIP: solitary lobulated, well-circumscribed mass lesion in the left breast.
b T1w precontrast slice image: well-circumscribed, lobulated, homogeneously hypointense lesion.
c IR T2w slice image: high signal intensity (water content). Depiction of several internal septations with lower signal intensity.
d Early subtraction slice image: inhomogeneous hypervascularization. Dark internal septations with lower vascularization.
e Zoomed subtraction image.
f TIC: rapid initial enhancement (max. 120%) and persistent postinitial enhancement.

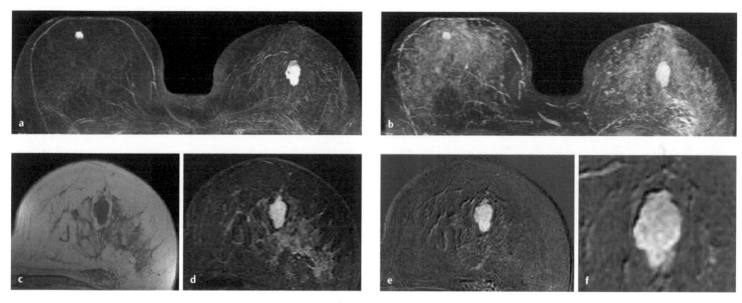

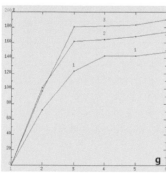

Fig. 8.3a–g Bilateral myxoid fibroadenomas. Left fibroadenoma displays a halo sign.
a Subtraction MIP: solitary lobulated (3 lobuli), well-circumscribed mass lesion in the left breast. Solitary oval, well-circumscribed mass lesion in the right breast.
b T2w MIP: high signal intensity (water content) of both lesions.
c T1w precontrast slice image (left): well-circumscribed, lobulated, homogeneously hypointense lesion with peritumoral border of fat-equivalent signal intensity (*halo sign*).
d IR T2w slice image: high signal intensity (water content). Depiction of multiple internal septations with lower signal intensity.
e Early subtraction slice image: inhomogeneous hypervascularization. Dark internal septations without vascularization.
f Zoomed subtraction image.
g TIC: rapid initial enhancement (max. 180%) and postinitial plateau.

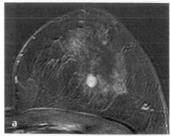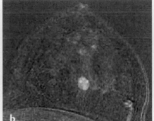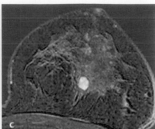

Fig. 8.4a–c Myxoid fibroadenoma. Unchanged in follow-up over several years.
a Subtraction slice image: sound, well-circumscribed mass lesion with strong hypervascularization and dark internal septations.
b Breast MRI 1 year later shows unchanged lesion characteristics.
c Breast MRI 2 years later continues to show unchanged lesion characteristics.

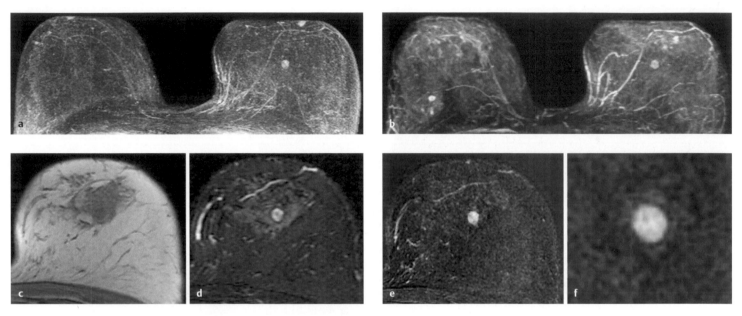

Fig. 8.5a–g Partially fibrotic fibroadenoma.
a Subtraction MIP: solitary round, well-circumscribed mass lesion in the left breast.
b T2w MIP: inhomogeneous high signal intensity (water content). Depiction of a few small cysts in both breasts.
c T1w precontrast slice image: well-circumscribed, partially hypointense, partially isointense (compared to surrounding parenchyma) lesion with halo sign.
d IR T2w slice image: partially high, partially low signal intensity.
e Early subtraction slice image: inhomogeneous hypervascularization.
f Zoomed subtraction image.
g TIC: moderate initial enhancement (max. 50%–80%) and persistent postinitial enhancement.

T1-Weighted Sequence (Contrast Enhanced)

The signal behavior of a fibroadenoma after contrast administration is dependent upon the histological composition of the tumor.

Myxoid fibroadenomas These are tumors with a high proportion of epithelial tissue, more frequent in younger women. Myxoid fibroadenomas are oval (**Fig. 8.1a, e, f**) or lobulated (**Fig. 8.2a**) lesions with well-circumscribed borders. The tumor matrix displays a rapid and strong enhancement. Dark internal septations often pass through the matrix and represent less vascularized fibrotic strands (**Figs. 8.2d, e, 8.3a, e, f**). Myxoid fibroadenomas typically have a strong CM uptake. The initial enhancement phase rarely shows a slow or medium (**Fig. 0.1 g**), often a rapid (**Fig. 8.2f**), and occasionally a very rapid enhancement (up to

several hundred percent), sometimes with values higher than those found in malignant tumors (**Fig. 8.3 g**). The postinitial signal phase usually displays a continuous increase (**Fig. 8.2f**) or plateau (**Fig. 8.1 g**). A postinitial signal washout is extremely rare (< 1% in our data collection). The transition from a myxoid to a fibrotic fibroadenoma usually takes many years (**Figs. 8.4, 8.5a, e, f**).

Fibrotic (hyalinized) fibroadenomas. These are tumors with a high proportion of fibrotic tissue, more frequent in older women. Fibrotic fibroadenomas are oval or lobulated lesions with well-circumscribed borders. Depending on the degree of fibrosis, there is little CM uptake (partially fibrotic fibroadenoma) (**Figs. 8.6a, d, e, 0.7a, e**) or no CM uptake (completely fibrotic fibroadenoma) (**Fig. 8.8a, d**). Only the less fibrous portion of a partially fibrotic

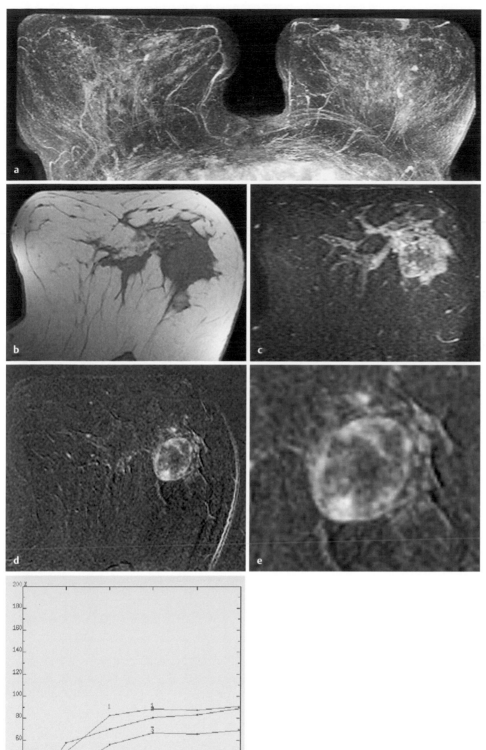

Fig. 8.6a–f Partially fibrotic fibroadenoma.
a Subtraction MIP: unremarkable findings in large breasts with strong parenchymal enhancement.
b T1w precontrast slice image: vague mass lesion with isointense signal in comparison with surrounding parenchyma.
c IR T2w slice image: indistinct mass lesion with higher signal intensity in peripheral tumor areas.
d Early subtraction slice image: well-circumscribed, oval mass lesion with peripheral hypervascularization and central areas without hypervascularization.
e. Zoomed subtraction image.
f TIC: moderate initial enhancement (max. 50%–80%) and persistent postinitial enhancement.

fibroadenoma will show hypervascularization. The classic fine internal septations seen in myxoid fibroadenomas are only rarely present. Instead there are wide areas of extensive sclerosis. If there is any enhancement at all, initial enhancement will be slow to moderate, and postinitial enhancement is persistent or shows a plateau (**Figs. 8.5 g, 8.6f**).

Special Types of Fibroadenomas

Juvenile fibroadenomas and giant fibroadenomas are variants that occur in addition to the common adult type of fibroadenoma. Apart from their greater size, they have the same image characteristics as the typical myxoid fibroadenoma. Despite the fact that they are benign lesions without an elevated risk of malignant transformation, they are usually excised because of their large size.

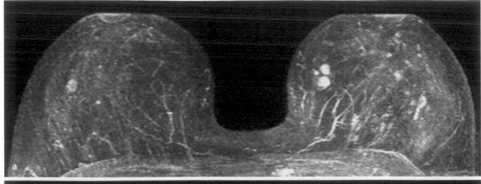

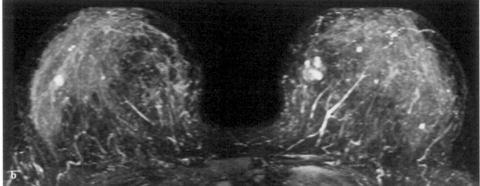

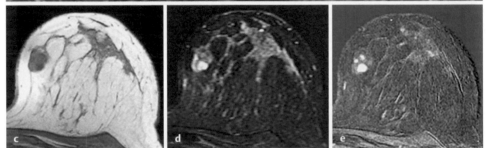

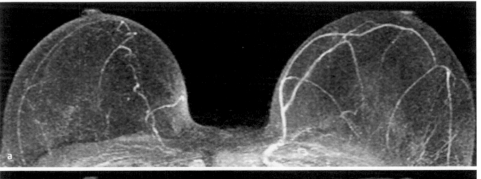

Fig. 8.7 a–e   Special case: Partially fibrotic fibroadenoma.

a Subtraction MIP: conglomerate of several foci and well-circumscribed mass lesions in the medial aspect of the left breast.

b T2w MIP: foci and masses display high signal intensity (water content).

c T1w precontrast slice image: the described conglomerate is localized within a larger lobulated, well-circumscribed lesion.

d IR T2w slice image: partially high, partially low signal intensity within larger lesion.

e Early subtraction slice image: homogeneous hypervascularization of areas with high water content.

Assessment: BI-RADS 2 lesion. The differential diagnosis includes a hamartoma and a fibroadenoma. *Histology* revealed a partially fibrotic fibroadenoma.

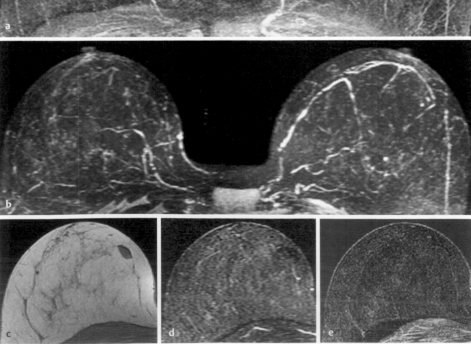

Fig. 8.8 a–e   Fibrotic fibroadenoma.

a Subtraction MIP: unremarkable findings.

b T2w MIP: unremarkable findings.

c T1w precontrast slice image: well-circumscribed, oval lesion easily identified within the fat tissue of the right breast.

d IR T2w slice image: no increased signal in the water-sensitive image.

e Early subtraction slice image: no enhancement.

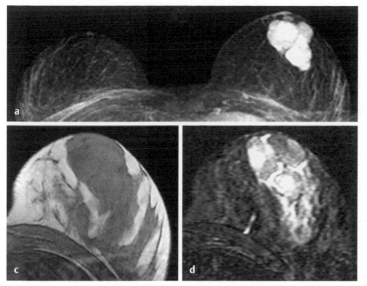

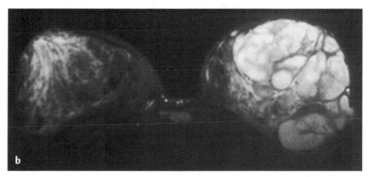

Fig. 8.9a–f Juvenile fibroadenoma. Conglomerate tumor. A 19-year-old woman with new palpable mass in the left breast.

a Subtraction MIP: conglomerate of several lobulated, well-circumscribed, hypervascularized mass lesions in the left breast.

b T2w MIP: high signal intensity (water content) of all lesions and surrounding parenchyma.

c T1w precontrast slice image: several well-circumscribed, isointense lesions.

d IR T2w slice image: lesions display partially high, partially low signal intensity.

e Early subtraction slice image: inhomogeneous enhancement.

f TIC: rapid initial enhancement (max. 100%–160%) and postinitial plateau.

The patient opted for the operative excision of the tumor.

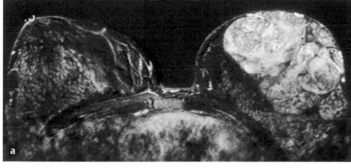

Fig. 8.10a, b Giant fibroadenoma. Massive volume increase of the left breast.

a Subtraction MIP: size asymmetry caused by extremely large, well-circumscribed, hypervascularized tumor with multiple dark internal septations in the left breast.

b IR T2w slice image: homogeneous high signal intensity with exception of the internal septations.

Operative excision of the tumor.

Juvenile fibroadenomas. These are rapidly growing lesions that appear during adolescence (i.e., puberty), and can reach a size of several centimeters. They make up ~0.5%–2% of all fibroadenomas (**Fig. 8.9**).

Giant fibroadenomas. These are large lesions with a diameter >5 cm. They appear with a higher frequency during pregnancy and the lactation period (**Fig. 8.10**).

 MR Mammography: Juvenile and Giant Fibroadenomas

T1-Weighted Sequence (Precontrast)

Round, oval, or lobulated lesion with an isointense or slightly hypointense signal in comparison with parenchyma (**Fig. 8.9c**).

T2-Weighted Sequence

Typically hyperintense signal (**Fig. 8.9b**). Internal septations or localized areas with a lower signal intensity are often seen (**Fig. 8.10b**).

T1-Weighted (Contrast Enhanced)

Strong, often inhomogeneous contrast enhancement (**Figs. 8.9a, 8.10a**). Dark internal septation and/or localized areas with reduced vascularization are typically seen (**Figs. 8.9e, 8.10b**). Sharp demarcation from surrounding tissue. TICs are uninformative, often showing a rapid initial enhancement and a postinitial plateau (**Fig. 8.9f**). They typically show no criteria that are suspicious for malignancy.

Adenomas

Adenomas of the breast are composed of benign epithelial elements with a sparse stromal component, features that differentiate them from fibroadenomas. Adenomas are commonly divided into two major groups: **tubular adenomas** and **lactating adenomas**. *Tubular adenomas* present in young women as well-circumscribed tumors composed of proliferating small tubular structures that are separated from adjacent breast tissue by an enveloping pseudocapsule. *Lactating adenomas* develop during pregnancy or the postpartum period and are composed of glands with an increased secretory activity.

The *nipple adenoma* is a rare, usually benign variant of intraductal papilloma involving the terminal portion of the nipple ducts. Microscopically there is a florid epithelial proliferation and adenosis, with a variable amount of sclerosis (**Fig. 8.15**).

Adenoma: General information	
Incidence:	Rare breast tumor.
Age peak:	Especially younger women.
Risk of malignant transformation:	No increased risk.
Multifocality:	Rare
Findings	
Clinical:	Small adenomas are clinically occult.
	Larger tumors are well-circumscribed, movable, painless nodules.
Mammography:	Small adenomas are mammographically occult.
	Larger tumors appear round, oval, or lobulated, well-circumscribed, and homogeneously dense, and may display a halo sign.
	Occasional macrocalcifications; less common than in fibroadenomas.
Ultrasonography:	Small adenomas are sonographically occult.
	Larger tumors appear round, oval, or lobulated, well-circumscribed, with a homogeneous internal echotexture.
	Moderate to strong posterior acoustic enhancement; possible bilateral acoustic shadowing. No or slight lesion compressibility.
	No criteria suspicious for malignancy.

Adenomas of the breast show similar characteristics to fibroadenomas in the various imaging techniques. If there is uncertainty about the histology, a percutaneous biopsy is indicated to rule out malignancy (preferably ultrasound-guided).

MR Mammography: Adenoma

T1-Weighted Sequence (Precontrast)

Small adenomas are not usually visible in the precontrast examination. Larger tumors, especially when located within lipomatous tissue are well-circumscribed, round (**Figs. 8.11b, 8.15a**), oval (**Fig. 8.13b**) or lobulated (**Figs. 8.12b, 8.14b**) lesions with an isointense or slightly hypointense signal. Sometimes a halo sign may be present.

T2-Weighted Sequence

Usually inhomogeneous (**Fig. 8.12c**) or high signal intensity (**Figs. 8.11c, 8.13c**), comparable to the signal intensity of myxoid fibroadenomas. Occasional internal septations.

T1-Weighted (Contrast Enhanced)

Hypervascularized focus or mass lesion with round, oval or lobulated shape (**Figs. 8.11a, 8.14a, d, e**) and well-circumscribed borders. Usually homogeneous contrast enhancement (**Figs. 8.11d, 8.13a, d**). Occasional inhomogeneous enhancement (**Fig. 8.12a, d**). Rare dark internal septations. No rim enhancement. In most cases rapid initial enhancement (**Fig. 8.11e**) with variable postinitial signal behavior (**Fig. 8.14f**: persistent postinitial signal increase, **Fig. 8.11e**: plateau, or **Figs. 8.13e** and **8.15e** washout).

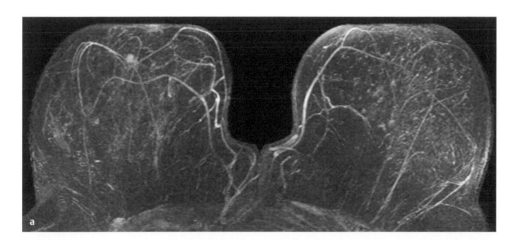

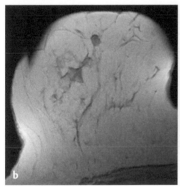
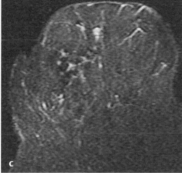
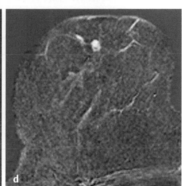
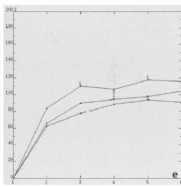

Fig. 8.11a–e   Small adenoma.
a Subtraction MIP: solitary focus (4 mm) in the retromamillary region of the right breast.
b T1w precontrast slice image: corresponding well-circumscribed, round, isointense lesion within surrounding lipomatous tissue.
c IR T2w slice image: homogeneous high signal intensity with horizontal septation (hamburger sign).
d Early subtraction slice image: homogeneous enhancement.
e TIC: unspecific dynamics with initial signal enhancement ~100% and postinitial plateau.

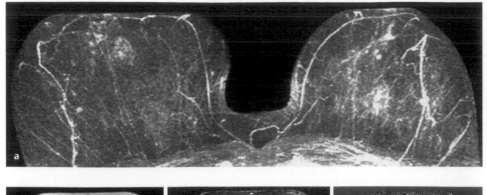

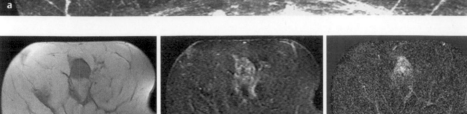

Fig. 8.12a–d Medium-sized adenoma.
a Subtraction MIP: solitary focus (4 mm) in the retromamillary region of the right breast.
b T1w precontrast slice image: corresponding well-circumscribed, round, isointense lesion within surrounding lipomatous tissue.
c IR T2w slice image: inhomogeneous, intermediary signal intensity.
d Early subtraction slice image: inhomogeneous enhancement. Because no suitable ROI placement is possible, no informative TIC can be plotted.

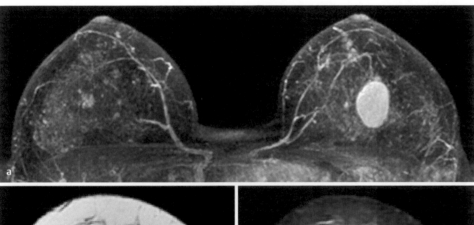

Fig. 8.13a–e Large adenoma.
a Subtraction MIP: well-circumscribed, oval, hypervascularized tumor in the left breast.
b T1w precontrast slice image: well-circumscribed, oval, isointense lesion.
c IR T2w slice image: inhomogeneous high signal intensity.
d Early subtraction slice image: homogeneous enhancement.
e TIC: rapid initial signal enhancement ~140% and postinitial washout.

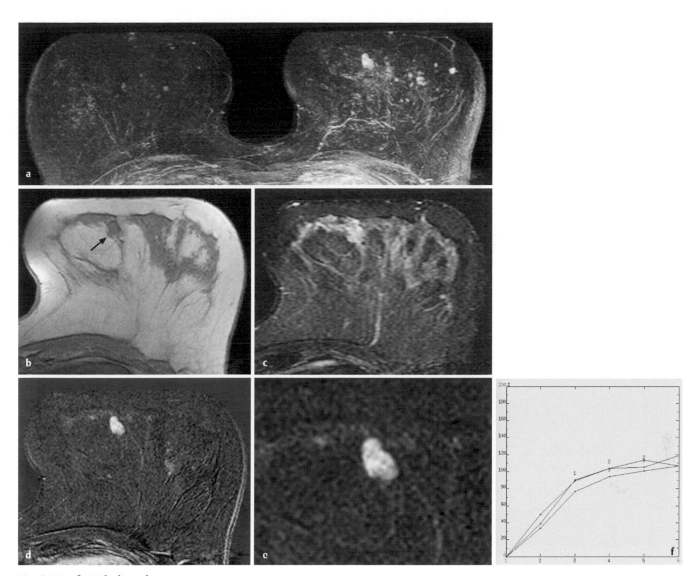

Fig. 8.14a–f   Tubular adenoma.

a Subtraction MIP: lobulated, hypervascularized mass lesions in the left breast. Additional bilateral harmless foci.

b T1w precontrast slice image: partially well-circumscribed, oval, isointense lesion within an area of parenchyma (arrow).

c IR T2w slice image: high signal intensity.

d Early subtraction slice image: inhomogeneous enhancement of a well-circumscribed, lobulated lesion.

e Zoomed subtraction image.

f TIC: moderate initial enhancement (max. 70%–90%) and persistent postinitial enhancement.

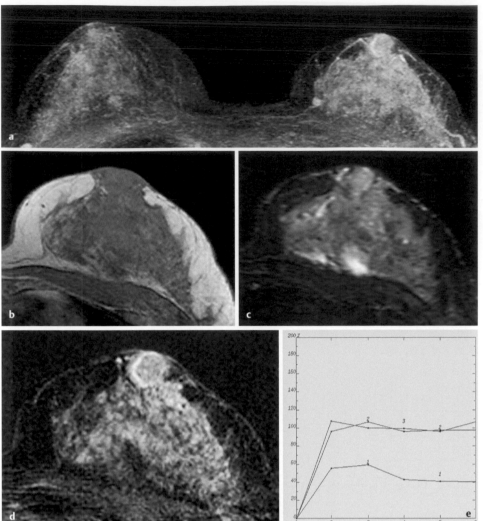

Fig. 8.15a–e   Nipple adenoma.

a Subtraction MIP: strong enhancement of parenchyma in both breasts. Round mass lesion with peripheral hypervascularization behind the left nipple.

b T1w precontrast slice image: widened iso-intense retromamillary region without clear demarcation of circumscribed lesion.

c IR T2w slice image: unremarkable findings.

d Early subtraction slice image: oval hyper-vascularized lesion behind the left nipple with thin rim-enhancement and intermediary vascularization of central tumor areas.

e TIC: varying curves due to difficult adequate placement of ROI. Conspicuous curve features are a rapid initial enhancement (> 100%) and a slight postinitial washout.

Benign Phyllodes Tumor

Synonyms: benign phyllodes tumor, fibroadenoma phyllodes.

The phyllodes tumor is a distinctive fibroepithelial tumor of the breast without counterpart in any other organ of the body. The benign form of this tumor is characterized by its structural similarity to the fibroadenoma, a low mitotic activity (0–4 mitoses/10 HPF at 400× magnification [HPF = high power field]), no nuclear atypia, and a tumor growth pattern that displaces the surrounding tissue. The tumor stroma can show fibrous, lipomatous, chondral, myxoid, and myoid differentiation. In addition, tumors often show signs of hemorrhage and ulceration.

 MR Mammography: Benign Phyllodes Tumor

T1-Weighted Sequence (Precontrast)
Benign phyllodes tumors are well-circumscribed round (**Fig. 8.17b**) or lobulated (**Figs. 8.16c, 8.18a**) lesions without pseudocapsular demarcation. Signal intensity is equivalent to that of parenchyma (isointense). Occasionally cystic or necrotic changes are seen as round inclusions with a comparatively hypointense signal.

T2-Weighted Sequence
Well-circumscribed round or lobulated lesion with iso- to hyperintense signal (**Fig. 8.16b, d**). Occasionally cystic or necrotic changes are seen as round inclusions with a hyperintense signal (**Figs. 8.17c, g, 8.18b**).

T1-Weighted (Contrast Enhanced)
The solid areas within a benign phyllodes tumor show a moderate to strong signal enhancement (**Figs. 8.16a, e, f, 8.17d**). In the course of the examination there is increasing demarcation of existing cystic or necrotic areas. Initial contrast enhancement is often > 100%. The postinitial signal phase usually displays a persistent increase or a plateau (**Figs. 8.17e, i, 8.18d**). If no liquid inclusions are seen, differentiation from a myxoid fibroadenoma is not possible.

Benign phyllodes tumor: General information

Incidence:	Rare breast tumor (~0.3% of all breast tumors).
Age peak:	30–50 years.
Risk of malignant transformation:	No increased risk. **Note**: High local recurrence rate of ~30%.

Findings

Clinical:	Rapidly growing, smooth or tuberous mass, diameter up to 10 cm or more.
	Larger tumors show skin changes (thinning and/or livid discoloration).
Mammography:	Round or lobulated, well-circumscribed, homogeneously dense mass (similar to a fibroadenoma).
	Occasionally displays a halo sign due to compression of surrounding tissue.
	Rarely has micro- or macrocalcifications.
Ultrasonography:	Round or lobulated, well-circumscribed mass with posterior acoustic enhancement.
	Cystic inclusions are a characteristic diagnostic attribute.

The differential diagnosis between a phyllodes tumor and a fibroadenoma is occasionally difficult. Rapid growth and the documentation of cystic inclusions are indicative of a phyllodes tumor. Benign and malignant forms cannot be differentiated on the basis of imaging characteristics. The term "cystosarcoma phyllodes" is historical and should no longer be used.

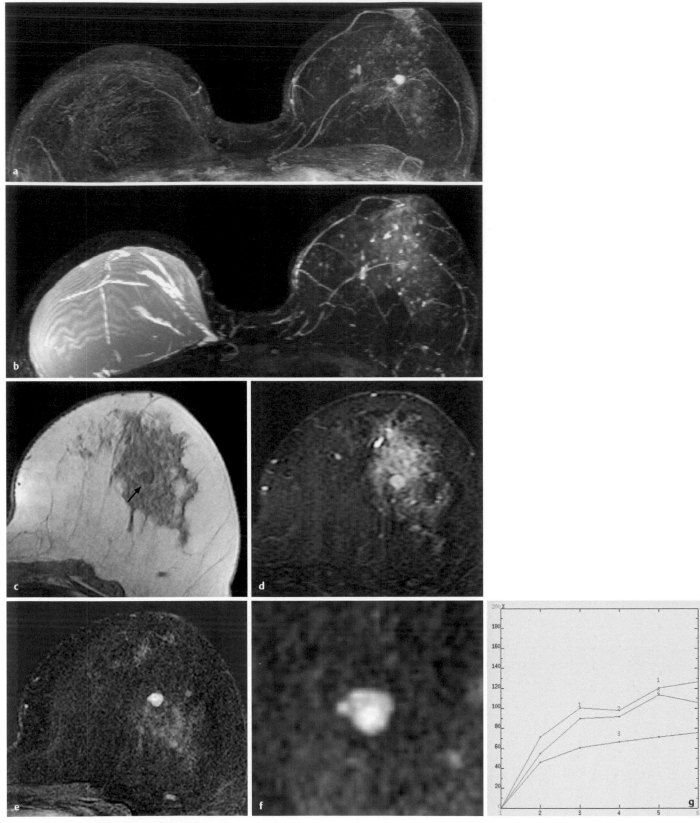

Fig. 8.16a–g   Benign phyllodes tumor.

a Subtraction MIP: hypervascularized, lobulated mass lesion in the left breast. Mastectomy and reconstruction with prosthesis implantation on the right after breast cancer.

b T2w MIP: relative high signal intensity (water content) of left lesion. Right silicone prosthesis shows harmless radial folds.

c T1w precontrast slice image (left breast): vague demarcation of a hypointense lesion.

d IR T2w slice image: lesion shows slightly elevated signal intensity relative to the surrounding parenchyma (water content).

e Early subtraction slice image: inhomogeneous hypervascularization within a well-circumscribed, lobulated lesion.

f Zoomed subtraction image.

g TIC: moderate initial enhancement (max. 50%–100%) and persistent postinitial enhancement.

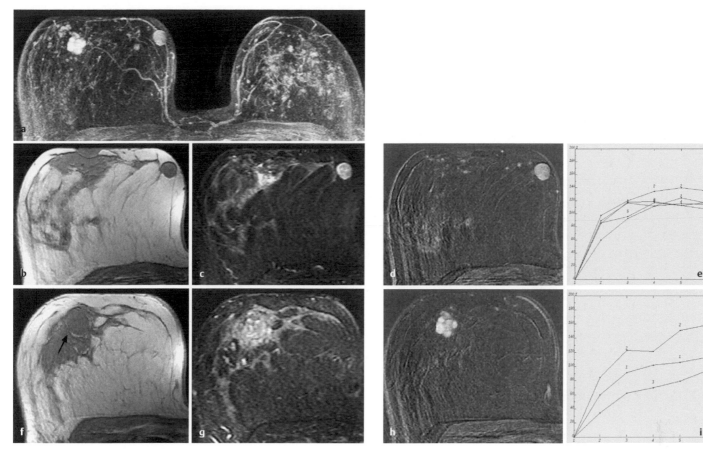

Fig. 8.17 a–i   Benign bifocal phyllodes tumor.

a Subtraction MIP: two hypervascularized mass lesions with different configurations in the right breast. Incidental finding: size asymmetry.

b T1w precontrast slice image (right medial lesion): round, well-circumscribed lesion.

c Corresponding IR T2w slice image: inhomogeneous water content.

d Corresponding early subtraction slice image: inhomogeneous hypervascularization.

e Unspecific TIC.

f T1w precontrast slice image (right central lesion): round lesion with halo sign (arrow).

g Corresponding IR T2w slice image: microcystic inclusions.

h Corresponding early subtraction slice image: inhomogeneous, confluent-nodular hypervascularization.

i TIC: moderate initial enhancement and persistent postinitial enhancement is indicative of a benign lesion.

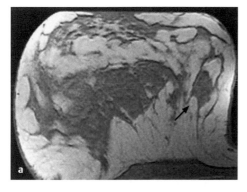
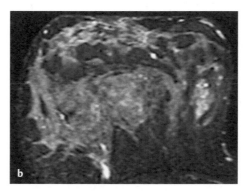
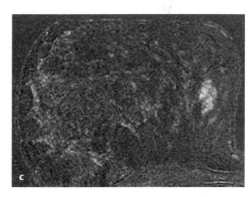

Fig. 8.18 a–d   Benign phyllodes tumor.

a T1w precontrast slice image: oval, microlobulated lesion within surrounding fatty tissue (high signal intensity) of the right breast (arrow).

b Corresponding IR T2w slice image: few microcystic inclusions within lesion with inhomogeneous intermediary signal intensity.

c Corresponding early subtraction slice image: inhomogeneous hypervascularization with dark internal septations.

d TIC: moderate initial enhancement and persistent postinitial enhancement.

Lipomas

Lipomas of the breast are composed of encapsulated nodules of mature fat cells. These rare lesions must be differentiated from mixed tumors with macroscopically visible adipose tissue.

Subcutaneous lipomas can be located in the breast, as well as in other body areas.

 MR Mammography: Lipomas

T1-Weighted Sequence (Precontrast)
Often oval, well-circumscribed lesion with hyperintense, fat-equivalent signal. Occasionally a thin, hypointense capsule can be seen (**Fig. 8.19b**). No nonadipose internal structures.

T2-Weighted Sequence
Often oval, well-circumscribed lesion with intermediary signal intensity equivalent to that of subcutaneous fat. In fat suppressed sequences (e.g. IR T2w) lipomas will appear hypointense due to suppression of the fat peak (*Note*: fat suppression is usually stronger in a lipoma than in normal fat tissue) (**Fig. 8.19c**).

T1-Weighted Sequence (Contrast Enhanced)
No contrast enhancement (**Fig. 8.19a, d**).

Lipoma: General information

Incidence:	Rare breast tumor.
Age peak:	All ages.
Risk of malignant transformation:	No increased risk.

Findings

Clinical:	Often occult.
	Occasionally soft, more rarely firm, movable nodule.
Mammography:	Well-circumscribed, fully or partially encapsulated radiolucent tumor.
Ultrasonography:	Large lesions are seen as well-circumscribed, highly compressible masses with an echogenicity similar to that of breast parenchyma.
	Note: Because the fat cells in lipomas are arranged differently than in normal fat tissue, they typically have a higher echogenicity.

Lipomas of the breast are rare, usually clinically occult lesions, often demonstrated solely in mammography as an incidental finding. The mammographic appearance is pathognomonic and no further diagnostic examinations are necessary.

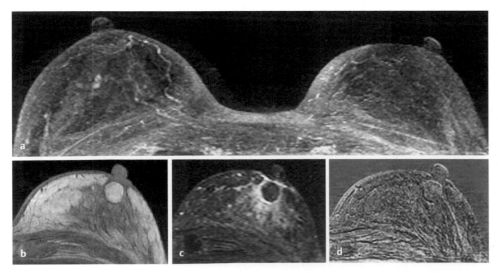

Fig. 8.19a–d Lipoma.
a Subtraction MIP: unremarkable findings with two harmless foci in the right breast (unchanged over years).
b T1w precontrast slice image: round, well-circumscribed hyperintense mass in the left retromamillary region.
c Corresponding IR T2w slice image: complete suppression of internal lesion signal in fat-suppressed water-sensitive sequence.
d Corresponding early subtraction slice image: no lesion enhancement.

Fibrocystic Breast Condition

The term fibrocystic breast condition, synonymous with fibrocystic breast disease, *fibrocystic changes*, and *mammary dysplasia*, is used to describe a proliferation of hormone-dependent mesenchymal and epithelial structures of the breast. Fibrocystic breast condition encompasses a heterogeneous group of abnormalities that may occur separately or together. The morphological components, present in various degrees, comprise cysts, lobular hyperplasia, adenosis, ductal and alveolar hyperplasia (papillomatosis or epitheliosis), and stromal fibrosis. The etiology of such changes is presumed to be a hormonal imbalance.

 MR Mammography: Fibrocystic Breast Condition

T1-Weighted Sequence (Precontrast)
Hypointense round lesions within breast parenchyma correlate with cystic component. No other specific changes (**Fig. 8.20c**) are seen.

T2-Weighted Sequence
Hyperintense lesions of various sizes (cysts) (**Fig. 8.20b**). Occasionally parenchyma displays a diffusely increased signal intensity (especially in the second half of the menstrual cycle and under hormonal stimulation).

T1-Weighted Sequence (Contrast Enhanced)
Breast parenchyma can display no, weak, or strong, sometimes patchy enhancement, leaving out the cystic lesions (**Fig. 8.20a, d**). Signal increases persistently within representative ROIs. Otherwise there are no specific changes. *Note*: Parenchymal enhancement in breast MRI does not correlate with the risk of malignant transformation.

Fibrocystic breast condition: General information

Incidence:	~50% of all women.
Age peak:	40–60 years.

Findings

Clinical:	Variable symptoms (small to middle-sized palpable lumps and increased diffuse breast firmness), usually symmetric.
	Symptoms fluctuate with the menstrual cycle, peaking premenstrually.
Mammography:	Often diffuse, rarely circumscribed structural hyperdensities, usually symmetric.
	Macro- and microcalcifications may be present, sometimes difficult to differentiate from malignancy.
Ultrasonography:	Increased hyperechoic structures.
	Multiple hypoechoic tubular patterns (dilated ductal structures).
	Often multiple anechoic lesions with posterior acoustic enhancement (cysts).
	Usually symmetric findings.

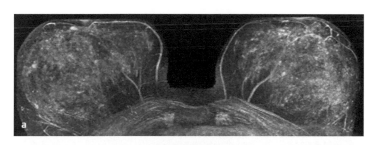
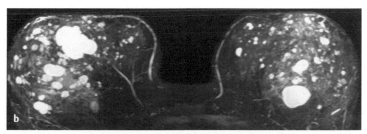
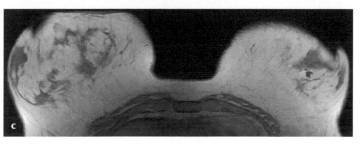
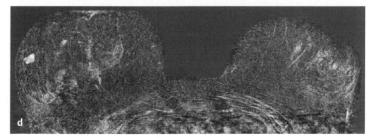

Fig. 8.20a–d   Fibrocystic breast condition.

a Subtraction MIP: confluent-stippled enhancement in both breasts. No suspicious abnormalities.

b T2w MIP: diffuse distribution of multiple small and large cysts in both breasts.

c T1w precontrast slice image: representative example with multiple lesions in both breasts.

d Corresponding early subtraction slice image: lesions display varying degrees of vascularization (none to high).

Adenosis

Synonym: adenosis mammae.

The term *adenosis* is used to describe clustered proliferations of small ductal and acinar structures in varying degrees, combined with an increase in the amount of lobular connective tissue. Histopathology differentiates adenosis into the following types: *sclerosing adenosis, blunt duct adenosis (microcystic adenosis)*, and the less common lesions *microglandular adenosis* and the *radial scar*, a borderline lesion that will be discussed separately.

> *!* Because a localized area of adenosis can be hypervascularized and have an irregular distribution, it is the most common cause of a false-positive finding in breast MRI. This is especially true for the nodular form of adenosis (**Fig. 8.24**).

 MR Mammography: Adenosis

T1-Weighted Sequence (Precontrast)
No specific changes (**Figs. 8.21 b, 8.23 b**). Occasionally hypointense changes that correlate with cysts (**Fig. 8.22 b**).

T2-Weighted Sequence
No specific changes (**Figs. 8.21 c, 8.23 c**). Occasionally associated with microcysts (**Fig. 8.22 c**).

T1-Weighted Sequence (Contrast Enhanced)
Focal areas of adenosis usually show a strong CM uptake, sometimes with a time–signal intensity curve (TIC) typical for malignancy, thus making the differentiation from an invasive carcinoma difficult to impossible (**Figs. 8.21 a, d–f, 8.22 a, d, 8.23 a, d–f**). Enhancement distribution is occasionally branching, making it then impossible to differentiate from an intraductal tumor. *Note:* There is a definite correlation between the degree of adenosis and the degree of contrast enhancement.

Adenosis: General information

Incidence:	Very common benign lesion.
Age peak:	All ages.
Risk of malignant transformation:	No increased risk. (exception: radial scar).

Findings

Clinical:	Usually clinically occult. Palpable mass may be present if proliferation is great or the area of adenosis is extensive.
Mammography:	Generally no specific findings.
	Often associated with monomorphic round, intralobular microcalcifications with regional or diffuse distribution.
Ultrasonography:	Generally no specific findings.
	Occasionally hypoechoic nodular areas within breast tissue, corresponding to areas of adenosis.

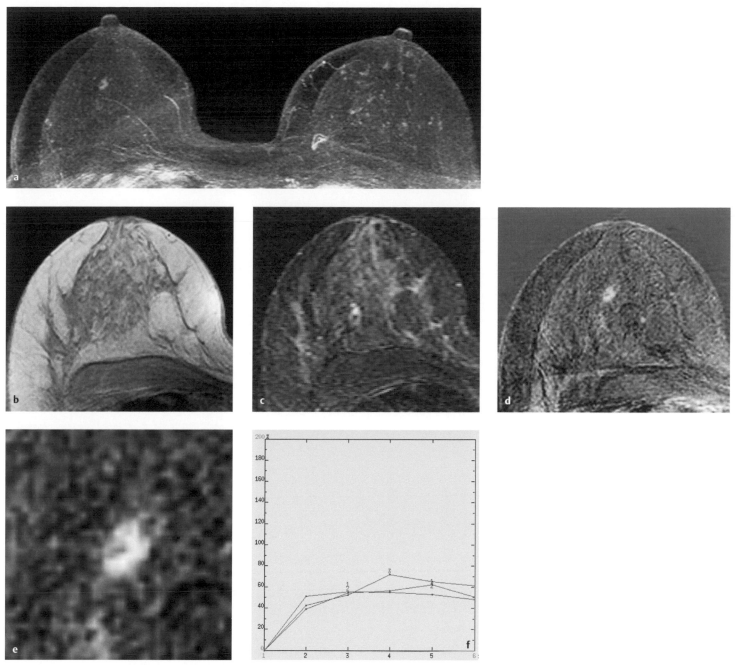

Fig. 8.21 a–f   Focal manifestation of a sclerosing adenosis.

a Subtraction MIP: localized area of enhancement in the central aspect of the right breast. No other conspicuous findings. *Note*: linear enhancement in the medial aspect of the left breast is a contrasted vein.

b Corresponding T1w precontrast slice image (right breast): unremarkable findings.

c Corresponding IR T2w slice image: unremarkable findings in area corresponding to enhancing lesion.

d Early subtraction slice image: irregularly shaped, nonmasslike lesion with inhomogeneous enhancement.

e Zoomed subtraction image.

f TIC: slow initial enhancement and postinitial plateau.

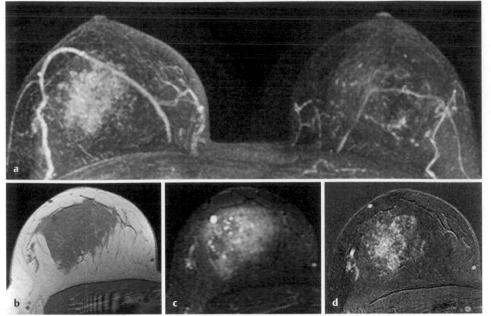

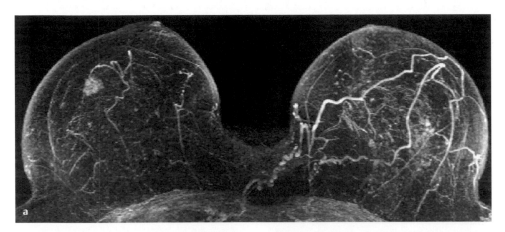

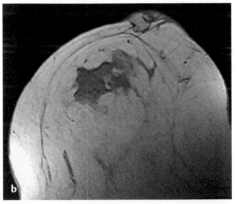
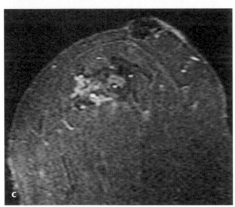
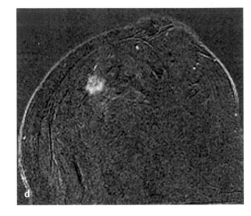

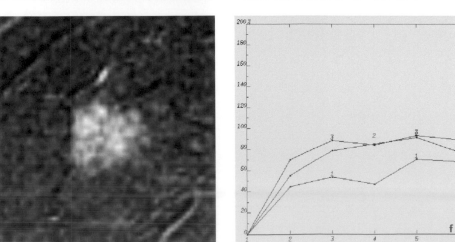

Fig. 8.22a–d Regional manifestation of a sclerosing adenosis.

a Subtraction MIP: asymmetric regional area of strong enhancement in the right breast.

b Corresponding T1w precontrast slice image (right breast): unremarkable findings.

c Corresponding IR T2w slice image: unremarkable findings apart from small cysts.

d Early subtraction slice image: nonmasslike, confluent-nodular enhancement pattern. Unspecific TIC (not shown).

Percutaneous biopsy-proven diagnosis.

Fig. 8.23a–f Blunt duct adenosis.

a Subtraction MIP: conspicuous enhancement in the right breast. Otherwise only slight enhancement asymmetry.

b Corresponding T1w precontrast slice image (right breast): unremarkable findings.

c Corresponding IR T2w slice image: unremarkable findings.

d Early subtraction slice image: lobulated, inhomogeneous nonmasslike enhancement.

e Zoomed subtraction image.

f Unspecific TIC: moderate initial enhancement (max. 50%–90%) and postinitial plateau.

Percutaneous biopsy-proven diagnosis.

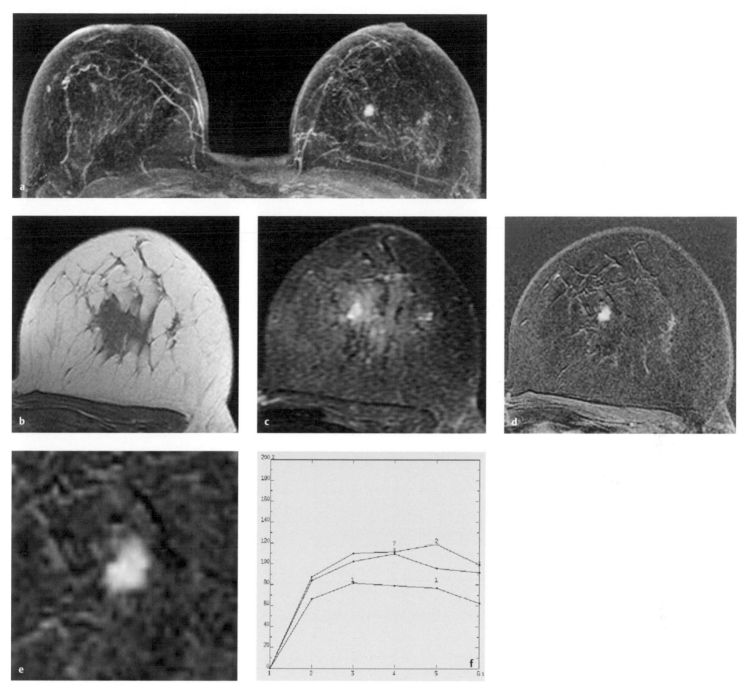

Fig. 8.24a–f Nodular adenosis.

a Subtraction MIP: solitary, round mass with ill-defined margins in the central aspect of the left breast.

b Corresponding T1w precontrast slice image (right breast): unremarkable findings.

c Corresponding IR T2w slice image: high signal intensity within lesion.

d Early subtraction slice image: hypervascularized mass lesion with irregular, partially ill-defined margins, and inhomogeneous enhancement.

e Zoomed subtraction image.

f TIC: Rapid initial enhancement (max. > 100%) and mild postinitial washout.

Percutaneous biopsy-proven diagnosis.

Stromal Fibrosis of the Breast

Stromal fibrosis of the breast is a proliferation of breast stroma with obliteration of mammary ducts and acini, resulting in areas of fibrous tissue associated with hypoplastic mammary ducts and lobules.

 MR Mammography: Stromal Fibrosis of the Breast

T1-Weighted Sequence (Precontrast)
No specific changes (**Figs. 8.25b, 8.26b**).

T2-Weighted Sequence
No specific changes (**Figs. 8.25c, 8.26c**).

T1-Weighted Sequence (Contrast Enhanced)
Generally stromal fibrosis of the breast will appear as a focal or regional area of nonmasslike enhancement (**Figs. 8.25a, 8.26a**), sometimes difficult or impossible to differentiate from a small intraductal carcinoma or an invasive lobular carcinoma (**Fig. 8.25d**). In rare cases, stromal fibrosis of the breast may appear as a mass lesion (**Fig. 8.26d**), often displaying an inhomogeneous internal enhancement, ill-defined borders, and an unspecific TIC (**Figs. 8.25e, 8.26e**).

Stromal fibrosis of the breast: General information

Incidence:	Common benign lesion.
Age peak:	All ages.
Risk of malignant transformation:	No increased risk.

Findings	
Clinical:	Usually clinically occult.
Mammography:	Generally no specific findings.
	Occasionally seen as asymmetry or density that is rarely associated with calcifications.
Ultrasonography:	Unspecific hypoechoic lesion.

Stromal fibrosis of the breast is a common incidental finding in biopsies performed for the diagnostic work-up of microcalcifications or a nonmasslike enhancement on breast MRI.

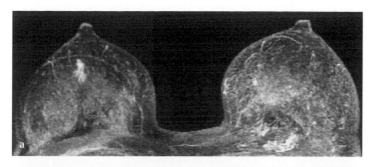

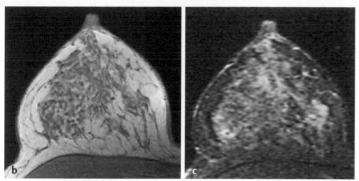

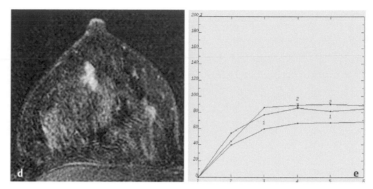

Fig. 8.25 a–f   Stromal fibrosis of the breast.

a Subtraction MIP: segmental enhancement along a mammary duct segment in the central aspect of the right breast. Harmless foci in the left breast.

b Corresponding T1w precontrast slice image (right breast): unremarkable findings.

c Corresponding IR T2w slice image: unremarkable findings.

d Early subtraction slice image: oblong, inhomogeneous nonmasslike enhancement.

e Unspecific TIC: moderate initial enhancement and postinitial plateau.

Percutaneous biopsy-proven diagnosis.

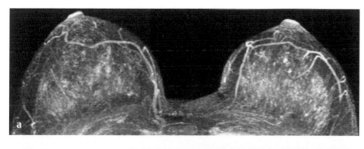

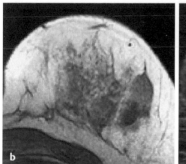

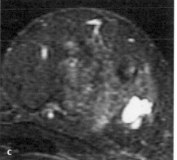

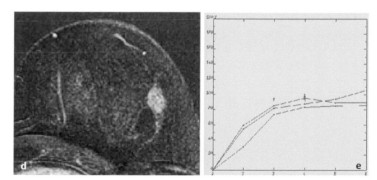

Fig. 8.26 a–e   Focal fibrosis of the nodular type.

a Subtraction MIP: regionally enhancing areas in both breasts. Several foci.

b T1w precontrast slice image (left breast): unremarkable findings.

c Corresponding IR T2w slice image: simple cyst. The area of fibrosis has intermediary signal intensity.

d Early subtraction slice image: hypervascularized mass with partially ill-defined margins and inhomogeneous enhancement.

e Unspecific TIC: moderate initial enhancement and postinitial plateau.

Percutaneous biopsy-proven diagnosis.

Pseudoangiomatous Stromal Hyperplasia

Pseudoangiomatous stromal hyperplasia (PASH) is a benign breast lesion characterized by proliferation of stromal spindle cells and associated with complex anastomosing, concentrically arranged clefts that are lined with CD 34-positive cells.

MR Mammography: Pseudoangiomatous Stromal Hyperplasia

T1-Weighted Sequence (Precontrast)
No specific changes (**Figs. 8.27c, 8.28b**). At most one might find a slight increase of parenchymal structures.

T2-Weighted Sequence
Variable findings. May display a high signal intensity (**Fig. 8.27 d**) or an isointense signal (**Fig. 8.28c**). No specific changes.

T1-Weighted Sequence (Contrast Enhanced)
May appear as a mass (**Fig. 8.27a**) or nonmasslike enhancement (**Fig. 8.28a**). Sometimes displays characteristics typical of malignancy and is therefore difficult or impossible to differentiate from a carcinoma (**Fig. 8.27e, f**). Enhancement distribution is occasionally branching (**Fig. 8.28 d**). The TIC is unspecific (**Fig. 8.28e**).

Pseudoangiomatous stromal hyperplasia: General information	
Incidence:	Rare.
Age peak:	All ages.
Risk of malignant transformation:	No increased risk.
Findings	
Clinical:	Usually clinically occult.
Mammography:	Usually mammographically occult.
Ultrasonography:	Usually sonographically occult.
PASH is a rare histopathological finding in biopsies performed for the diagnostic work-up of hypervascularized lesions on breast MRI.	

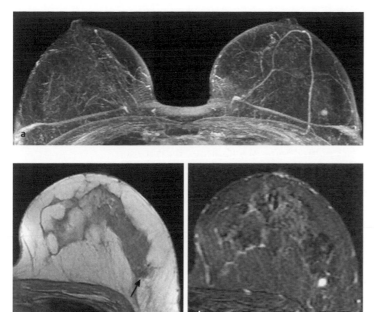
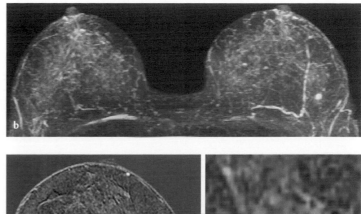
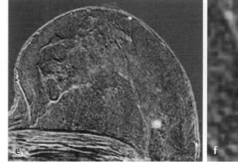
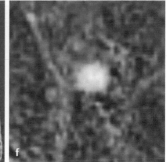

Fig. 8.27 a–f Pseudoangiomatous stromal hyperplasia.

a Subtraction MIP: hypervascularized focus with 4 mm diameter in the lateral aspect of the left breast.

b T2w MIP: focus displays a high intensity signal (water-content).

c Corresponding T1w precontrast slice image (left breast): isointense corresponding structure (arrow).

d Corresponding IR T2w slice image: high intensity signal (water-content).

e Early subtraction slice image: inhomogeneous enhancement and ill-defined margins.

f Zoomed subtraction image: unspecific TIC (not shown).

Percutaneous biopsy-proven diagnosis.

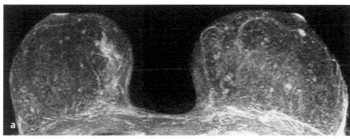
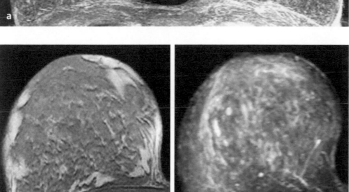
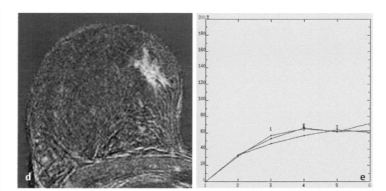

Fig. 8.28 a–e Pseudoangiomatous stromal hyperplasia.

a Subtraction MIP: asymmetric enhancement with irregular distribution in the medial aspect of the right breast.

b Corresponding T1w precontrast slice image (right breast): no corresponding lesion.

c Corresponding IR T2w slice image: unremarkable findings.

d Early subtraction slice image: nonmasslike enhancement with dendritic pattern.

e TIC: slow initial enhancement and persistent postinitial enhancement.

Percutaneous biopsy-proven diagnosis.

Hemangioma

Hemangiomas of the breast are intramammary, thin-walled, blood-filled vascular spaces. They can be differentiated into the cavernous and capillary types.

 MR Mammography: Breast Hemangioma

T1-Weighted Sequence (Precontrast)
When located within fat tissue of the breast, hemangiomas are seen as isointense, clustered or convoluted round structures (**Fig. 8.29b**). When located within breast parenchyma, they are often unremarkable (**Fig. 8.30b**). Signal extinction may be seen if macrocalcifications are present (**Fig. 8.31c**). Susceptibility artifacts may be caused by the ferromagnetic influence of blood components in a thrombus (**Fig. 8.29b**).

T2-Weighted Sequence
Usually displays a hyperintense signal (**Figs. 8.30c, 8.31d**). Susceptibility artifacts may also be seen (**Fig. 8.29c**).

T1-Weighted Sequence (Contrast Enhanced)
Breast hemangiomas show a delayed, inhomogeneous contrast enhancement that does not always involve the entire lesion (**Figs. 8.29a, d, 8.31a, e**). Occasionally they display a strong contrast enhancement (**Fig. 8.30a, d**). Blocked-out areas without enhancement may be seen when calcifications are present (**Fig. 8.29d**). The TICs are usually unspecific but may occasionally show a postinitial washout (**Fig. 8.30e**).

Breast hemangioma: General information

Incidence:	Rare.
Age peak:	All ages, more frequently >25 years.
Risk of malignant transformation:	No increased risk.

Findings	
Clinical:	Usually clinically occult.
Mammography:	Unspecific. Sometimes seen as density that may be associated with round microcalcifications.
Ultrasonography:	Unspecific. Occasionally seen as hypoechoic lesion with inhomogeneous internal echo-pattern. Possibly shows increased blood flow in duplex-sonography.

Hemangiomas are rare histopathological findings in biopsies performed for the diagnostic work-up of hypervascularized lesions on breast MRI.

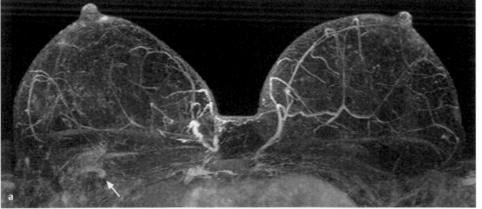
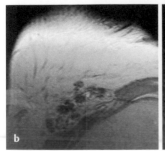
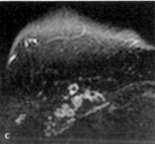
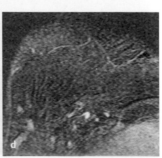

Fig. 8.29a–d Hemangioma.
a Subtraction MIP: hypervascularized area near the chest wall of the right breast (arrow).
b T1w precontrast slice image (right breast): convolution of numerous round isointense structures.
c Corresponding IR T2w slice image: decreased signal intensity in the center of some of these structures.
d Early subtraction slice image: partial enhancement of these round and oblong structures, some with blocked out enhancement in the center (calcifications).

Percutaneous biopsy-proven diagnosis.

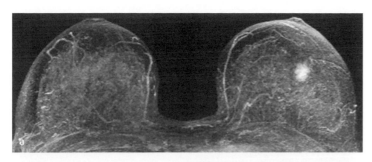

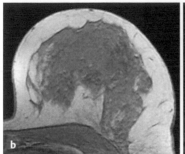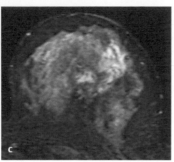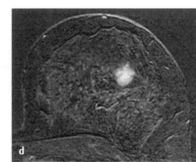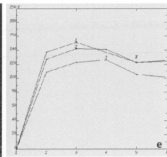

Fig. 8.30a–e   Hemangioma.

a Subtraction MIP: hypervascularized lesion in the central aspect of the left breast.

b T1w precontrast slice image (left breast): unremarkable findings.

c Corresponding IR T2w slice image: unremarkable findings.

d Early subtraction slice image: inhomogeneous enhancement of partially ill-defined, nonmasslike lesion.

e TIC: rapid, strong initial enhancement and postinitial washout.

Percutaneous biopsy-proven diagnosis.

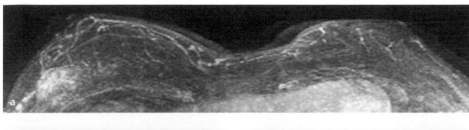

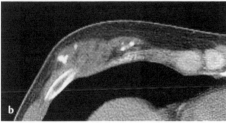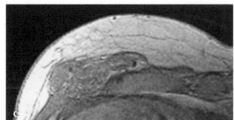

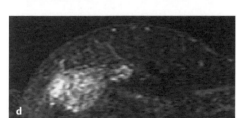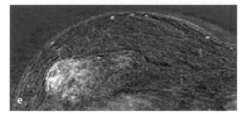

Fig. 8.31a–e   Hemangioma in a male breast.

a Subtraction MIP: regional enhancement in the lateral aspect of the right breast.

b CT (without contrast): soft-tissue, isodense structure with calcified inclusions.

c T1w precontrast slice image (right breast, adjacent to the chest wall): well-circumscribed, isointense lesion with internal areas of signal loss (calcifications) and numerous internal fat lamellae.

d Corresponding IR T2w slice image: inhomogeneous, increased water signal.

e Early subtraction slice image: inhomogeneous enhancement, the lateral aspects showing better blood flow than the medial aspects.

Adenomyoepithelioma

An adenomyoepithelioma is a well-circumscribed tumor composed of a solid proliferation of myoepithelial cells.

 MR Mammography: Adenomyoepithelioma

T1-Weighted Sequence (Precontrast)
No specific changes (**Fig. 8.32b**).

T2-Weighted Sequence
No specific changes (**Fig. 8.32c**).

T1-Weighted Sequence (Contrast Enhanced)
Adenomyoepitheliomas usually appear as hypervascularized foci or masses of small size (a few millimeters) (**Fig. 8.32a, d, e**). They usually display a moderate or rapid initial contrast enhancement and may show a postinitial washout (**Fig. 8.32f**).

Adenomyoepithelioma: General information

Incidence:	Very rare.
Age peak:	All ages.
Risk of malignant transformation:	No increased risk.

Findings

Clinical:	Usually clinically occult.
Mammography:	Usually mammographically occult.
Ultrasonography:	Usually sonographically occult.

An adenomyoepithelioma is a rare histopathological finding in biopsies performed for the diagnostic work-up of hypervascularized lesions on breast MRI.

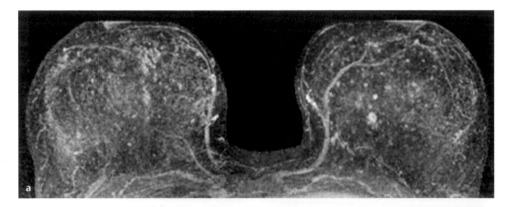

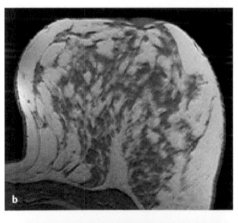

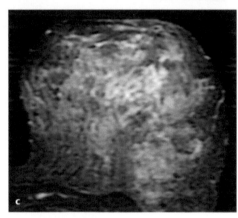

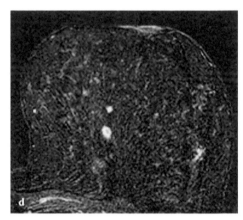

Fig. 8.32a–f Adenomyoepithelioma.
a Subtraction MIP: multiple bilateral foci of 1–3 mm diameter. Hypervascularized focus of 4 mm diameter in the central aspect of the left breast.
b Corresponding T1w precontrast slice image (left breast): unremarkable findings.
c Corresponding IR T2w slice image: unremarkable findings.

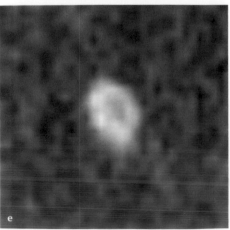

d Early subtraction slice image: hypervascularized, ill-defined focus of 4 mm in diameter with increased vascularization in peripheral lesion aspects (rim sign). Additional focus of 2 mm in diameter is seen ventral to the primary lesion.
e Zoomed subtraction image.
f TIC (ROI placed in rim): moderate initial signal enhancement and postinitial washout.

Percutaneous biopsy-proven diagnosis.

Simple Cysts

Cysts are fluid-filled round to ovoid structures that vary in size from microscopic to grossly evident as a palpable mass. Histopathology shows that the lining epithelium usually consists of two layers: an inner epithelial layer and an outer myoepithelial layer. Occasionally there may be fine intracystic septations. Cysts may occur as a singular lesion or be multiple in number and are a typical component of the fibrocystic breast condition.

 MR Mammography: Simple Cyst

T1-Weighted Sequence (Precontrast)
Well-circumscribed, round, oval (**Fig. 8.34a**), or lobulated (**Fig. 8.33a**), hypointense lesion. Good demarcation of cysts located within adipose tissue. Poor demarcation of cysts located within breast parenchyma. Occasional halo sign (**Fig. 8.33a**).

T2-Weighted Sequence
Well-circumscribed, round, oval (**Fig. 8.34b**), or lobulated (**Fig. 8.33b**), hyperintense lesion with homogeneous internal structure. Occasional intracystic septations. Detection is possible from a diameter of 1–2 mm (**Fig. 8.35**). Comprehensive presentation as a T2w MIP image (**Fig. 8.36**).

T1-Weighted Sequence (Contrast Enhanced)
Improved demarcation of cystic lesions within parenchyma due to CM-uptake in surrounding breast tissue. No significant improvement of cyst demarcation when located in fat tissue. No CM-uptake within simple mammary cysts (**Figs. 8.33c, 8.34c**).

Simple cyst: General information

Incidence:	Very common (up to 50% of all women).
Age peak:	All ages, decreasing prevalence in postmenopausal women.
Risk of malignant transformation:	No increased risk.

Findings

Clinical:	Small cysts: clinically occult.
	Larger cysts: firm-elastic, well-circumscribed, movable nodules.
	Occasional mastodynia.
Mammography:	Small cysts: mammographically occult.
	Larger cysts: well-circumscribed, homogeneous mass.
	May display halo sign.
Ultrasonography:	Well-circumscribed, anechoic mass with posterior acoustic enhancement.
	May be detected as small as 1–2 mm in diameter.
	No criteria suspicious for malignancy.

Gross cysts can cause breast pain and be clinically relevant. In such cases, percutaneous aspiration may be performed to relieve symptoms. Small asymptomatic cysts are incidental findings.

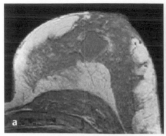
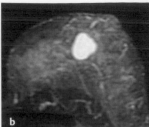
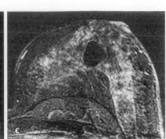

Fig. 8.33a–c Simple cyst.
a T1w precontrast slice image: well-circum-scribed, lobulated, isointense lesion with halo sign (fine fat lamella around circumference of lesion). Internal pattern is more homogeneous than that of the surrounding parenchyma (no interspersed fat).
b Corresponding IR T2w slice image: high homogeneous signal intensity.
c Corresponding early subtraction slice image: no contrast enhancement within cyst.

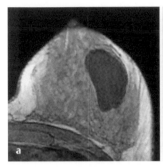
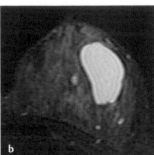
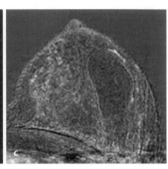

Fig. 8.34a–c Large simple cyst (macrocyst).
a T1w precontrast slice image: well-circum-scribed, oval, isointense lesion with a maximum diameter of 4 cm.
b Corresponding IR T2w slice image: high homogeneous signal intensity.
c Corresponding early subtraction slice image: no internal contrast enhancement.

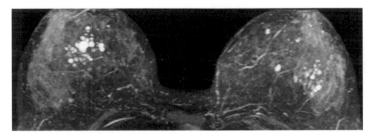
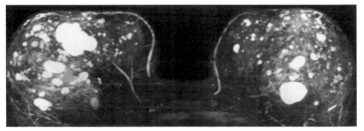

Fig. 8.35 Conglomerate of microcysts. Regionally distributed simple cysts in both breasts (IR T2w MIP).

Fig. 8.36 Cystic breasts. Diffuse distribution of numerous simple cysts in both breasts (IR T2w MIP).

Inflamed Cysts

Inflamed mammary cysts differ from simple mammary cysts in that inflammatory changes are present in the cyst wall.

 Inflammatory changes in a cyst wall are harmless incidental findings. Intracystic proliferations, on the other hand, should always be histologically examined to exclude malignancy.

MR Mammography: Inflamed Cyst

T1-Weighted Sequence (Precontrast)
Well-circumscribed, occasionally ill-defined hypointense lesion (**Fig. 8.39c**). Good demarcation of cysts located within adipose tissue. Poor demarcation between cysts and breast parenchyma (**Fig. 8.38c**). Inflammation of a cyst wall usually causes no visible changes and cannot be differentiated from a simple cyst (**Fig. 8.37c**).

T2-Weighted Sequence
Usually well-circumscribed, occasionally ill-defined hyperintense lesion (**Figs. 8.37b, d, 8.38b, d, 8.39b, d**).

T1-Weighted Sequence (Contrast-Enhanced)
Cyst wall is usually of normal caliber, occasionally thickened, and shows an increased CM-uptake (wall enhancement). No enhancement of internal cyst contents (**Figs. 8.37e, 8.38e**). When numerous cysts are present, repeat examinations often show differences in which lesions enhance. Occasionally surrounding breast tissue may be involved in the inflammatory process and show reactive pericystic enhancement (**Fig. 8.39a**). TICs usually show a persistent signal increase (**Fig. 8.38f**), or are unspecific and display a postinitial plateau (**Fig. 8.39f**).

The "rim-enhancement" seen in inflamed cysts is not a sign of malignancy. It should be assessed as a harmless incidental finding and is therefore better termed *wall-enhancement*.

Inflamed cyst: General information

Incidence:	Occasional finding in women with simple cysts.
Age peak:	All ages, decreasing prevalence in postmenopausal women.
Risk of malignant transformation:	No increased risk.

Findings

Clinical:	Small cysts: clinically occult.
	Larger cysts: Often cause mastodynia or pain upon applied pressure.
	If palpable: firm-elastic, well-circumscribed, movable nodule.
Mammography:	Small cysts: mammographically occult
	Larger cysts: well-circumscribed, homogeneous mass.
	Note: (Partially) ill-defined margins more likely indicate a complicated cyst.
Ultrasonography:	Anechoic mass with posterior acoustic enhancement.
	Occasionally ill-defined margins.

Hamartoma of the Breast

Synonyms: fibroadenolipoma, lipofibroadenoma.

Hamartomas of the breast are well-defined lesions with organoid structure and fissurelike or pseudocapsular borders. They are composed of variable amounts of adipose tissue, fibrous stroma, and breast parenchyma (with or without cystic inclusions).

! Figuratively: "Breast within the breast" (Kronsbein and Bässler 1982).

 MR Mammography: Breast Hamartoma

T1-Weighted Sequence (Precontrast)
Well-circumscribed, round, or oval lesion with surrounding pseudocapsular demarcation (**Fig. 8.44b**) and organoid internal structures: Parenchymal components with intermediary signal intensity, lipomatous components with high signal intensity, and cystic components with low signal intensity (**Figs. 8.45b, 8.46b**).

T2-Weighted Sequence
Well-circumscribed, round, or oval lesion with surrounding pseudocapsular demarcation, and organoid internal structures: Parenchymal components with intermediate signal intensity (**Fig. 8.45c**), lipomatous components with high signal intensity (T2-SE), or suppressed signal (IR T2w) (**Fig. 8.46c**), and cystic components with high signal intensity (**Fig. 8.44c**).

T1-Weighted Sequence (Contrast Enhanced)
Very variable internal enhancement pattern of the parenchymal component, from no enhancement to strongly increased enhancement. The internal enhancement pattern of a breast hamartoma may be very different from that of the surrounding parenchyma (**Fig. 8.45a, d**). No CM uptake in lipomatous (**Fig. 8.46a, d**) and cystic (**Fig. 8.44a, d**) tumor areas.

Hamartoma of the breast: General information

Incidence:	Rare breast tumor (1:1000).
Age peak:	40–60 years.
Risk of malignant transformation:	No increased risk.

Findings	
Clinical:	Occult if the adipose component is large.
	Palpable nodule if the fibrous component is large and depending on size.
Mammography:	Well-circumscribed mass with lipomatous and nonlipomatous inclusions surrounded by a pseudocapsule.
	May display a halo sign due to compression of surrounding tissue.
Ultrasonography:	Well-circumscribed lesion with parenchymal and cystic inclusions.

Incidental finding without therapeutic consequences if no signs of malignancy are present.

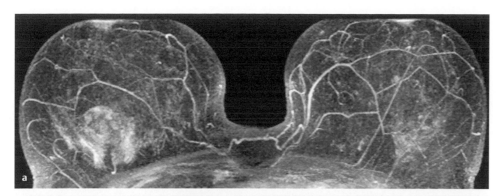

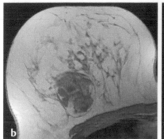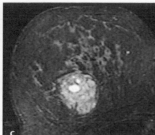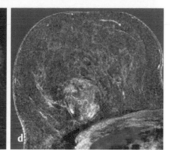

Fig. 8.44 a–d   Hamartoma with typical pseudocapsule.

a Subtraction MIP: lesion with inhomogeneous enhancement in the central aspect of the right breast.

b Corresponding T1w precontrast slice image (right breast): round, inhomogeneous lesion with internal areas of fat-equivalent and parenchyma-equivalent signal intensity. Lesion is separated from surrounding fat tissue by a thin pseudocapsule.

c Corresponding IR T2w slice image: inhomogeneous internal signal intensity with a few cystic inclusions.

d Early subtraction slice image: mild enhancement of nonadipose/noncystic internal tumor areas. Slight pseudocapsule enhancement.

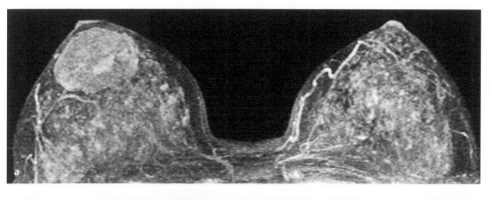

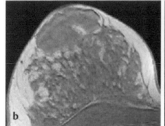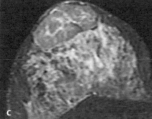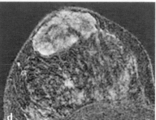

Fig. 8.45 a–d   Hamartoma with predominant glandular component.

a Subtraction MIP: large, oval, hypervascularized lesion in the retroareolar aspect of the right breast.

b Corresponding T1w precontrast slice image (right breast): lobulated, well-circumscribed, lesion with predominantly parenchyma-equivalent signal intensity, partially surrounded by thin fat lamella and pseudocapsule.

c Corresponding IR T2w slice image: inhomogeneous, intermediary internal signal intensity with streaks of high (water) signal intensity. Suppression of fat lamella signal.

d Early subtraction slice image: Diffuse enhancement of internal tumor areas with the exception of the fat lamella and fluid streaks.

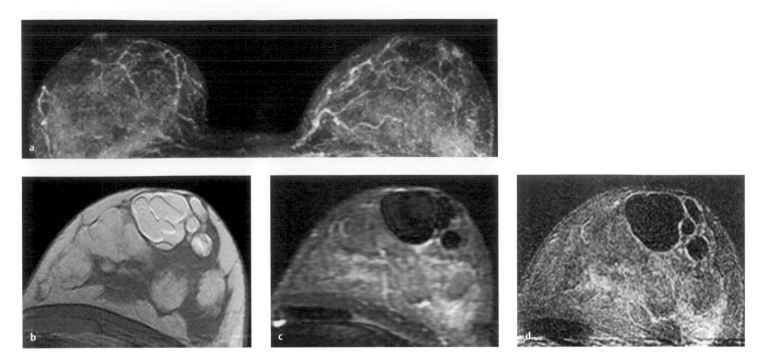

Fig. 8.46a–d   Hamartoma with predominant lipomatous component.

a Subtraction MIP: unremarkable findings.

b Corresponding T1w precontrast slice image (left breast): conglomerate of well-circumscribed, septated lesions in the retroareolar aspect of the left breast. The internal fat signal is of higher intensity than that of normal intramammary fat.

c Corresponding IR T2w slice image: greater suppression of internal fat signal than of normal intramammary fat signal.

d Early subtraction slice image: enhancement of thin capsular structures. No internal enhancement.

Stability of lesion characteristics was documented over many years.

Acute Nonpuerperal Mastitis

The term *acute mastitis* is used to describe an infection of the breast with interstitial and intraductal spreading. Mastitis occurring during the lactational period is designated *puerperal mastitis.* If it occurs outside this period, it is called *nonpuerperal mastitis.* Conditions that predispose to nonpuerperal mastitis are immunosuppressive therapy and diabetes.

> When antibiotic therapy fails to remedy signs and symptoms of a nonpuerperal mastitis, (percutaneous or open) biopsy must be performed to rule out malignancy.

 MR Mammography: Acute Nonpuerperal Mastitis

T1-Weighted Sequence (Precontrast)
Often no specific changes (**Figs. 8.47b, 8.48c**). Occasionally there may be dilated milk ducts with signal-intense contents (**Fig. 8.49c**) and/or thickening of the skin (**Fig. 8.49c**).

T2-Weighted Sequence
Increased signal intensity in area of inflammation (**Figs. 8.47c, 8.48d**). Occasionally there may be dilated milk ducts with signal-intense contents (**Fig. 8.49b**). A liquid center indicates abscess formation (**Fig. 8.50c**). Thickened skin appears hyperintense (**Fig. 8.49b**).

T1-Weighted Sequence (Contrast Enhanced)
Nonmasslike enhancement with linear, segmental, or diffuse distribution (**Figs. 8.47a, d, 8.48a**). Occasional *track phenomenon* due to enhancement of duct walls separated by nonenhancing duct contents (**Fig. 8.48e**). Uninformative TIC (**Fig. 8.47e**). Associated abscesses show strong wall-enhancement and signal-free contents (**Fig. 8.50d**). Thickened skin appears hyperintense (**Fig. 8.49a, d**).

Acute nonpuerperal mastitis: General information

Incidence:	Rare.
Age peak:	All ages.
Complications:	Abscess formation, fistula formation.

Findings	
Clinical:	Pain, erythema, hyperthermia (classical triad indicating inflammation), swelling, skin thickening, abscess formation, swollen lymph nodes, fever, elevated laboratory parameters indicating inflammation.
Exfoliative cytology:	Confirmation of pathogenic organisms in pus.
Mammography:	Diffuse reduction of transparency (indistinct structures) in comparison with the contralateral breast, skin thickening, lymphadenopathy.
Ultrasonography:	Edema with indistinct structures. Increased echogenicity of subcutaneous structures, skin thickening.

Clinical examination and breast imaging techniques do not allow a reliable differentiation between nonpuerperal mastitis and inflammatory breast cancer.

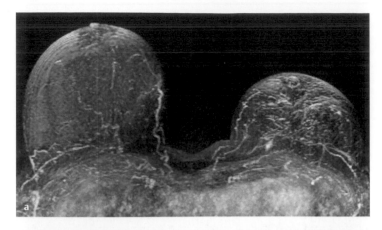

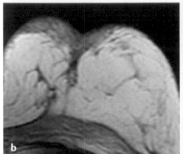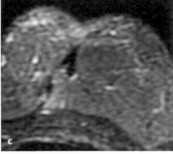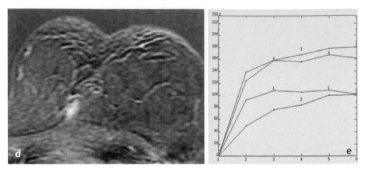

Fig. 8.47 a–e Focal mastitis after open biopsy.

a Subtraction MIP: new linear enhancement near the chest wall in the medial aspect of the left breast. Status 4 years after breast-conserving therapy, and 2 years after local recurrence in the left breast.

b T1w precontrast slice image (left breast): postoperative changes with skin retraction and fat necrosis. No specific inflammatory changes.

c IR T2w slice image: no specific inflammatory changes.

d Early subtraction slice image: spindle-shaped enhancement near the chest wall.

e TIC: rapid initial enhancement (up to 150%) and postinitial plateau.

Percutaneous vacuum-assisted biopsy revealed focal mastitis.

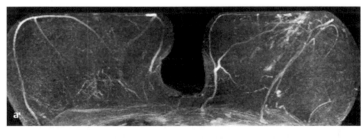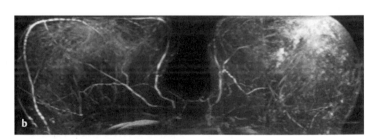

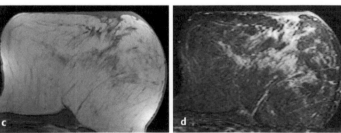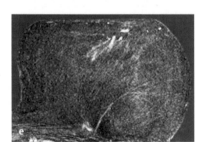

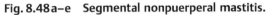

Fig. 8.48 a–e Segmental nonpuerperal mastitis.

a Subtraction MIP: reticular enhancement with segmental distribution reaching from the nipple to the chest wall in the left breast.

b T2w MIP: pronounced edematous changes in the retroareolar region.

c T1w precontrast slice image (left breast): only slightly ectatic milk ducts. Otherwise no specific inflammatory changes.

d IR T2w slice image: linear and dendritic pattern of increased signal intensity in the retroareolar region.

e Early subtraction slice image: dendritic enhancement pattern, conforming to the milk ducts' anatomical arrangement.

Percutaneous vacuum-assisted biopsy revealed nonpuerperal mastitis. Complete remission after antibiotic therapy.

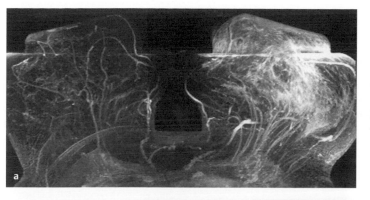
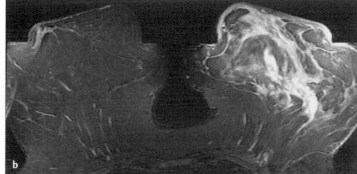
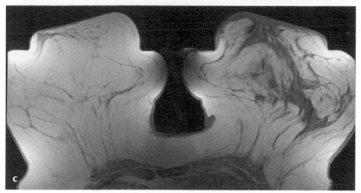
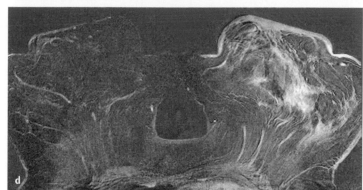

Fig. 8.49a–d Diffuse nonpuerperal mastitis.

a Subtraction MIP: macromastia. Diffuse enhancement of the entire left breast and thickened skin.

b IR T2w slice image: correspondingly increased signal intensity.

c T1w precontrast slice image: skin thickening and asymmetric nonadipose structures in the left breast.

d Early subtraction slice image: diffuse enhancement of all nonadipose structures, and complete skin circumference of the left breast.

Percutaneous vacuum-assisted biopsy revealed nonpuerperal mastitis.

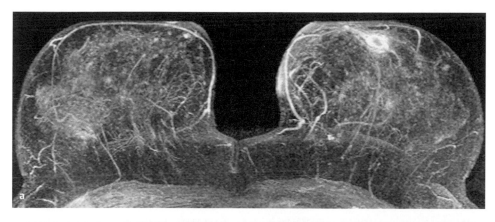
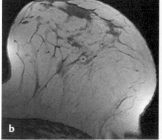
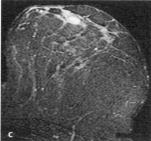
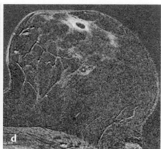

Fig. 8.50a–d Nonpuerperal mastitis with abscess formation.

a Subtraction MIP: "rim-enhancement" in the left retromamillary region. Diffuse, stippled enhancement of parenchyma in both breasts.

b T1w precontrast slice image (left breast): at most, discretely reduced signal intensity in the left retromamillary region.

c IR T2w slice image: high signal intensity corresponding to abscess.

d Early subtraction slice image: strong wall-enhancement with hypervascularization of surrounding parenchymal areas. TIC unspecific (not shown).

Complete remission after antibiotic therapy.

Abscess

A breast abscess is a localized, intramammary collection of pus in a cavity formed by an inflammatory disintegration of tissue. It is typically seen as a complication of (usually puerperal) mastitis or after breast surgery.

 MR Mammography: Abscess

T1-Weighted Sequence (Precontrast)
Hypointense lesion. Good demarcation when located within adipose tissue (**Fig. 8.51a**). When located within parenchyma, it presents as an isointense lesion with a center of lesser signal intensity (pus) (**Fig. 8.52b**).

T2-Weighted Sequence
Hyperintense signal in the abscess center correlating with pus accumulation (**Figs. 8.51b, 8.52b**).

T1-Weighted Sequence (Contrast Enhanced)
Strong contrast enhancement in thickened abscess wall (wall-enhancement) (**Figs. 8.51c, 8.52a, d**). Occasional hyperemia of surrounding parenchymal tissue (**Fig. 8.52d**).

Abscess: General information

Incidence:	Rare.
Risk of malignant transformation:	No increased risk.

Findings	
Clinical:	Local swelling, pain, erythema. Enlarged lymph nodes.
Mammography:	Round, oval, or irregular mass with homogeneous, increased density.
Ultrasonography:	Hypoechoic mass with internal echoes. May be ill-defined or have surrounding capsule.

Abscess formation is usually associated with mastitis, injury, or surgery.

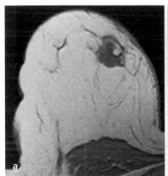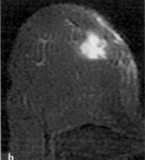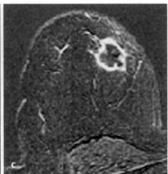

Fig. 8.51a–c Abscess.
a T1w precontrast slice image: hypointense, round lesion with signal-intense, protein-containing inclusion.
b IR T2w slice image: high signal intensity corresponding to an abscess.
c Early subtraction slice image: strong wall-enhancement. No internal enhancement.

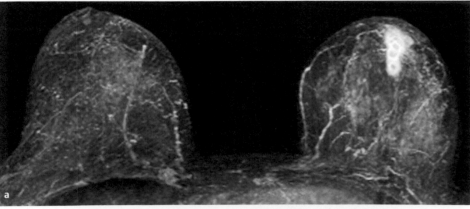

Fig. 8.52a–d Abscess.
a Subtraction MIP: "rim-enhancements" in the left retromamillary region, distributed along a milk duct.
b T1w precontrast slice image (left breast): hypointense milk duct lumen.
c IR T2w slice image: corresponding high signal intensity in the milk duct lumen.
d Early subtraction slice image: strong wall-enhancement of thickened, inflamed milk duct wall. No central enhancement. Mild periductal enhancement.

Confirmation of diagnosis by fine-needle aspiration biopsy.

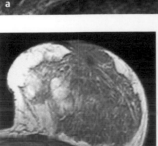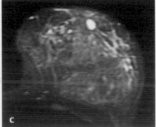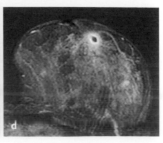

Chronic Nonpuerperal Mastitis

Chronic nonpuerperal mastitis is a chronic, aseptic, inflammatory process that occurs in and around the terminal ducts and lobuli of the breast. Three forms are differentiated according to histology and pathogenesis: **Galactophoritis** and **granulomatous lobular mastitis** (galactostatic and obliterative) are characterized by retention of secretory products, duct ectasia, and periductal mastitis. The pathogenesis of **lobular mastitis**, also a granulomatous and obliterative inflammation, is unclear. In the final stage one typically finds hyaline changes of the ducts with calcification deposits (**plasma cell mastitis**).

 MR Mammography: Chronic Nonpuerperal Mastitis

T1-Weighted Sequence (Precontrast)
Occasionally duct ectasia with signal-intense contents may be seen (**Fig. 8.53b**). Otherwise no specific changes (**Fig. 8.54c**).

T2-Weighted Sequence
Increased signal intensity in areas of inflammation (**Fig. 8.54b**). Occasionally duct ectasia with signal-intense contents may be seen (**Fig. 8.54d**). If intraductal fluids contain fat/proteins, contents will appear signal-free (**Fig. 8.53c**).

T1-Weighted Sequence (Contrast Enhanced)
Linear, segmental, or diffuse, nonmasslike contrast enhancement (**Fig. 8.54a, g**). Duct wall-enhancement (*track phenomenon*) (**Figs. 8.53d, 8.54e**). TICs are uninformative (**Fig. 8.54f**).

Chronic nonpuerperal mastitis: General information

Incidence:	5%–25% of all women (depending on the precise definition). In daily practice: ~5%. Often bilateral finding.
Age peak:	30–90 years (max. 40–49 years).
Complications (rare):	Fistula formation. Abscess formation.

Findings

Clinical:	Nipple discharge (rarely bloody). Breast pain (rare). Nipple retraction or fistula (rare).
Mammography:	No specific changes if breast parenchyma is dense. Dilated retromamillary ducts. Microcalcifications are rare in early stages of the disease. In later stages, typical spherical and tubular calcifications with lucent centers, and linear microcalcifications with orientation toward the nipple.
Galactography:	Subareolar duct ectasia. CM depicts cystic dilatation of ductal structures.
Ultrasonography:	Hypoechoic tubular structures in the retromamillary region (duct ectasia). Occasionally hypoechoic (granulomas) or anechoic (cystlike) lesions.

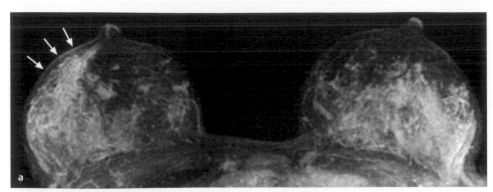

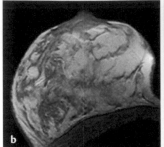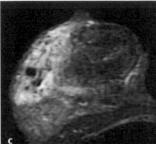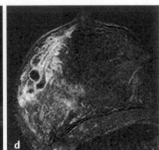

Fig. 8.53a–d Galactostatic mastitis.

a Subtraction MIP: strong early enhancement of parenchyma in both breasts. Segmental hypervascularization of milk duct structures in the lateral aspect of the right breast (arrows).

b T1w precontrast slice image (right breast): dilated milk duct with multiple round, cystic extensions in the lateral aspect of the right breast. Hyperintense contents due to protein/fat.

c IR T2w fat-suppressed slice image: suppressed signal intensity of fat-containing milk duct contents.

d Early subtraction slice image: parallel, linear enhancement of affected duct walls, separated by nonenhancing duct contents (track phenomenon).

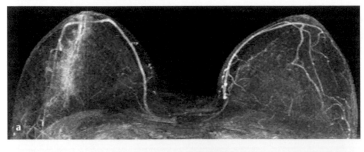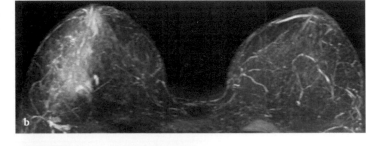

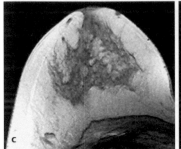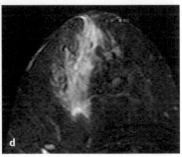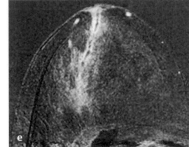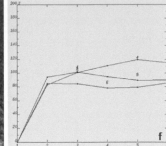

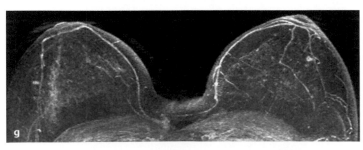

Fig. 8.54a–g Chronic recurring nonpuerperal mastitis.

a Subtraction MIP: segmental hypervascularization along ectatic milk duct in the right breast. No remarkable findings in the left breast.

b IR T2w MIP: high water content in segmental area with mastitis.

c T1w precontrast slice image (right breast): No corresponding findings.

d IR T2w slice image: depiction of fluids within ectatic duct and edema in surrounding tissues.

e Early subtraction slice image: parallel, linear enhancement of affected duct walls, separated by nonenhancing duct lumen (track phenomenon). Increased periductal vascularization.

f Uninformative TIC: moderate initial enhancement and postinitial plateau.

g Subtraction MIP after antibiotic therapy: significant improvement of inflammatory changes.

This patient opted for surgical excision of the affected milk duct in a symptom-free interval after several recurrences. Histology revealed fibrocystic breast condition with multiple small papillomas.

Mondor Disease

Mondor disease is a thrombophlebitis of the superficial breast and/or anterior chest wall veins. The pathogenesis is based on the stagnation of blood flow in the affected veins. No specific therapy is recommended, and symptoms usually subside spontaneously within weeks to months.

! Mondor disease is not usually associated with breast cancer. In spite of this, a diagnostic work-up of the affected breast must be performed to exclude breast cancer.

 MR Mammography: Mondor Disease

T1-Weighted Sequence (Precontrast)
Usually no characteristic changes (**Fig. 8.56 c**). Occasionally a prominent vein may be seen along the lateral periphery of the breast (**Fig. 8.55 c**).

T2-Weighted Sequence
Possible depiction of a vein ectasia along the lateral periphery of the breast. Increased signal intensity if acute thrombophlebitis is present (**Fig. 8.55 d**). No increased signal intensity if thrombosis is present (**Fig. 8.56 d**). Increasing signal intensity with increasing recanalization.

T1-Weighted Sequence (Contrast Enhanced)
Usually no contrast enhancement within the vessel if thrombophlebitis is acute (**Fig. 8.55 e**). No contrast enhancement if thrombosis occurs. Increasing enhancement with increasing recanalization/perfusion of affected vein (**Fig. 8.56 e**). TICs are uninformative.

Mondor disease: General information

Incidence:	Very rare.
	Unilateral finding in the lateral (!) breast quadrant.
Predisposition:	Recent breast surgery. Trauma. Long flight.
Age peak:	All ages.
Risk of malignant transformation:	No increased risk.
Complications:	None.

Findings

Clinical:	Linear skin retraction in an outer quadrant of the breast. May extend from the upper outer quadrant, over the lower outer quadrant, and run medially over the caudal breast half. Often palpable, tubular hardening along skin retraction.
Mammography:	No specific findings. Occasionally visible skin fold or thrombosed vein in the lateral aspect of one breast.
Ultrasonography:	Hypoechoic, tubular structure in the lateral aspect of one breast as correlation to thrombosed vein. No flow phenomenon on color Doppler.

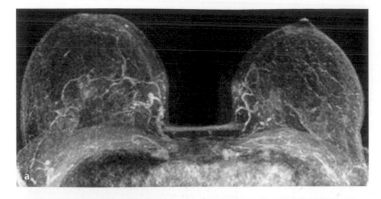
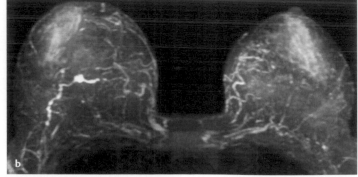

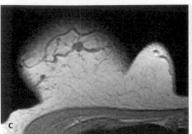
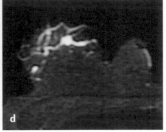

Fig. 8.55a–e   Mondor disease (acute phase).
a Subtraction MIP: unremarkable findings.
b IR T2w MIP: large caliber, varicose vein with high signal intensity in the central aspect of the right breast.
c T1w precontrast slice image (right breast): normal depiction of varicose vein in the caudal aspect of the right breast.
d IR T2w slice image: high signal intensity of vein contents.

e Early subtraction slice image: no enhancement of varicose vein as indication of thrombosis in this vein segment. Normal enhancement of another vein seen in the same slice image.

Patient with classical clinical symptoms of Mondor disease. Complete regression within 4 weeks.

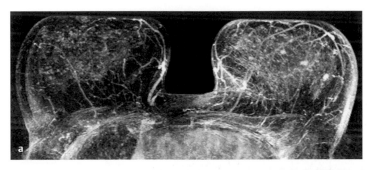
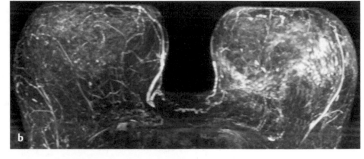

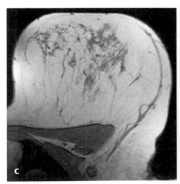
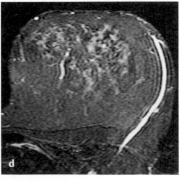
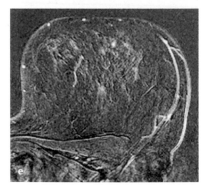

Fig. 8.56a–e   Mondor disease (in regression).
a Subtraction MIP: mild, harmless enhancement asymmetry. Strong enhancement of a subcutaneous vein in the lateral aspect of the left breast. Physiological enhancement of vein convolutes in the medial aspects of both breasts.
b IR T2w MIP: normal depiction of breast veins with high signal intensity.
c T1w precontrast slice image (left breast): normal depiction of a large-caliber vein in the lateral aspect of the left breast.
d IR T2w slice image: high signal intensity of the lumen of the vein. No other visible veins.

e Early subtraction slice image: linear enhancement of the vein described above. In addition, inhomogeneous enhancement of a subcutaneous vein that branches from the first described vein and is the imaging representation of a partially recanalized vein after thrombophlebitis.

The patient 2 weeks after presenting with classical clinical symptoms of a superficial thrombophlebitis. Partial regression.

Cutaneous Changes in Breast MRI

Cutaneous changes that can be visualized on breast MRI include angiomas (**Figs. 8.57, 8.58**) and skin nevi (**Fig. 8.59**).

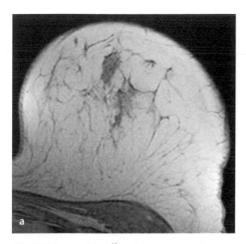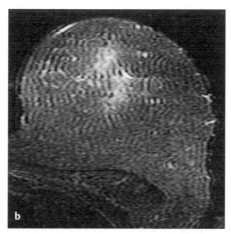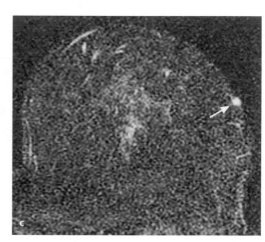

Fig. 8.57a–c Small cutaneous angioma.
a T1w precontrast slice image (left breast): unremarkable findings.
b IR T2w slice image: unremarkable findings.

c Early subtraction slice image: depiction of round, hypervascularized lesion 3 mm in diameter within the skin on the lateral side of the left breast (arrow).

The patient has a typical angioma in the skin at this location.

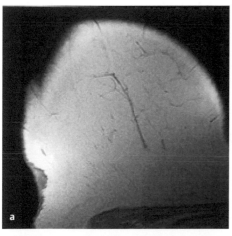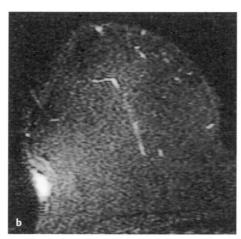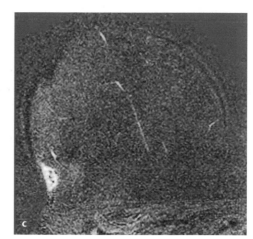

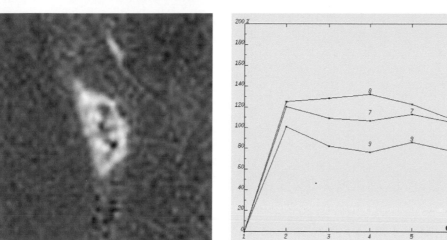

Fig. 8.58a–e Large cutaneous angioma.
a T1w precontrast slice image (right breast): localized, inward thickening of the skin on the lateral side of the right breast.
b IR T2w slice image: lesion displays a high water content.
c Early subtraction slice image: the lesion displays peripheral contrast enhancement without enhancement of central tumor portions.
d Zoomed image of lesion from the early subtraction slice image.
e TIC: rapid initial enhancement and post-initial washout.

The patient has a typical angioma in the skin at this location.

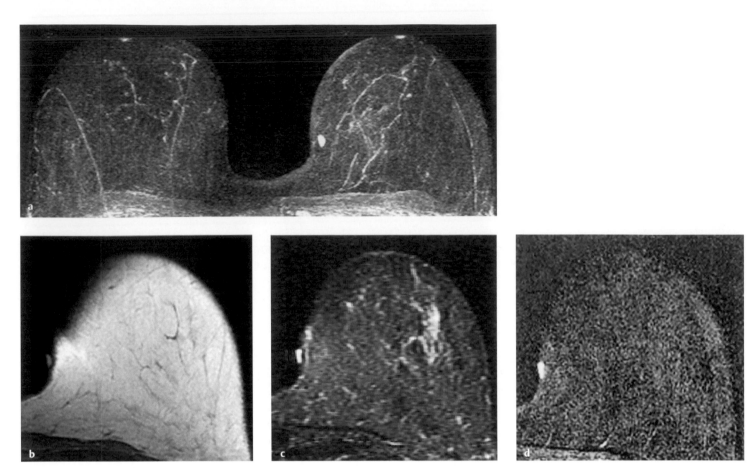

Fig. 8.59a–d   Skin nevus.

a Subtraction MIP: hypervascularized mass lesion projected into the medial aspect of the left breast.

b. T1w precontrast slice image (left breast): hyperintense lesion can be localized in the skin.

c IR T2w slice image: lesion displays a high water content.

d Early subtraction slice image: oval, homogeneously hypervascularized lesion in the skin on the medial side of the left breast.

The patient has a typical benign nevus in the skin at this location.

9 Postoperative/Posttraumatic Changes

Fat Necrosis

Synonyms: liponecrosis microcystica calcificata.

Fat necrosis is a localized area of dead adipose tissue characterized by morphological changes resulting from progressive enzymatic degradation. Leukocytic and histiocytic infiltrates are encountered in new areas of fat necrosis. Gradually, well-vascularized granulation tissue develops. The transformation into scar tissue is usually complete in a matter of weeks. The coalescence of liquefied adipose tissue can lead to formation of so-called *oil cysts*.

! A fresh fat necrosis can be very difficult to differentiate from breast cancer, i.e., breast cancer recurrence in breast MRI, as well as in mammography and breast ultrasound.

 MR Mammography: Fat Necrosis

T1-Weighted Sequence (Precontrast)
Signal intensity equivalent to that of parenchyma (**Fig. 9.1b**). *Oil cysts* present as rounded lesions with a hyperintense (fat-equivalent) signal (**Figs. 9.2b, 9.3b**). Possible signal loss due to macrocalcifications (**Figs. 9.4b, 9.5a**).

T2-Weighted Sequence
A fresh fat necrosis presents as an ill-defined, hyperintense area (**Fig. 9.1c**). Later, when oil cysts are present, round lesions with central, fat-equivalent signal intensity are seen (signal-free in IR T2w sequence due to fat suppression) (**Figs. 9.3c, 9.4c**). Otherwise no characteristic changes after 6 months.

T1-Weighted Sequence (Contrast Enhanced)
In the early phase when capillary sprouting takes place (first 6 months after trauma/surgery), fat necrosis presents as a localized, sometimes well-defined (**Fig. 9.1a, d**), but usually ill-defined (**Fig. 9.2a, d**) area with increased CM uptake (**Fig. 9.1a, d**). Initial signal enhancement is usually moderate (**Fig. 9.1e**). The postinitial signal increase is typically persistent or displays a plateau. In the late phase (>6 months) there is usually no more contrast enhancement (**Figs. 9.3a, d, 9.5b**). Mild enhancement may be seen when there is an additional inflammatory component (**Fig. 9.4d**).

Fat necrosis: General information

Etiology:	Posttraumatic (e.g., injury, surgery, needle biopsy), inflammation, foreign body reaction (e.g., silicone, paraffin).
Risk of malignant transformation:	No increased risk.

Findings

Clinical:	Usually occult. Large findings may present as a mass or thickening.
Mammography:	Round, oval, or irregular mass lesion. Homogeneous and hyperdense. No specific findings.
	New fat necrosis: ill-defined area of increased density.
	Older fat necrosis: improving demarcation of density.
	Oil cysts: rounded, centrally radiolucent lesions possibly containing bizarre or rim calcifications.
Ultrasonography:	Great variability: from round, well-defined lesions to irregularly shaped lesions showing echo texture typical of malignancy.

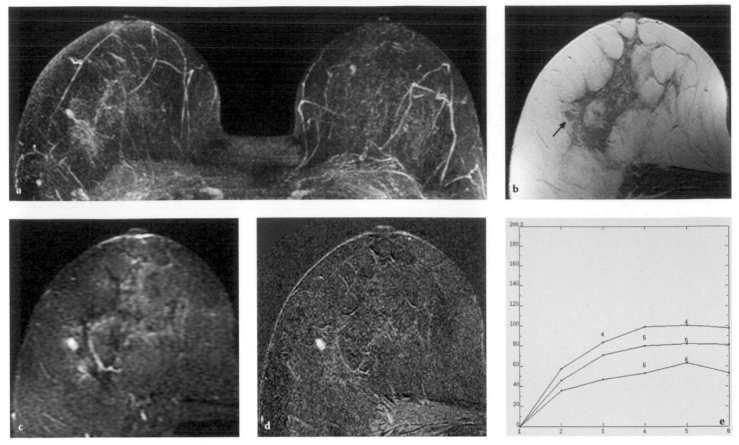

Fig. 9.1 a–e Fresh fat necrosis.

a Subtraction MIP: oval, hypervascularized focus in the lateral aspect of the right breast.

b T1w precontrast slice image: corresponding oval focus (4 mm, arrow) within the lipomatous breast tissue lateral to the parenchymal body.

c IR T2w slice image: lesion displays a high signal intensity, i.e., water content.

d Early subtraction slice image: strong contrast enhancement.

e Unspecific TIC.

Percutaneous biopsy-proven diagnosis.

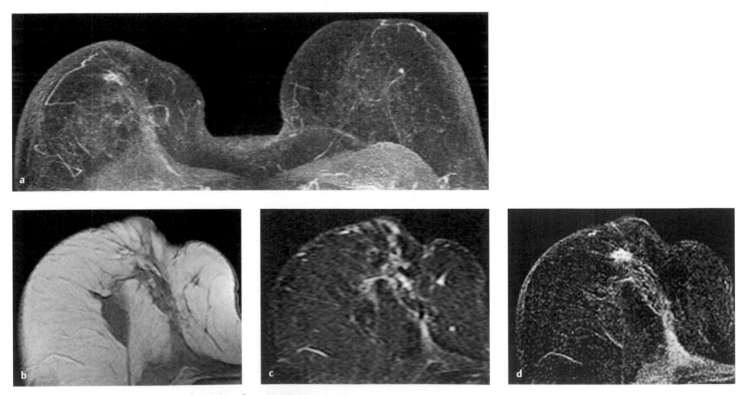

Fig. 9.2 a–d Fat necrosis: several weeks after surgery.

a Subtraction MIP: irregular, hypervascularized lesion in the scar tissue area of the right breast, 8 weeks after breast-conserving therapy.

b T1w precontrast slice image: morphologic distortion in the right breast due to scar tissue. Slight signal increase in fat necrosis.

c IR T2w slice image (fat saturated): mild reactive edematous changes in scar tissue area.

d Early subtraction slice image: rim-enhancement around discrete central liquid inclusions.

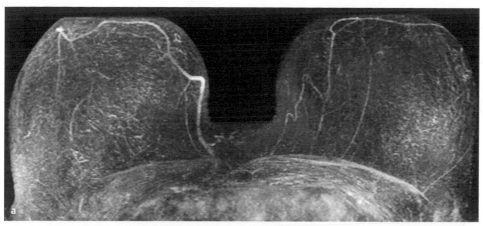

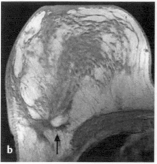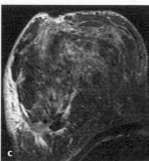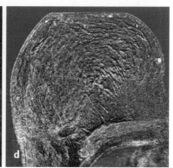

Fig. 9.3a–d   Old fat necrosis.
a Subtraction MIP: unremarkable findings 2 years after breast-conserving therapy.
b T1w precontrast slice image: localized area of scar tissue with oval, fat-containing area (arrow). Skin thickening.
c IR T2w slice image (fat saturated): reactive edematous changes of cutaneous and subcutaneous areas after radiation therapy. Complete signal suppression of oval fat necrosis.
d Early subtraction slice image: fat necrosis displays no contrast enhancement.

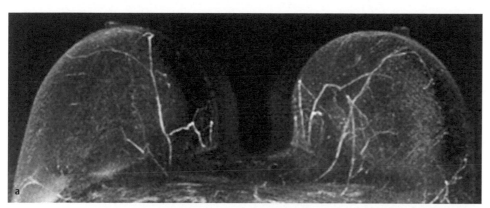

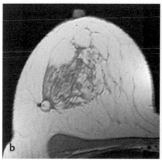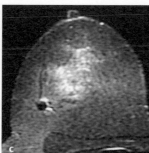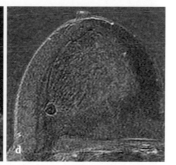

Fig. 9.4a–d   Oil cyst.
a Subtraction MIP: unremarkable findings several years after diagnostic excision.
b T1w precontrast slice image: round lesion with fat-equivalent internal signal and peripheral punctate signal extinction due to calcification.
c IR T2w slice image (fat saturated): mildly elevated signal intensity (water content) of parenchyma. Signal suppression of the lesion's internal liquefied fat.
d Early subtraction slice image: very discrete rim-enhancement.

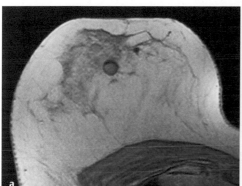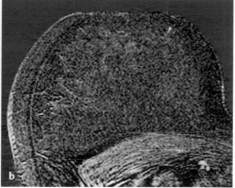

Fig. 9.5a, b   Oil cyst.
a T1w precontrast slice image: round oil cyst with slightly elevated internal signal and peripheral signal extinction due to calcification.
b Early subtraction slice image: fat necrosis displays no contrast enhancement.

Seroma

A seroma is a localized collection of wound serum in the tissues, for example after surgery.

 MR Mammography: Seroma

T1-Weighted Sequence (Precontrast)
More or less circumscribed area usually demonstrating a slightly hypointense signal in comparison with surrounding parenchyma

(**Fig. 9.7a**). Occasionally cushionlike or villuslike internal structures along or stemming from internal seroma wall (**Fig. 9.6a**).

T2-Weighted Sequence
Hyperintense fluid within seroma (**Figs. 9.6b, 9.7b**).

T1-Weighted Sequence (Contrast Enhanced)
Immediately after surgery CM uptake is usually slight, after several days it is stronger in areas immediately surrounding the seroma (**Figs. 9.6c, 9.7c**).

Seroma: General information

Age peak:	No age dependence. Postoperative.
Risk of malignant transformation:	No increased risk.

Findings

Clinical:	Small seromas are clinically occult. Large findings may present as an elastic mass.
Mammography:	Seromas within dense parenchymal areas are often mammographically occult. Within lipomatous areas: round, hyperdense mass.
Ultrasonography:	Well-circumscribed, liquid-filled mass (similar to a cyst). Occasionally villuslike, noncystic internal structures on the seroma wall.

Seroma is a frequent postoperative finding without major clinical significance. Large seromas may be an indication for fine-needle aspiration.

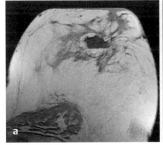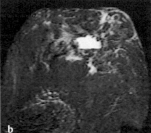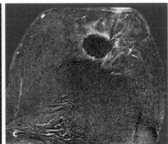

Fig. 9.6a–c Postoperative seroma.
a T1w precontrast slice image: round lesion with surrounding capsule and polypous structures adhering to the internal wall.
b IR T2w slice image: high signal intensity (water content) within the seroma.
c Early subtraction slice image: discrete enhancement of seroma wall. Polypous structures display no perfusion.

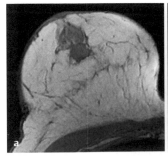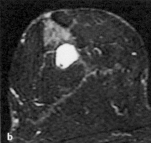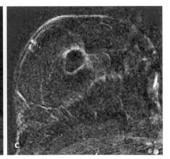

Fig. 9.7a–c Postoperative seroma.
a T1w precontrast slice image: lobulated, hypointense lesion with surrounding capsule.
b IR T2w slice image: high signal intensity (water content) within the seroma.
c Early subtraction slice image: discrete enhancement of seroma wall.

Hematoma

A breast hematoma is an intramammary hemorrhage, for example, due to intervention or surgery.

 MR Mammography: Hematoma

T1-Weighted Sequence (Precontrast)
A hematoma shows a typical signal intensity, as in other regions of the body, depending on the time elapsed since its development. A fresh hemorrhage demonstrates a homogeneous high signal intensity (**Fig. 9.8**). A subacute hematoma shows a low internal signal with a hyperintense peripheral ring (**Fig. 9.9**). An old hematoma may be hyperintense (**Fig. 9.10a**).

T2-Weighted Sequence
A fresh hematoma displays a homogeneous low signal intensity. With increasing age, a hypointense peripheral ring develops (**Fig. 9.10b**).

T1-Weighted Sequence (Contrast Enhanced)
Diffuse reactive CM uptake occurs in the parenchyma surrounding a subacute hematoma. With increasing age, the reactive changes decrease and usually disappear completely (**Fig. 9.10c**).

Hematoma: General information

Incidence:	Often after intervention. Occasionally after surgery. Rare after other trauma.
Risk of malignant transformation:	No increased risk.

Findings

Clinical:	Small hematomas are clinically occult.
	Large findings may present as a palpable mass.
	Later visible skin pigmentation.
Mammography:	Hematomas within dense parenchymal areas are often mammographically occult.
	Within lipomatous areas: round, hyperdense mass.
Ultrasonography:	Well-circumscribed, hypoechoic structure.

Incidental finding without major clinical significance. Large hematomas may be an indication for fine-needle aspiration.

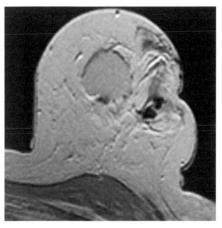

Fig. 9.8 Acute hematoma. Hyperintense, fat-equivalent lesion in the T1w precontrast image immediately after percutaneous vacuum-assisted biopsy.

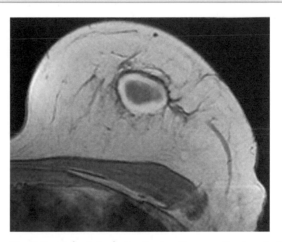

Fig. 9.9 Subacute hematoma. Same patient as in **Fig. 9.8**, several days later. Hyperintense rim in the peripheral areas of the hematoma due to hemosiderin precipitation and lower signal intensity in the center of the hematoma (T1w precontrast image).

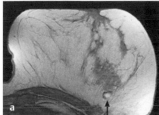 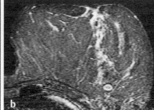 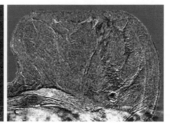

Fig. 9.10a–c Old hematoma. Breast MRI 6 months after percutaneous vacuum-assisted biopsy.
a T1w precontrast slice image: small hematoma with high central signal intensity and hypointense rim.
b IR T2w slice image: opposite signal intensities (low central signal intensity and hyperintense rim).
c Early subtraction slice image: no enhancement.

Scar Tissue

In the course of wound healing, scar tissue develops from granulation tissue ~3 to 6 months after tissue injury (e.g., vacuum-assisted biopsy, surgery, trauma). Scar tissue is then mostly composed of collagen with a smaller amount of cells and blood vessels.

 The absence of contrast enhancement in an area of scar tissue rules out a recurrence/breast cancer with high reliability. Not every contrast enhancement in an area of scar tissue, however, is proof of a recurrence or breast cancer.

📚 MR Mammography: Scar Tissue

T1-Weighted Sequence (Precontrast)
Hypointense, usually ill-defined or stellate finding (**Figs. 9.11a, 9.12a, 9.13a**). More difficult to detect when located within parenchyma (**Figs. 9.14b, 9.15b**). If located within lipomatous tissue, identification as high contrast stellate lesion. Often associated with susceptibility artifacts due to cauterization during surgery (**Figs. 9.11a, 9.13a**).

T2-Weighted Sequence
Variable, unspecific findings with a low (**Fig. 9.12b**) or increased water content (**Figs. 9.14c, 9.15c**) in the scar tissue area.

T1-Weighted Sequence (Contrast Enhanced)
Ideally there is no contrast enhancement in a scar tissue area (**Figs. 9.11b, 9.12c**). Occasionally enhancement in a scar tissue area can last over 6 months (**Fig. 9.16b–e**), for example as focal or diffuse enhancement in the case of prolonged wound healing, or as a regional enhancement in the case of localized granulomatous-inflammatory changes (**Figs. 9.13b, 9.14a, d, 9.15a, d**). In these cases the differential diagnosis between scar tissue and a recurrence or cancer of other etiology is difficult. The time–signal intensity curves (TICs) are uninformative (**Fig. 9.15e**).

Scar tissue: General information

Incidence:	After surgery.
Risk of malignant transformation:	No increased risk.

Findings	
Clinical:	Small scars and those deep within the parenchyma are clinically occult.
	Large scars and/or those near the skin may present as a palpable hardening.
	Possible skin retraction.
Mammography:	Architectural distortion or irregular/spiculated mass.
	May initially be associated with microcalcifications. Later macrocalcifications represent regressive changes.
Ultrasonography:	Irregular or spiculated, hypoechoic structure, often displaying dorsal acoustic shadowing. No flow phenomena in the CCDS.

A postoperative scar is difficult to differentiate from malignancy using morphologic criteria (mammography, ultrasonography).

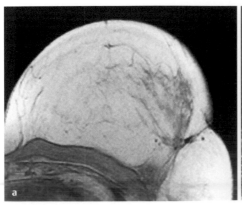 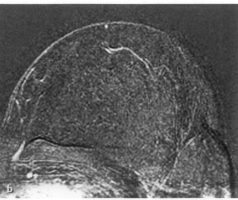

Fig. 9.11a, b   Typical findings of a postoperative scar.
a T1w precontrast slice image (left breast): architectural distortion and susceptibility artifacts.
b Early subtraction slice image (left breast): no enhancement in entire scar area.

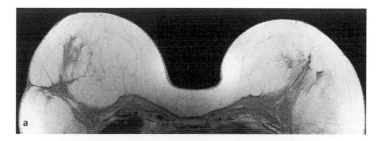

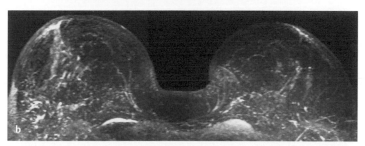

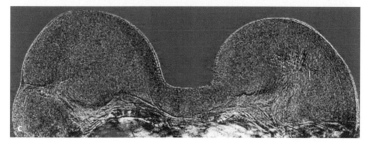

Fig. 9.12a–c Typical findings: bilateral postoperative scars.
a T1w precontrast slice image: bilateral scar structures after bilateral breast-conserving therapy.
b IR T2w slice image: discrete edematous changes in both breasts after radiotherapy.
c Early subtraction slice image: no enhancement in both scar areas.

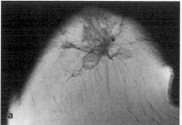

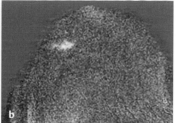

Fig. 9.13a, b Postoperative scar with mild inflammatory component.
a T1w precontrast slice image: architectural distortion and susceptibility artifacts after breast-conserving therapy.
b Early subtraction slice image: localized enhancement in the lateral aspect of the surgical scar area.

Histology after vacuum-assisted biopsy: scar tissue with mild granulomatous inflammation.

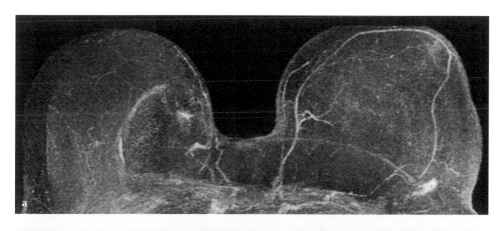

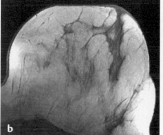

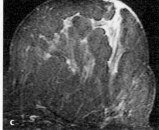

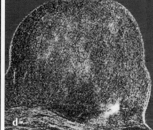

Fig. 9.14a–d Postoperative scar with significant inflammatory component. Breast-conserving therapy of the left breast 4 years before examination.
a Subtraction MIP: localized enhancement in the scar area in the lateral aspect of the left breast.
b T1w precontrast slice image (left breast): typical structural changes associated with a scar area.
c IR T2w slice image (left breast): very discrete increased water content in the scar area.
d Early subtraction slice image (left breast): regional enhancement in the center of the scar area.

Histology after vacuum-assisted biopsy: granulomatous mastitis in scar tissue area.

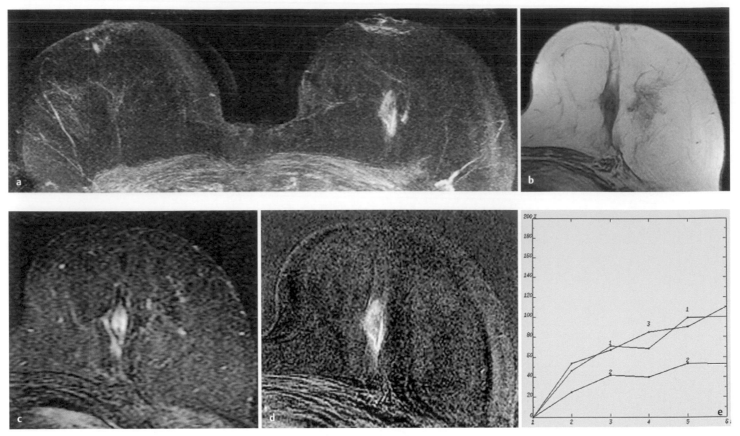

Fig. 9.15a–e **Postoperative scar with significant inflammatory component.** Breast-conserving therapy of the left breast 3 years before examination.

a Subtraction MIP: oblong enhancement area in the scar area of the left breast.

b T1w precontrast slice image (left breast): oblong scar area.

c IR T2w slice image (left breast): increased water content in scar area.

d Early subtraction slice image (left breast): strong enhancement of the entire scar area.

e TIC: moderate initial enhancement and persistent postinitial enhancement.

Histology after vacuum-assisted biopsy: granulomatous inflammation within scar tissue.

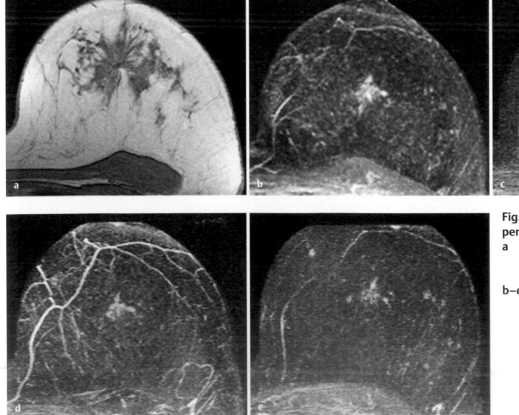

Fig. 9.16a–e **Postoperative scar with persistent inflammatory component.**

a T1w precontrast slice image (left breast): architectural distortion after diagnostic excision.

b–e T1w precontrast slice images (left breast): increased vascularization of scar area. Examination images at yearly intervals.

Changes following Breast-Conserving Therapy plus Radiotherapy/Mastectomy

Breast-conserving surgery (BCS) for invasive breast cancer is generally followed by radiation therapy. In the course of years following BCS with radiotherapy, increased vascularization and reactive/edematous changes show variable, sometimes complete remission (**Figs. 9.17, 9.18, 9.19**).

Remaining areas of parenchyma must be reckoned with even after mastectomy. Often small islands of breast tissue can be detected despite the assumed complete excision of all breast parenchyma (**Fig. 9.21**). In rare cases these can be difficult to differentiate from a chest wall recurrence (**Fig. 9.22**).

 MR Mammography: BCS plus Radiotherapy/Mastectomy

T1-Weighted Sequence (Precontrast)
Skin thickening asymmetric, occasionally lasting several years.

T2-Weighted Sequence
Asymmetry with pronounced increase of signal intensity in the parenchyma of the irradiated breast, usually lasting several years (**Figs. 9.17b, 9.18b,** and **9.20b**). Occasionally the signal intensity of irradiated breast may revert to its original state or to a decreased signal intensity in comparison with the contralateral breast (**Fig. 9.19b**).

T1-Weighted Sequence (Contrast Enhanced)
Regional or diffuse enhancement of irradiated parenchyma and thickened skin (**Fig. 9.20a**). Great interindividual variability with changes slowly decreasing over a period of years (**Figs. 9.17a, 9.18a**). Occasional "reversal effect" due to reduced proliferation of healthy, irradiated breast tissue with ensuing diminishment of its vascularization several years after radiation therapy (**Fig. 9.19a**).

Breast-conserving therapy plus radiotherapy: General information	
Clinical:	Acute reaction: hyperthermia, edema, and a feeling of increased pressure. This phase usually lasts several weeks, occasionally months (great variability).
	Possible late changes: hyperpigmentation of the skin, increased breast firmness, deformation of breast shape.
Mammography:	Edema and trabecular and skin thickening are common changes.
Ultrasonography:	Asymmetric edema and skin thickening are common changes.

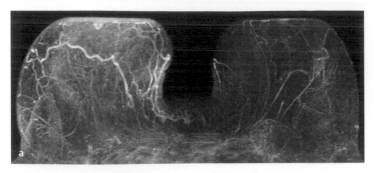

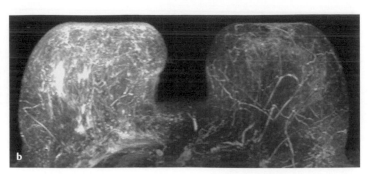

Fig. 9.17a, b   Early findings after radiation therapy.

a Subtraction MIP: breast MRI 6 months after completion of radiation therapy of the right breast. Increased, early vascularization of the right breast.

b IR T2w MIP: interstitial edema of the irradiated right breast.

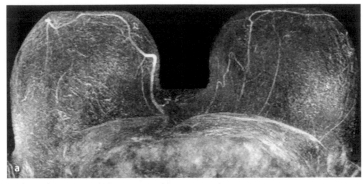

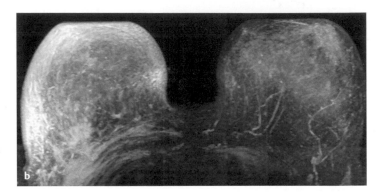

Fig. 9.18a, b   Findings 10 months after radiation therapy.

a Subtraction MIP: breast MRI 10 months after completion of radiation therapy of the right breast. Discretely increased vascularization of the right breast.

b IR T2w MIP: interstitial edema of the irradiated right breast is still pronounced.

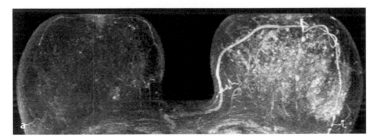

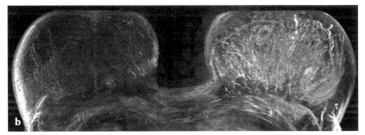

Fig. 9.19a, b   Older findings after radiation therapy.

a Subtraction MIP: breast MRI 24 months after completion of radiation therapy of the right breast. Reduced vascularization of the right breast.

b IR T2w MIP: reduced signal intensity (water content) and no visible cysts in the irradiated right breast in comparison with the healthy left breast.

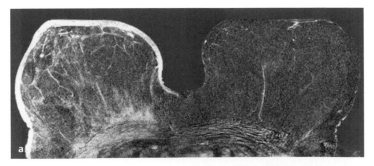

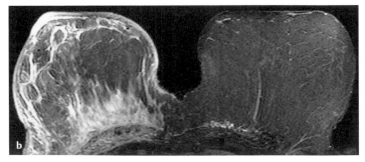

Fig. 9.20a, b   Radiogenic, abacterial mastitis after radiation therapy.

a Subtraction MIP: breast MRI 14 months after completion of radiation therapy of the right breast. Pronounced skin thickening and increased vascularization of the right breast.

b IR T2w MIP: increased signal intensity (water content) of thickened skin and parenchyma in the irradiated right breast in comparison with the healthy left breast.

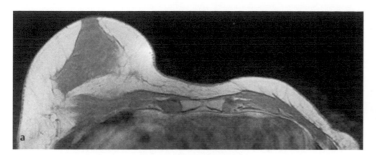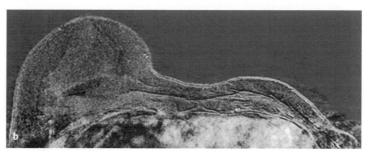

Fig. 9.21a, b   Chest wall after mastectomy.

a T1w precontrast slice image: no conspicuous findings after mastectomy of the left breast.

b Early subtraction slice image: no conspicuous findings after contrast administration.

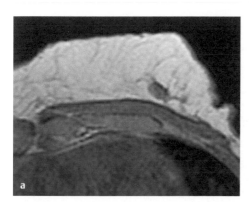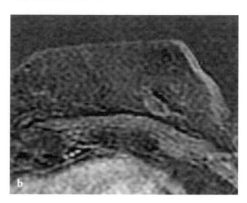

Fig. 9.22a, b   Residual parenchyma after mastectomy.

a T1w precontrast slice image (left chest wall): residual parenchyma near the chest wall after mastectomy of the left breast.

b Early subtraction slice image (left chest wall): residual parenchyma near the chest wall after contrast administration.

R1 Resection

After surgical removal of a breast cancer, the meticulous pathological examination of the resected breast tissue is crucial in determining whether the tumor has been excised completely or not, and what margins between the tumor and the border of excision have been achieved.

Due to the interfering changes caused by surgery, breast imaging is significantly compromised postoperatively. This is also true for breast MRI since reactive, hyperemic changes due to the healing process limit its informative value. According to experience, it will therefore only be possible to attain evidence indicating the localization of residual carcinoma in a few, individual cases (**Fig. 9.23**).

> ! It is strongly advisable to avoid an R1 resection situation, making the identification and localization of residual carcinoma tissue necessary. It is therefore prudent to routinely perform preoperative breast MRI to facilitate planning of the appropriate course of action for excising the target volume.

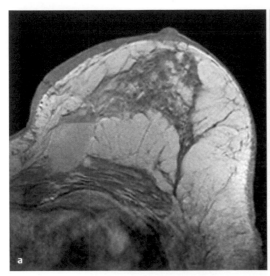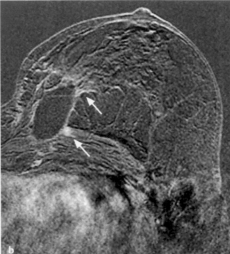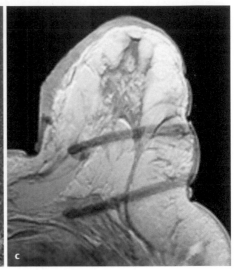

Fig. 9.23a–c R1 resection after breast-conserving therapy. Breast MRI 2 weeks after breast-conserving therapy. Histology indicated macroscopic residual carcinoma.

a T1w precontrast slice image (left breast): skin thickening and large seroma in the medial aspect of the left breast.

b Early subtraction slice image (left breast): nodular area of contrast enhancement at the lateral and ventral (less conspicuous) edges of the seroma (arrows).

c T1w postcontrast slice image (left breast): documentation of localization wires after MRI-guided localization of both lesions.

Histology: residual carcinoma tissue at both locations.

Recurrence after Breast-Conserving Therapy/Mastectomy/Breast Reconstruction

The local breast cancer recurrence rate after breast-conserving therapy and radiotherapy is estimated to be ~1% per year for the first 3–5 years. The recurrence rate after mastectomy, with and without breast reconstruction, depends on the patient's initial tumor stage.

Breast MRI can detect **skin metastases** but its utility is very limited in the detection of small metastases (**Fig. 9.24**). In any case, conspicuous findings in the skin must be correlated with clinical findings and targeted high-resolution ultrasound findings (**Fig. 9.25**).

In contrast, breast MRI is much more sensitive in the detection of **recurrences within the breast**. Generally, any enhancement in

the scar area occurring at least 1 year after breast-conserving therapy is suspicious for breast cancer recurrence (**Fig. 9.27**). Within 1 year after breast-conserving therapy, scar enhancement may be due to reactive hyperemia, limiting the informative value of the examination (**Fig. 9.26**).

Recurrences after **mastectomy, with and without breast reconstruction**, are reliably detected in the T1 w precontrast images, in which they are easily seen within the subcutaneous lipomatous tissue (**Figs. 9.28a, 9.29a**). After contrast administration they usually display typical enhancement pattern (**Figs. 9.28b, 9.29b**).

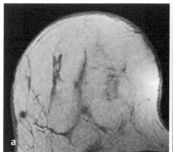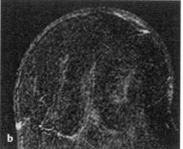

Fig. 9.24a, b Cutaneous metastasis after breast-conserving therapy. Breast MRI 3 years after breast-conserving therapy of the right breast.
a T1w precontrast slice image (right breast): circular skin thickening after radiotherapy. No other conspicuous findings.
b Early subtraction slice image (right breast): retrospective reevaluation after later appearance of skin nodule. Skin recurrence in the lateral aspect of the right breast.

Histology: skin metastasis.

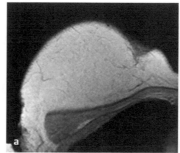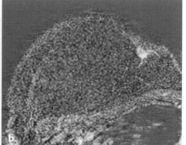

Fig. 9.25a, b Cutaneous metastasis after breast-conserving therapy. Breast MRI 3 years after breast-conserving therapy of the right breast.
a T1w precontrast slice image (right breast): skin thickening and retraction in the medial aspect of the right breast after surgery.
b Early subtraction slice image (right breast): localized hypervascularized nodule in the thickened skin of the scar.

Histology: skin metastasis.

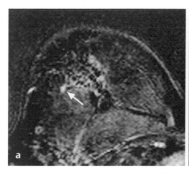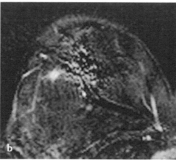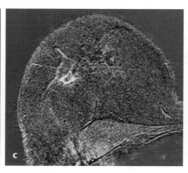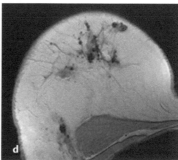

Fig. 9.26a–d Progression of breast cancer recurrence in the breast after breast-conserving therapy. Breast MRI as part of tumor follow-up examination 2 years after breast-conserving therapy. The patient had not undergone recommended adjuvant radiotherapy.
a Early subtraction slice image (left breast, external examination): diffuse enhancement in the scar area. Discrete focal enhancing area (arrow). Valid categorization as MRI BI-RADS 3.
b Follow-up early subtraction slice image 6 months after a (left breast, external examination): focus size increase to a mass lesion with slight rim-enhancement. Incorrect categorization as MRI BI-RADS 3.
c Follow-up early subtraction slice image another 6 months later in high-resolution technique (12 months after a, left breast): size increase of mass lesion with rim-enhancement. Categorization as MRI BI-RADS 5.
d Corresponding T1w slice image (left breast): the entire scar area is displayed.

Histology after second breast-conserving therapy: breast cancer recurrence.

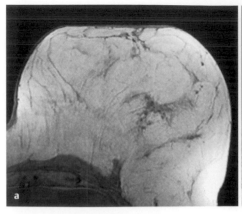
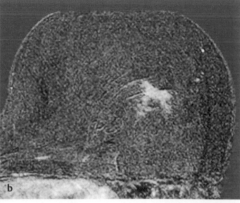

Fig. 9.27a, b   Local breast cancer recurrence after breast-conserving therapy (segmentectomy). Breast MRI as part of tumor follow-up examination 2 years after breast-conserving therapy of the left breast.
a T1w precontrast slice image (left breast): slight architectural changes due to surgery.
b Early subtraction slice image (left breast): regional enhancement in the scar area (nonmasslike lesion).

Histology: breast cancer recurrence.

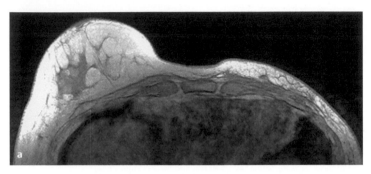
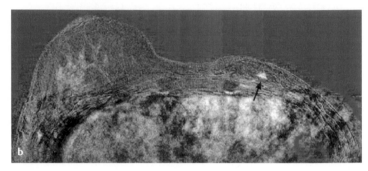

Fig. 9.28a, b   Breast cancer recurrence in the chest wall after mastectomy.
a T1w precontrast slice image: new mass lesion in the ventral aspect of the chest wall after mastectomy of the left breast.
b Early subtraction slice image: mass displays increased enhancement (arrow).

Histology: breast cancer recurrence.

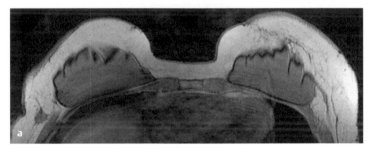
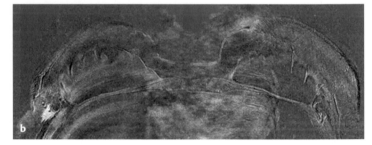

Fig. 9.29a, b   Periprosthetic breast cancer recurrence on the right side. Breast MRI after bilateral mastectomy and implantation of breast prostheses.
a T1w precontrast slice image: conspicuous, nonlipomatous mass far laterally of the right prosthesis.
b Early subtraction slice image with the phase-encoding gradient swapped to the ventrodorsal direction: strong enhancement of this very suspicious lesion.

Histology: breast cancer recurrence.

10 Borderline Lesions

Papilloma

Papillomas are characterized histopathologically as intraductal tumors composed of benign epithelial cells covering a central branching fibrovascular core. They are generally differentiated to include **solitary intraductal papillomas**, which are typically located in the retromamillary region, and the small, usually multiple, **peripheral intraductal papillomas**.

Papillomas must be distinguished from *pseudopapillary lesions*, which are intraductal hyperplasias with a papillary architecture that occur without the presence of a central fibrous core, and from the **papillary adenoma of the nipple**, with its combination of papillary and tubular structures. The pseudopapillary lesions include **papillomatosis** and **juvenile papillomatosis**, the latter of which commonly occurs in adolescents and young women between 10 and 40 years of age.

> ! Papillomas are considered to be borderline epithelial lesions with an increased lifetime risk for the development of DCIS or invasive papillary breast cancer.

If the histopathological results of a percutaneous breast biopsy reveal a papilloma or papillomatosis, they are usually classified into the pathological B3 category (see **Table 16.1**). Because of the increased tumor transformation risk, a pathological–radiological tumor conference is held to decide whether surgical excision is required. The decision is usually dependent upon the primary lesion size on imaging, and the extent of tissue sampling. If it must be assumed that the papilloma has not been sufficiently removed, surgical excision should be recommended to attempt complete excision.

 MR Mammography: Papilloma

T1-Weighted Sequence (Precontrast)
Small solitary intraductal papilloma. Usually not detectable (**Figs. 10.1b, 10.2b**).

Larger solitary intraductal papilloma (>1 cm). Round or oval lesion with isointense signal to parenchyma (**Fig. 10.3b**).

Peripheral intraductal papillomas. Usually not detectable (**Figs. 10.4b, 10.5b**).

T2-Weighted Sequence
Small solitary intraductal papilloma. Often occult. Otherwise usually intermediate (**Fig. 10.2c**) or high signal intensity (**Fig. 10.1c**).

Larger solitary intraductal papilloma (>1 cm). Often occult. Otherwise round or oval lesion with intermediate or high signal intensity (**Fig. 10.3c**).

Peripheral intraductal papillomas. Usually not detectable. Occasionally high water signal within ductal structure (**Figs. 10.4c, 10.5c**).

T1-Weighted Sequence (Contrast Enhanced)
Small solitary intraductal papilloma. A focus or mass with increased enhancement can be detected from a size of 4–5 mm diameter (**Fig. 10.1a, d**). It usually has a round or oval shape, is well-circumscribed, and typically displays a homogeneous enhancement. Occasionally, displays a rim-enhancement. TIC is uninformative (**Fig. 10.1e**).

Larger solitary intraductal papilloma (>1 cm). Round or oval lesion that typically displays a homogeneous enhancement. Occasionally displays rim-enhancement (**Fig. 10.3a, d**). TIC is uninformative (**Fig. 10.3e**).

Peripheral intraductal papillomas. Linear (**Fig. 10.5d**), linear-branching (**Fig. 10.4d**), or regional enhancement (nonmasslike) (**Fig. 10.6a, d**). TIC may be uninformative (**Figs. 10.4e, 10.5e**) or typical for malignancy (**Fig. 10.6e**).

> ! Breast MRI does not allow a reliable differentiation between a benign papilloma and a papilloma in which malignant transformation has taken place (**Figs. 10.7, 10.8, 10.9**).

Papilloma: General information

Incidence:	Rare, 1%–2% of all benign tumors.
Age peak:	40–50 years.
Risk of malignant transformation:	Solitary papilloma: slightly increased lifetime risk (comparable with that of ADH).
	Multiple peripheral papillomas: increased lifetime risk of ~10%.

Findings

Clinical:	Often clinically occult.
	Spontaneous or provokable nipple discharge (exfoliative cytology).
	Rarely presents as palpable mass (e.g., large retromamillary papillomas).
Mammography:	Usually mammographically occult.
	Larger tumors appear well-circumscribed, homogeneously dense, round or oval.
Galactography:	Intraductal exclusion(s) or abrupt duct truncation(s).
	Indication: pathological secretion.
Ultrasonography:	Usually occult.
	Rarely seen as round, retromamillary lesion.

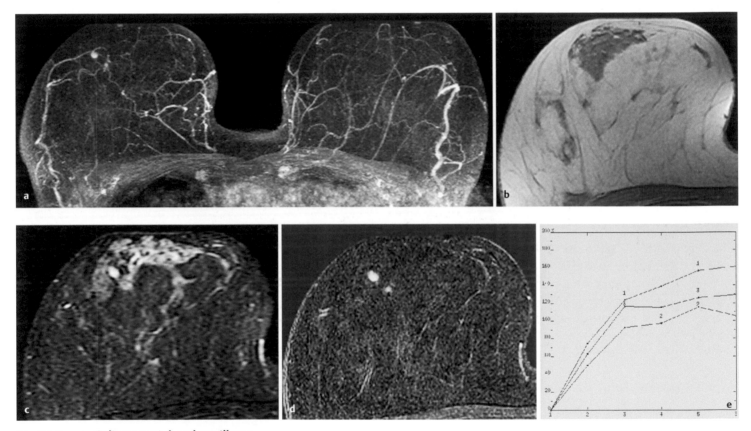

Fig. 10.1 a–e   Solitary peripheral papilloma.
a Subtraction MIP: solitary, small focus in the right breast.
b T1w precontrast slice image: unremarkable findings.
c IR T2w slice image: focus displays high water content.

d Early subtraction slice image: well-circumscribed, hypervascularized focus of 4 mm diameter.
e Time–signal intensity curve (TIC): uninformative.

Histology: papilloma of 4 mm diameter.

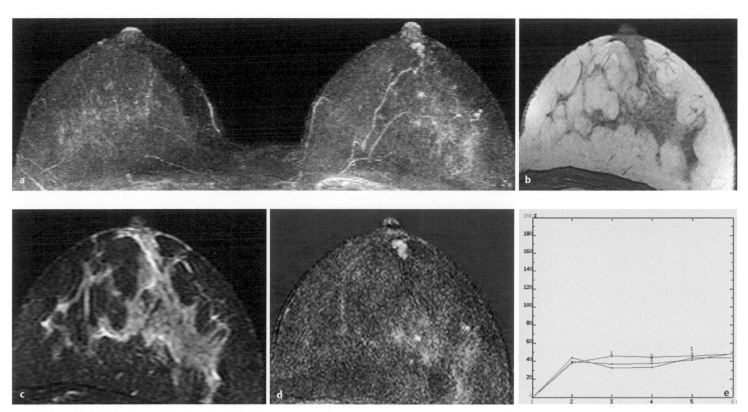

Fig. 10.2a–e Solitary retromamillary papilloma.

a Subtraction MIP: hypervascularized lesion with meandering shape in the retromamillary aspect of the left breast.

b T1w precontrast slice image: unremarkable findings.

c IR T2w slice image: intermediate signal intensity of lesion.

d Early subtraction slice image: hypervascularized, elongated, lobular finding in the retromamillary aspect of the left breast.

e TIC: uninformative.

Histology: papilloma of 7 mm diameter.

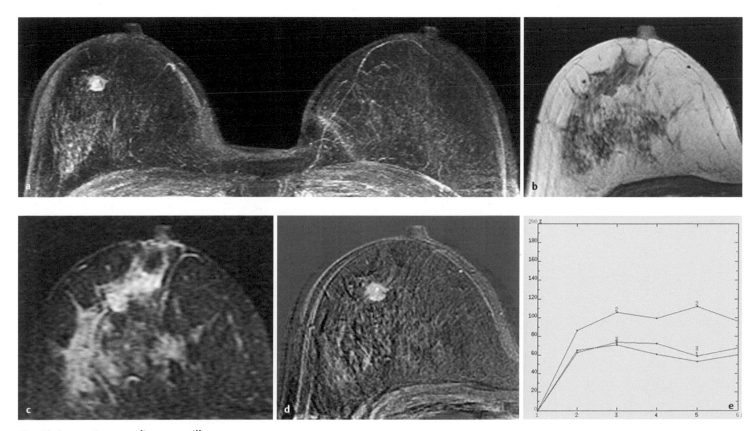

Fig. 10.3a–e Large solitary papilloma.

a Subtraction MIP: hypervascularized mass in the right breast.

b T1w precontrast slice image: unremarkable findings.

c IR T2w slice image: mass displays slightly increased signal intensity.

d Early subtraction slice image: mass of 10 mm diameter displays rim and central enhancement.

e TIC: strong initial enhancement and postinitial plateau.

Histology: papilloma of 10 mm diameter.

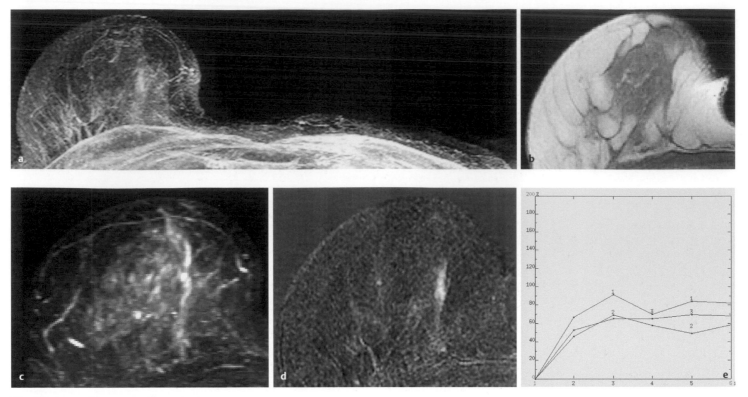

Fig. 10.4a–e   Linear papillomatosis.

a Subtraction MIP: linear hypervascularization in the central aspect of the right breast. Status after mastectomy of the left breast.

b T1w precontrast slice image (right breast): unremarkable findings.

c IR T2w slice image (right breast): increased signal intensity in affected milk duct.

d Early subtraction slice image (right breast): linear-branching enhancement in the central aspect.

e TIC: uninformative.

Histology: papillomatosis.

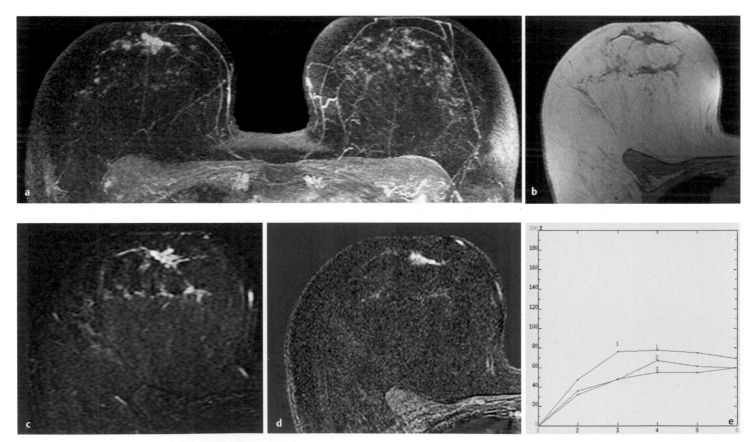

Fig. 10.5a–e   Segmental peripheral papillomatosis.

a Subtraction MIP: segmental hypervascularization in the retromammillary aspect of the right breast. Multiple foci in the left breast.

b T1w precontrast slice image (right breast): discrete duct ectasia.

c IR T2w slice image (right breast): increased signal intensity in affected milk duct.

d Representative early subtraction slice image (right breast): linear enhancement along milk duct.

e TIC: uninformative.

Histology: papillomatosis.

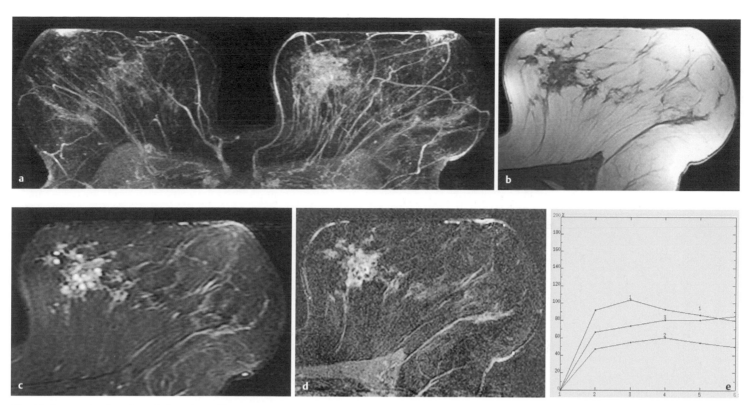

Fig. 10.6a–e   Regional peripheral papillomatosis.

a Subtraction MIP: regional hypervascularization in the medial aspect of the left breast. Unremarkable right breast.

b T1w precontrast slice image (left breast): hypointense region containing several round lesions in the medial aspect of the left breast.

c IR T2w slice image (left breast): increased signal intensity of these round lesions.

d Representative early subtraction slice image (left breast): round lesions within regional area of enhancement display no enhancement.

e TIC: suspicious curve with mild postinitial washout.

Histology: papillomatosis. No associated malignancy.

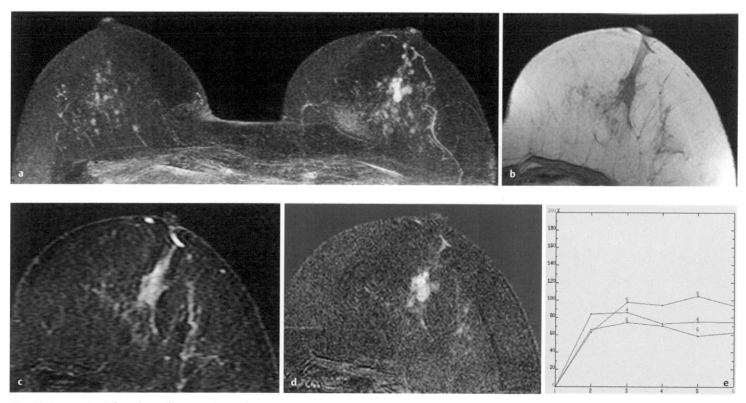

Fig. 10.7a–e   Peripheral papillomatosis with ADH.

a Subtraction MIP: convolute of hypervascularized, round lesions in the central aspect of the left breast. Multiple foci in the right breast.

b T1w precontrast slice image (left breast): isointense, masslike region in the central aspect of the left breast.

c IR T2w slice image (left breast): slightly increased signal intensity in this region.

d Representative early subtraction slice image (left breast): conglomerate of hypervascularized foci and masses in the central aspect of the left breast.

e TIC: suspicious curve with mild postinitial washout.

Histology: papillomatosis with ADH.

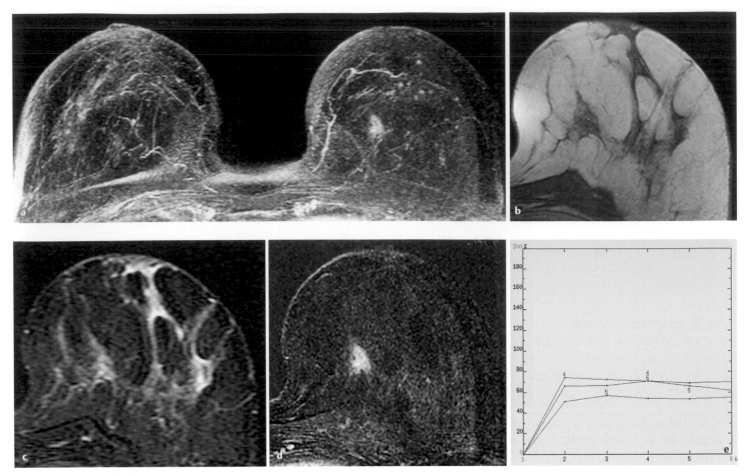

Fig. 10.10 a–e   Radial scar.

a Subtraction MIP: regional hypervascularization in the left breast. Unremarkable right breast.

b T1w precontrast slice image (left breast): unremarkable findings.

c IR T2w slice image (left breast): unremarkable findings.

d Early subtraction slice image (left breast): nonmasslike enhancement.

e TIC: uninformative.

Histology: radial scar. No malignancy.

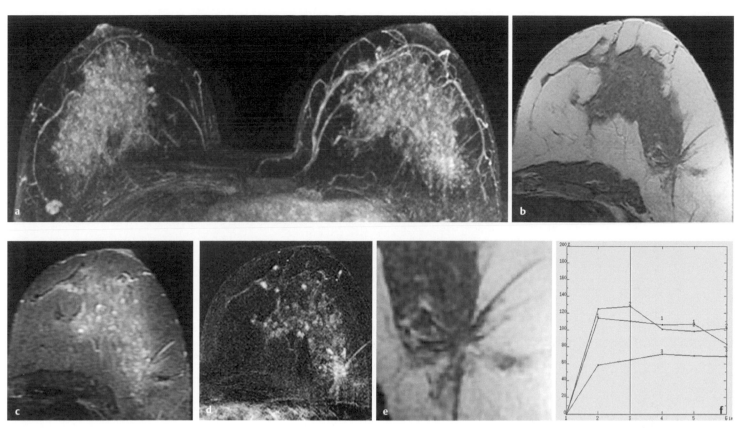

Fig. 10.11 a–f   Radial scar.

a Subtraction MIP: early, strong enhancement of breast parenchyma.

b T1w precontrast slice image (left breast): pronounced architectural distortion in the lateral aspect of the left breast.

c IR T2w slice image (left breast): unremarkable findings.

d Early subtraction slice image (left breast): strong enhancement in the central aspect of the architectural distortion and in the peripheral spiculations.

e Zoomed T1w precontrast slice image (left breast).

f TIC: uninformative curve with postinitial washout.

Histology: radial scar. No malignancy.

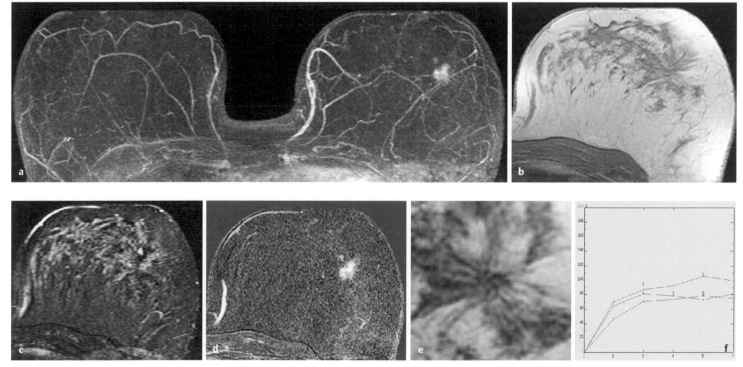

Fig. 10.12 a–f   Radial scar with associated DCIS.

a Subtraction MIP: nonmasslike, hypervascularized, spiculated lesion in the left breast. Unremarkable right breast.

b T1w precontrast slice image (left breast): architectural distortion in the lateral aspect of the left breast.

c IR T2w slice image (left breast): discrete architectural distortion.

d Early subtraction slice image (left breast): strong enhancement in the center of a spiculated lesion without enhancement of peripheral spiculations.

e Zoomed T1w precontrast slice image (left breast).

f TIC: curve with postinitial plateau.

Histology: radial scar with associated DCIS.

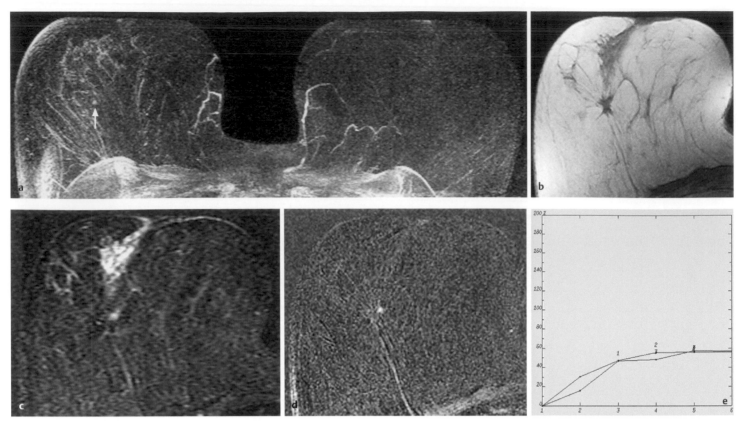

Fig. 10.13 a–e   Radial scar with associated IDC.

a Subtraction MIP: slight motion artifacts in the right breast. Hypervascularized focus in the central aspect of the right breast (arrow). Unremarkable left breast.

b T1w precontrast slice image (right breast): hypointense lesion with fine spiculations in the central aspect of the right breast.

c IR T2w slice image (right breast): uninformative signal increase in the center of the spiculated lesion.

d Early subtraction slice image (right breast): hypervascularized focus (2 mm diameter) in the center of the spiculated lesion.

e TIC: uninformative.

Histology: radial scar with central IDC (pT1a).

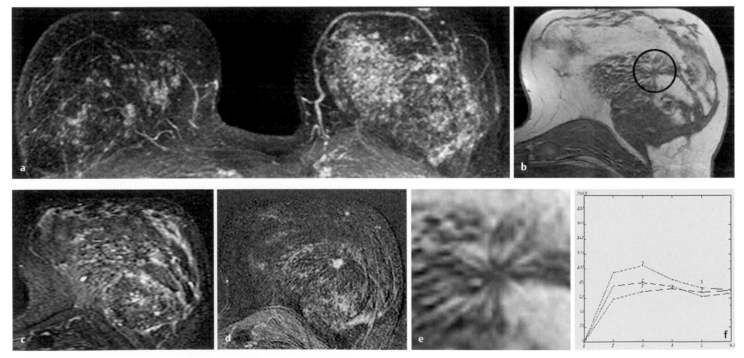

Fig. 10.14 a–f   Radial scar with central tubular breast carcinoma.

a Subtraction MIP: early stippled parenchymal enhancement with asymmetry toward the left breast.

b T1w precontrast slice image (left breast): architectural distortion in the central aspect of the left breast with radial lipomatous and nonlipomatous spiculations (circle).

c IR T2w slice image (left breast): uninformative signal increase in the center of the spiculated lesion.

d Early subtraction slice image (left breast): hypervascularized lesion (6 mm diameter) in the center of the architectural distortion.

e Zoomed T1w precontrast slice image (left breast).

f TIC: suspicious curve with postinitial washout.

Histology: radial scar with central tubular breast carcinoma (pT1b).

Lobular Carcinoma in Situ (LCIS)

Lobular carcinoma in situ is characterized by a proliferation of tumor cells present in the terminal duct-lobular units of the breast without light-microscopic evidence of invasion through the basement membrane into the surrounding stroma.

> **!** LCIS is not considered a precancerous lesion as it does not develop into an invasive lobular carcinoma. Instead it is a noninvasive condition that increases the risk of developing invasive cancer in either or both breasts in the future.

If the histopathological results of a percutaneous breast biopsy reveal LCIS, the lesion is usually classified into the pathological B3 category (see **Table 16.1**). A pathological–radiological tumor conference is held to decide on further management. A small LCIS lesion is typically an incidental finding in a biopsy performed for other reasons and can usually be followed up. Larger LCIS lesions, on the other hand, should be surgically excised. Generally, women who have been histologically diagnosed with LCIS should receive individually adapted, high-quality breast imaging at yearly intervals.

 MR Mammography: LCIS

T1-Weighted Sequence (Precontrast)
No characteristic findings (**Figs. 10.15b, 10.16b**).

T2-Weighted Sequence
No characteristic findings (**Figs. 10.15c, 10.16c**).

T1-Weighted Sequence (Contrast Enhanced)
Focal, punctate or lobulated hypervascularized findings (**Figs. 10.15a,d, 10.16a, d**). No characteristic TIC (**Figs. 10.15e, 10.16e**).

Lobular carcinoma in situ: General information

Incidence:	In ~1% of all breast biopsies.
Age peak:	40–50 years. (often premenopausal).
Multicentricity:	>50%.
Bilaterality:	~50%.

Findings

Clinical:	Usually clinically occult.
Mammography:	Usually mammographically occult. Occasionally unspecific microcalcifications.
Ultrasonography:	No specific findings.

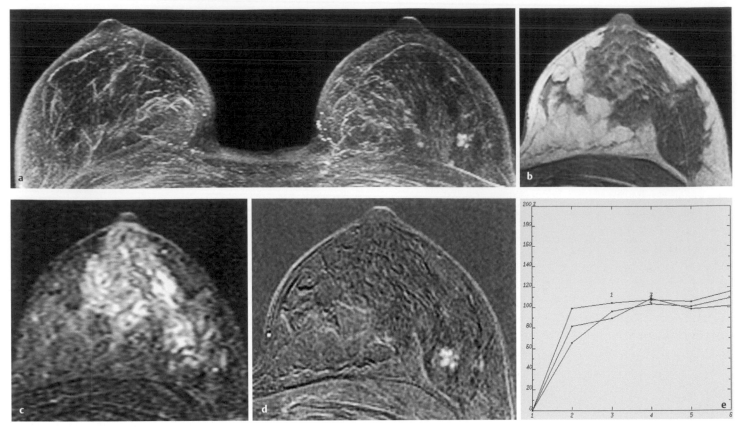

Fig. 10.15a–e   LCIS.
a Subtraction MIP: area of clumped enhancement in the lateral aspect of the left breast. Unremarkable right breast.
b T1w precontrast slice image (left breast): unremarkable findings.
c IR T2w slice image (left breast): unremarkable findings.

d Early subtraction slice image (left breast): conglomerate of punctate hypervascularizations.
e TIC: uninformative.

Histology after vacuum-assisted biopsy: LCIS. Follow-up at yearly intervals as a consequence.

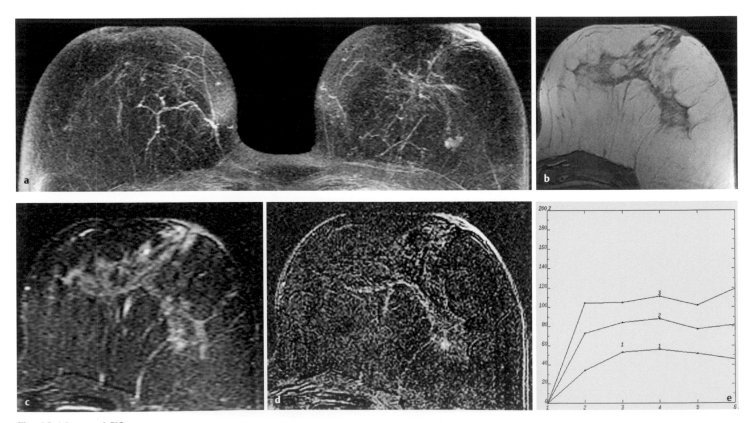

Fig. 10.16a–e   LCIS.
a Subtraction MIP: localized area of enhancement in the lateral aspect of the left breast. Unremarkable right breast.
b T1w precontrast slice image (left breast): unremarkable findings.
c IR T2w slice image (left breast): unremarkable findings.

d Early subtraction slice image (left breast): focus.
e TIC: uninformative.

Histology after vacuum-assisted biopsy: LCIS. Follow-up at yearly intervals as a consequence.

Atypical Ductal Hyperplasia

The term atypical ductal hyperplasia (ADH) is used to denote a lesion with marked epithelial proliferation (more than four cell layers) in structures of ductal type associated with atypia, but not fulfilling the criteria for carcinoma in situ. ADH rarely has dimensions greater than 2–3 mm.

! ADH is considered to be a precancerous lesion with a 5-fold increased risk for developing breast cancer. ADH may be the last step in tumor transformation to DCIS.

If the histopathological results of a percutaneous breast biopsy reveal ADH, the lesion is usually classified into the pathological B3 category (see **Table 16.1**). A pathological–radiological tumor conference is held to decide on further management. Generally, surgical excision will be recommended to exclude or excise any potentially existing areas with intraductal or invasive carcinoma.

 MR Mammography: ADH

T1-Weighted Sequence (Precontrast)
No characteristic findings (**Figs. 10.17b, 10.18b**).

T2-Weighted Sequence
No characteristic findings (**Figs. 10.17c, 10.18c**).

T1-Weighted Sequence (Contrast Enhanced)
Focus or small hypervascularized mass (**Figs. 10.17a, d, e, 10.18a, d, e**). No characteristic TIC (**Figs. 10.17f, 10.18f**).

Atypical ductal hyperplasia: General information	
Incidence:	In ~1% of all breast biopsies.
Age peak:	Usually 40–60 years.
Findings	
Clinical:	Usually clinically occult.
Mammography:	Usually mammographically occult. Occasionally unspecific microcalcifications.
Ultrasonography:	No specific findings.

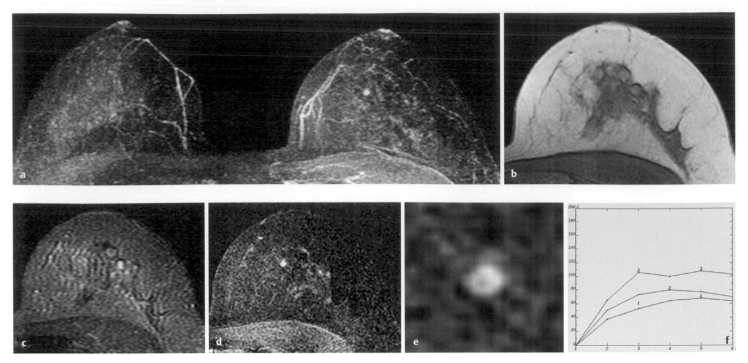

Fig. 10.17a–f ADH.

a Subtraction MIP: solitary hypervascularized focus in the left breast.

b T1w precontrast slice image (left breast): unremarkable findings.

c IR T2w slice image (left breast): unremarkable findings.

d Early subtraction slice image (left breast): focus.

e Zoomed early subtraction slice image (left breast): possible rim-enhancement.

f TIC: uninformative.

Histology after vacuum-assisted biopsy: ADH. Surgical excision revealed no additional areas with atypia or malignancy.

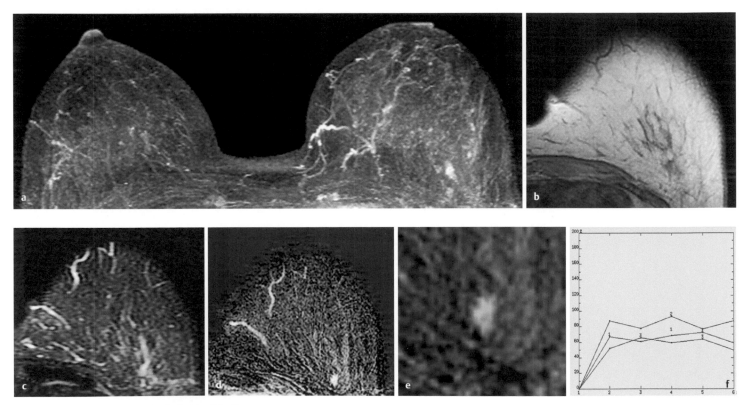

Fig. 10.18a–f Flat epithelial atypia (FEA).

a Subtraction MIP: localized area of enhancement in the lateral aspect of the left breast. Unremarkable right breast.

b T1w precontrast slice image (left breast): Unremarkable findings.

c IR T2w slice image (left breast): Unremarkable findings.

d Early subtraction slice image (left breast): hypervascularized mass lesion of 5 mm diameter. Indistinct borders and possible rim-enhancement.

e Zoomed early subtraction slice image (left breast).

f TIC: uninformative.

Histology after vacuum-assisted biopsy: FEA. Surgical excision revealed no additional areas with atypia or malignancy.

Breast Cysts with Intracystic Proliferation

Because intracystic proliferations are potentially early malignant lesions, cysts with internal nonliquid structures can be considered to be borderline lesions in the broadest sense.

> ! Intracystic proliferations should always be histologically verified to rule out malignancy.

 MR Mammography: Intracystic Proliferations

T1-Weighted Sequence (Precontrast)
Well-circumscribed, hypointense mass with internal signal-intense structure (**Figs. 10.19b, 10.20b**).

T2-Weighted Sequence
Well-circumscribed, hyperintense mass (**Fig. 10.20c**). Occasionally internal isointense structure can be seen (**Fig. 10.19c**).

T1-Weighted Sequence (Contrast Enhanced)
Occasional cyst wall-enhancement (**Figs. 10.19d, 10.20d**). In addition, contrast enhancement of internal proliferation (**Figs. 10.19a, d, 10.20a, d**).

Intracystic proliferation: General information	
Incidence:	Rare. Can occur in any cyst.
Age peak:	All ages. Incidence increases with age.
Risk of malignant transformation:	10%–20%.

Findings	
Clinical:	Small cysts: clinically occult.
	Large cysts: firm-elastic, well-circumscribed, movable nodules.
	Differentiation of simple cysts from cysts with internal proliferations is not usually clinically possible.
Mammography:	Mammographic findings are like those of simple cysts.
	Rare documentation of internal microcalcifications.
	Mammographic differentiation of simple cysts from cysts with internal proliferations is not usually possible.
Ultrasonography:	Reliable detection of intracystic proliferations.

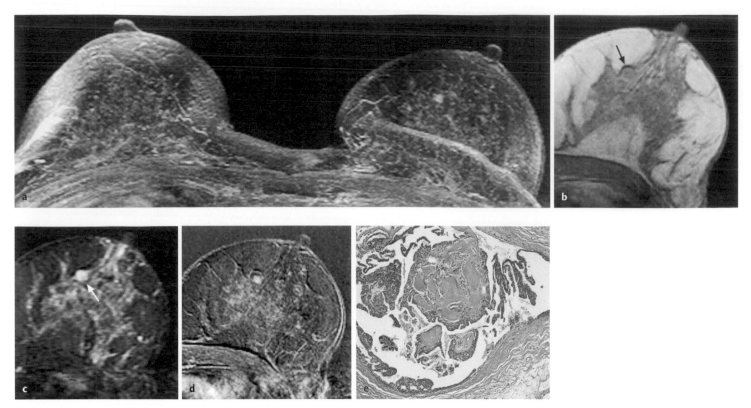

Fig. 10.19a–e   Complicated cyst with intracystic proliferation: low-grade DCIS.

a Subtraction MIP: solitary hypervascularized focus in the central aspect of the left breast. Motion artifacts in the right breast.

b T1w precontrast slice image (left breast): round, well-circumscribed mass with isointense internal signal intensity (arrow).

c IR T2w slice image (left breast): high signal intensity with vague nonliquid internal structure (arrow).

d Early subtraction slice image (left breast): pronounced enhancement of intracystic proliferation and discrete cyst wall-enhancement.

e Hematoxylin and eosin stain (H&E stain): primary open surgery.

Histology: intracystic low-grade DCIS.

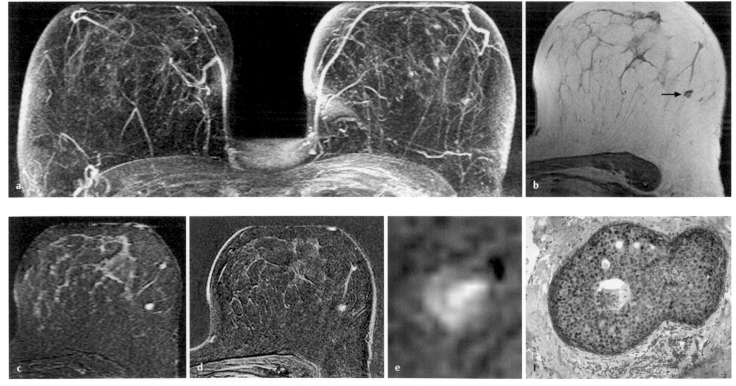

Fig. 10.20a–f   Complicated cyst with intracystic proliferation: high-grade DCIS.

a Subtraction MIP: unremarkable findings with foci in the left breast.

b T1w precontrast slice image (left breast): round, hypointense small mass within lipomatous tissue in the lateral aspect of the left breast.

c IR T2w slice image (left breast): homogeneous high signal intensity within the cyst.

d Early subtraction slice image (left breast): discrete cyst wall-enhancement. Hypervascularized area within the cyst.

e Zoomed early subtraction slice image (left breast): a region of interest for calculation of a TIC cannot be reasonably placed due to the small lesion size.

f Hematoxylin and eosin stain (H&E stain): percutaneous biopsy.

Histology: intracystic high-grade DCIS.

11 Intraductal Carcinomas

Synonyms: ductal carcinoma in situ, DCIS.

DCIS is characterized by a proliferation of malignant tumor cells that are confined to the ductal units of the breast and show no light-microscopic evidence of invasion through the basement membrane into the surrounding stroma. The term ductal carcinoma in situ encompasses a pathologically heterogeneous group of lesions. The **comedo type** of DCIS (high-grade DCIS) is characterized by prominent necrosis in the center of the involved ducts.

The **noncomedo type** of DCIS (intermediate type, low-grade DCIS) is further differentiated into *solid*, *cribriform*, *micropapillary*, *papillary*, and *clinging* types with different histological patterns. Coexistence of several patterns in any one case is common.

> Apparent discrepancy: DCIS is an early diagnosis, but not always small.

Intraductal carcinomas: General information

Incidence:	Up to 20% of all breast carcinomas, depending on image quality. Comedo type accounts for 50% of all DCIS.
Age peak:	40–60 years.
Multifocality:	~30%.
Bilaterality:	Not significantly increased.
Risk of invasion:	Comedo type: ~50%. Noncomedo type: <50%.

Findings

Clinical:	Often clinically occult. Palpable mass in extensive cases (~10%). Rarely presents with pathologic secretion or mamillary changes (Paget disease).
Mammography:	Suspicious microcalcifications (pleomorphic with linear, segmental, or clustered distribution). Rarely presents as architectural distortion or spiculated density.
Ultrasonography:	Usually occult. Intraductal proliferations rarely display dorsal acoustic shadowing/extinction.

Classification

Among other matters, the new WHO classification deals with current issues pertaining to traditional DCIS terminology and recommends additional use of the "ductal intraepithelial neoplasia" (DIN) classification system. The morphological variants of DCIS are divided into three main classes (DIN 1, DIN 2, DIN 3) and several subclasses.

The complete extent of a DCIS lesion is occasionally difficult to determine on breast imaging. The therapy of DCIS is still a subject of much debate.

> DCIS lesions are heterogeneous and considered to be precancerous lesions that can develop into invasive breast cancer. On the other hand, some DCIS lesions never become invasive.
> DCIS is a disease limited to the breast, not a systemic disease.

 MR Mammography: Intraductal Carcinoma

T1-Weighted Sequence (Precontrast)
Normally there are no specific findings associated with DCIS because of its nonmass configuration (**Figs. 11.2b, 11.6b, 11.9b**). The spatial resolution of breast MRI is not sufficient for the visualization of microcalcifications. Rarely, DCIS may appear as a mass lesion (**Figs. 11.4b, 11.11b**).

T2-Weighted Sequence
No characteristic findings (**Figs. 11.1c, 11.3c, 11.5c**). Occasionally affected milk duct displays high signal intensity (**Fig. 11.6c**).

T1-Weighted Sequence (Contrast Enhanced)
Nonmasslike focal (**Fig. 11.4a, d**), linear (**Fig. 11.1a, d**), diffuse (**Figs. 11.3a, d, 11.7a, c**), rarely regional (**Fig. 11.2a, d**), frequently segmental (**Figs. 11.6a, d, 11.8a, d, 11.12a, d**) enhancement along the course of one or several milk ducts. Linear-branching en-

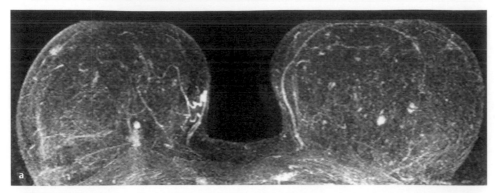

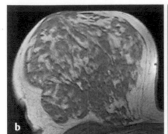 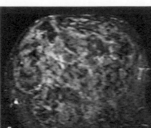 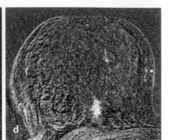

Fig. 11.1 a–d Low-grade DCIS, linear.
a Subtraction MIP: a broad linear enhancing area is projected dorsally of a fibroadenoma in the right breast. Coincidental fibroadenoma in the left breast.
b T1w precontrast slice image (right breast): unremarkable findings.
c IR T2w slice image (right breast): unremarkable findings.
d Early subtraction slice image (right breast): better visualization of ill-defined, linear enhancement.

Histology: DCIS, grade 1.

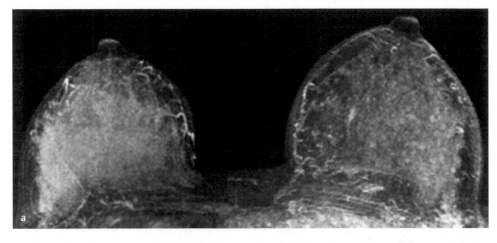

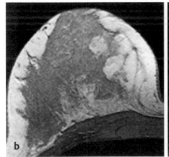 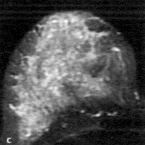 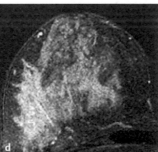

Fig. 11.2 a–d Low-grade DCIS, regional.
a Subtraction MIP: early hypervascularization of breast parenchyma in both breasts with asymmetry toward the right breast, especially in the lateral aspect.
b T1w precontrast slice image (right breast): unremarkable findings.
c IR T2w slice image (right breast): unremarkable findings.
d Early subtraction slice image (right breast): better visualization of the regionally increased vascularization of the lateral aspect of the right breast.

Histology: DCIS, grade 1.

hancement pattern (**Figs. 11.9a, d, 11.10a, d**). Rare presentation as mass lesion (**Fig. 11.11a, d**), occasionally with rim-enhancement. TIC analysis of nonmasslike enhancement is of little value. Linear enhancement seen bordering on or near a suspicious mass lesion potentially represents an extensive intraductal component (EIC) (**Fig. 11.13**). Enhancing nodular areas within or in the periphery of a nonmasslike lesion potentially represents beginning tumor invasion, i.e., minimally invasive tumor stage (**Fig. 11.14**).

!
• A reliable differentiation of low-, intermediate-, and high-grade DCIS lesions cannot be made on the basis of their enhancing pattern or distribution.

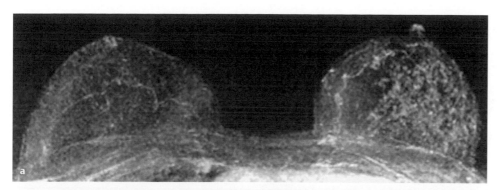

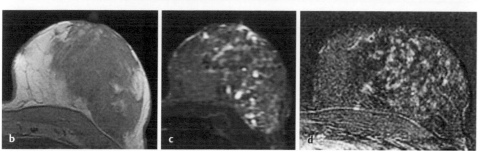

Fig. 11.3a–d   Low-grade DCIS, diffuse.
a Subtraction MIP: asymmetric, diffuse enhancement of the left breast.
b T1w precontrast slice image (left breast): unremarkable findings.
c IR T2w slice image (left breast): unremarkable findings.
d Early subtraction slice image (left breast): diffuse, linear-branching enhancement pattern (nonmasslike lesion).

Histology: DCIS, grade 1.

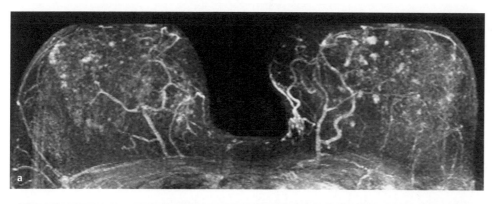

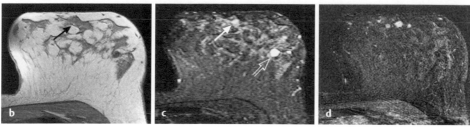

Fig. 11.4a–d   Intermediate-grade DCIS, focal.
a Subtraction MIP: bilateral foci and small mass lesions.
b T1w precontrast slice image (left breast): vague, space-occupying lesion (arrow).
c IR T2w slice image (left breast): increased signal intensity of this lesion (arrow). Coincidental hyperintense cyst (double arrow).
d Early subtraction slice image (left breast): 5 mm spiculated mass with decreased central perfusion (rim sign).

Histology: DCIS, grade 2.

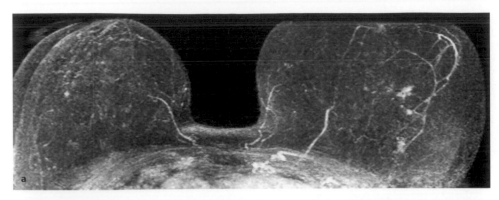

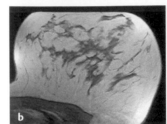
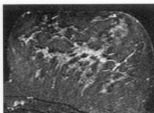
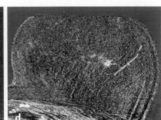

Fig. 11.5 a–d Intermediate-grade DCIS, linear.

a Subtraction MIP: discontinuous linear enhancement along the course of a milk duct in the left breast. Benign focus in the right breast.

b T1w precontrast slice image (left breast): unremarkable findings.

c IR T2w slice image (left breast): unremarkable findings.

d Early subtraction slice image (left breast): ventral segment of the lesion is a 3 mm spiculated focus with subtle linear-branching, peripheral enhancement, and decreased central perfusion (rim sign).

Histology: DCIS, grade 2.

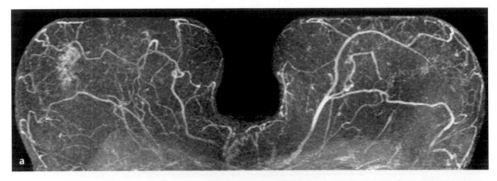

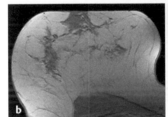
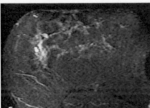
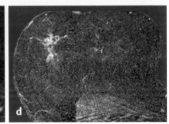

Fig. 11.6 a–d Intermediate-grade DCIS, segmental.

a Subtraction MIP: segmental enhancement in the lateral aspect of the right breast. Unremarkable findings in the left breast.

b T1w precontrast slice image (right breast): unremarkable findings.

c IR T2w slice image (right breast): increased signal intensity (water content) in the duct lumen within the area corresponding to the enhancing segment.

d Early subtraction slice image (right breast): nonmasslike enhancement with dendritic pattern in the lateral aspect of the right breast. No enhancement within the duct lumen seen in **c**.

Histology: DCIS, grade 2.

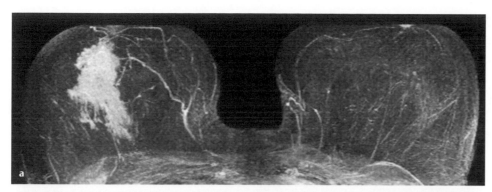

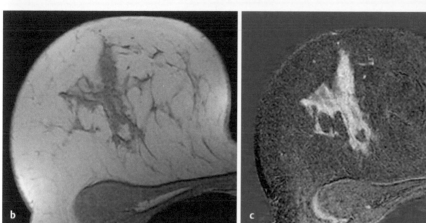

Fig. 11.7 a–c   Intermediate-grade DCIS, diffuse.
a Subtraction MIP: pronounced enhancement of all nonlipomatous structures in the right breast. Normal left breast findings.
b T1w precontrast slice image (right breast): no significant findings.
c Early subtraction slice image (right breast): nonmasslike enhancement of all nonlipomatous tissues in the right breast.

Histology: DCIS, grade 2.

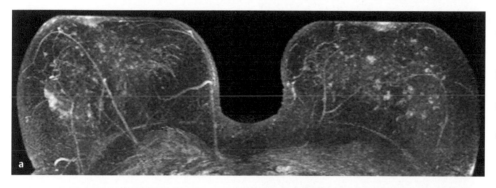

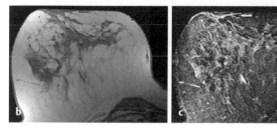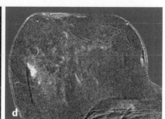

Fig. 11.8 a–d   High-grade DCIS, regional.
a Subtraction MIP: regional enhancement in the lateral aspect of the right breast. Bilateral foci.
b T1w precontrast slice image (right breast): no significant findings.
c IR T2w slice image (right breast): no significant findings.
d Early subtraction slice image (right breast): regional, enhancement in the lateral aspect of the right breast.

Histology: DCIS, grade 3.

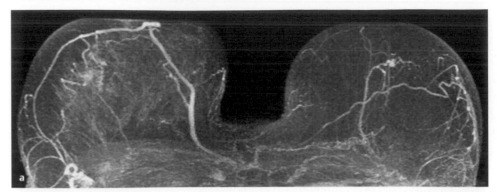
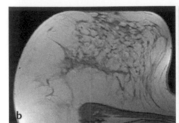
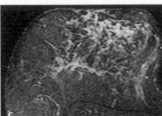
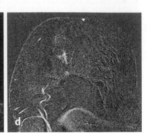

Fig. 11.9a–d High-grade DCIS, linear-branching.

a Subtraction MIP: area of dendritic enhancement in the lateral aspect of the right breast. Unremarkable findings in the left breast.

b T1w precontrast slice image (right breast): no significant findings.

c IR T2w slice image (right breast): no significant findings.

d Early subtraction slice image (right breast): linear-branching, ductal enhancement pattern.

Histology: DCIS, grade 3.

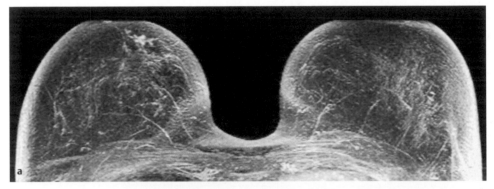
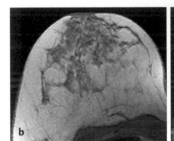
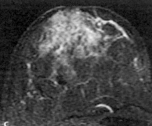
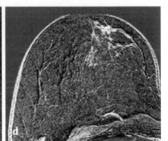

Fig. 11.10a–d High-grade DCIS, linear-branching.

a Subtraction MIP: area of dendritic enhancement in the retromamillary aspect of the right breast. Unremarkable findings in the left breast.

b T1w precontrast slice image (right breast): no significant findings.

c IR T2w slice image (right breast): no significant findings.

d Early subtraction slice image (right breast): linear-branching, ductal enhancement pattern.

Histology: DCIS, grade 3.

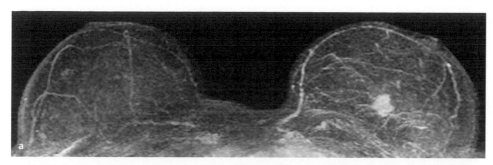

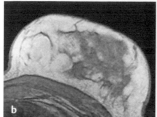 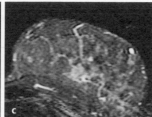 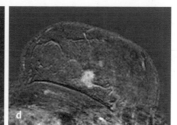

Fig. 11.11 a–d   High-grade DCIS, mass lesion.

a Subtraction MIP: hypervascularized mass lesion in the central aspect of the left breast.

b T1w precontrast slice image (left breast): isointense mass lesion.

c IR T2w slice image (left breast): increased signal intensity of mass lesion.

d Early subtraction slice image (left breast): round, ill-defined lesion with rim-enhancement. Findings suspicious for invasive breast cancer.

Histology: DCIS, grade 3.

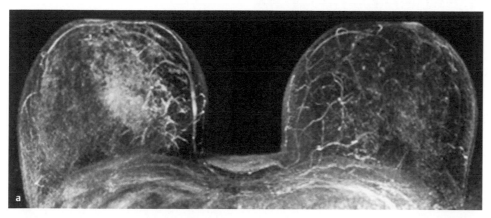

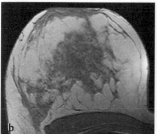 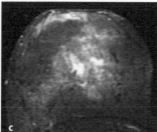 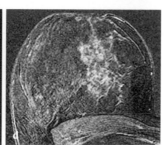

Fig. 11.12 a–d   High-grade DCIS, segmental.

a Subtraction MIP: nonmass area of dendritic enhancement affecting several medial segments of the right breast. Benign foci in the left breast.

b T1w precontrast slice image (right breast): no significant findings.

c IR T2w slice image (right breast): no significant findings.

d Early subtraction slice image (right breast): dendritic enhancement pattern with segmental distribution.

Histology: DCIS, grade 3.

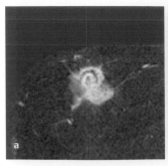
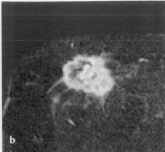
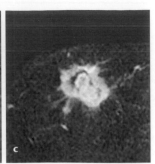

Fig. 11.13a–c Peritumoral extensive intra-ductal component (EIC). Early subtraction slice images through a 2 cm index carcinoma with pathomorphology typical of malignancy. All slices show peritumoral fine-linear enhancement up to several centimeters long as an indication of EIC (histologically confirmed).

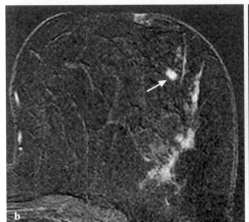

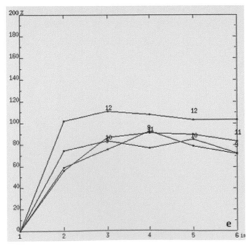
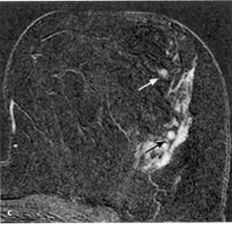
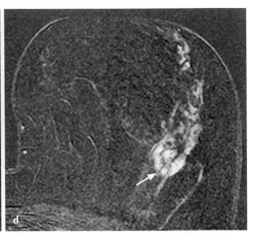

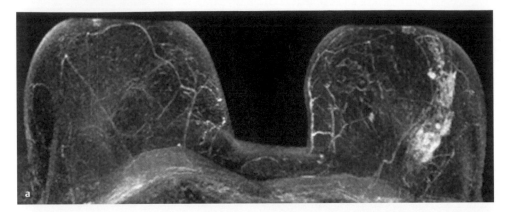

Fig. 11.14a–g DCIS with minimal invasion.

a Subtraction MIP: nonmasslike enhancement with segmental distribution in the lateral aspect of the left breast. No other significant findings.

b–d Early subtraction slice images (left breast): nonmasslike lesion with dendritic, branching enhancement pattern. Enhancing nodular areas within and in the periphery of the lesion (arrows) indicate increased tumor angiogenesis after invasion through the basement membrane (minimal invasion).

e–g Time–signal intensity curves measured in different ROIs with unspecific (**e**), typically benign (**f**), and typically malignant (**g**) configuration.

Histology: breast carcinoma pT1mic (minimal invasion).

Study Results

Breast MRI and DCIS. Study results in recent years substantiate that breast MRI has a higher sensitivity for the detection of intraductal carcinomas than x-ray mammography (**Table 11.1**). This is especially true for high-grade DCIS tumors that are judged to have a poorer prognosis. In addition it is important to note that palpation and ultrasonography have no significant value in the detection of DCIS lesions.

! The excellent results achieved by breast MRI in the detection of DCIS lesions are only possible when MRI is performed in HR technique and with adequate breast compression.

Table 11.1 Sensitivity of breast MRI in the detection of DCIS compared with that of x-ray mammography

Author	Year	DCIS cases	DCIS total				HG DCIS	
			Mx (%)	MRI (%)	CE (%)	US (%)	Mx (%)	MRI (%)
Berg et al.	2004	111	55	89	n.a.	47		
Kuhl et al.	2007	167	56	92	n.a.	n.a.	52	100
Fischer et al.	2009	144	73[a]	88[b]	15	18		

HG: high-grade.
Mx: x-ray mammography.
CE: clinical examination.
US: ultrasonography.
n.a.: not applicable.
[a] False-negative findings on Mx: 70% of high-grade DCIS, 30% of low-grade DCIS.
[b] False negative findings on breast MRI: 25% of intermediate-grade DCIS, 75% of low-grade DCIS.

12 Malignant Changes

Invasive Ductal Carcinoma

Synonyms: not otherwise specified (NOS).

Invasive ductal carcinoma (IDC) is defined as a malignant tumor of the breast partially or wholly lacking specific histological differentiation patterns and therefore not falling into any of the other categories for invasive mammary carcinoma. The tumor cells initially develop in the terminal ducts, and tumor cells infiltrate the basal membrane continuously or in several distinct locations. Invasive ductal carcinomas possess a strong fibrotic component. In addition, an extensive intraductal component, which can comprise an area more than one-quarter the size of the primary invasive tumor, is often present.

! IDC is the most common and morphologically heterogeneous malignant tumor of the breast.

 MR Mammography: Invasive Ductal Carcinoma

T1-Weighted Sequence (Precontrast)
Isointense signal in comparison with the surrounding breast parenchyma and therefore no specific changes allowing demarcation of lesion when located within breast parenchyma (**Fig. 12.1b**). Lesions surrounded by adipose tissue are seen as hypointense, occasionally round (**Fig. 12.3b**) or ovoid, more often spiculated masses (**Fig. 12.2b**). The spatial resolution of MR mammography does not allow the depiction of pleomorphic microcalcifications.

T2-Weighted Sequence
Typically intermediate or slightly decreased signal intensity in comparison with the surrounding breast parenchyma. Occasional hyperintense zone of peritumoral edema (**Figs. 12.2c, 12.3c**). Tumor matrix shows increased signal intensity (water content) in ~20% of cases (**Fig. 12.8b**). High signal intensity in the center of the tumor if central necrosis is present (**Fig. 12.7b**).

T1-Weighted Sequence (Contrast Enhanced)
Enhancement is obligatory. Depending upon size, lesions are focal (**Fig. 12.1a, d**), mass (**Figs. 12.3a, d, 12.4a, d, 12.6b**), or rarely nonmasslike (**Fig. 12.2a, d**). Tumor borders are often ill-defined or spiculated (**Figs. 12.2d, 12.8a**). Enhancement is inhomogeneous (**Fig. 12.3d**), or stronger in the tumor periphery (rim-enhancement) (**Fig. 12.7a**). Peritumoral linear enhancement is a potential indication of an EIC (**Fig. 12.5a, d**).

Time–signal intensity analysis is recommended for mass lesions. Initial signal increase is often intermediate or rapid (>100%) (**Figs. 12.3e, 12.4e**). A slow initial signal increase is very rare (<5%). The postinitial signal course is often an unspecific plateau or suspicious washout (**Figs. 12.3e, 12.4e**). A persistent signal increase is very rare. Nodular carcinomas never display "late enhancement." This expression originated from historic measurement protocols and there is no pathophysiological explanation for such enhancement dynamics.

Invasive ductal carcinoma: General information

Incidence:	Most common form of invasive breast cancer (65%–75%).
Age peak:	All ages, peak between 50th and 60th years.
Grading:	*Histological grade*: well-differentiated (G1), intermediate (G2), poorly differentiated (G3).
Prognosis:	Dependent upon size, grading, N-stage, and receptor status among other factors.
Multifocality:	15%.
Bilaterality:	5%.

Findings

Clinical:	Small tumors are clinically occult. Average diameter of palpable tumor: 2.3 cm.
	Typical criteria of breast cancer (usually not early signs): hard, ill-defined mass, poorly movable, indolent, skin or nipple retraction.
Mammography:	Tumors not associated with microcalcifications located within dense breast tissue are often mammographically occult. Tumors associated with microcalcifications or located within lipomatous breast areas are reliably detected.
	Typical mammographic criteria of breast cancer: irregular shape, ill-defined or spiculated, high radiodensity.
	Associated clustered, pleomorphic microcalcifications in ~30% of all invasive breast cancers.
Ultrasonography:	Small tumors are often sonographically occult. Tumor detectability increases with size from a minimum diameter of approx. 5 mm.
	Examples of typical sonographic criteria of breast cancer: ill-defined, hypoechoic mass with hyperechoic margins. Central or peripheral posterior acoustic shadowing.

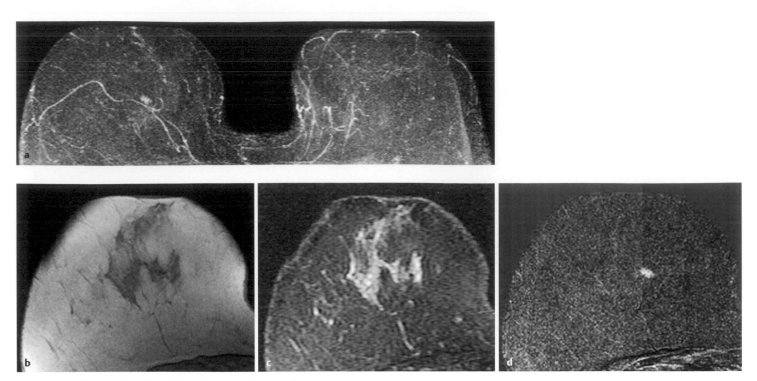

Fig. 12.1 a–d   Invasive ductal carcinoma of 4 mm diameter.

a Subtraction MIP: hypervascularized focus in the right breast. Unremarkable findings in the left breast.

b T1w precontrast slice image (right breast): unremarkable findings.

c IR T2w slice image (right breast): slightly decreased signal intensity (water content).

d Early subtraction slice image: oval, ill-defined focus. TICs are unspecific (not shown).

Histology: IDC (pT1a).

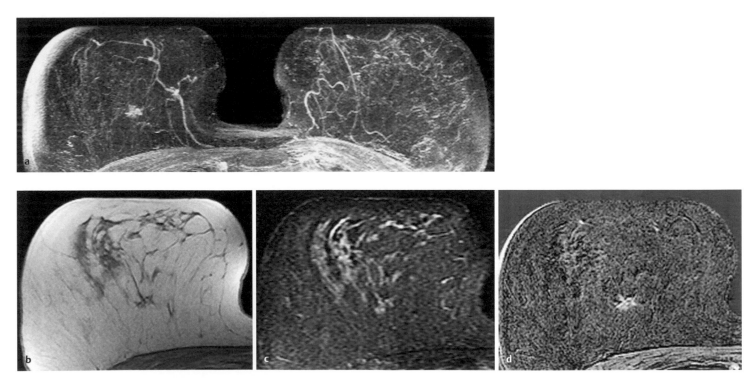

Fig. 12.2 a–d   Invasive ductal carcinoma (pT1 b).

a Subtraction MIP: spiculated hypervascularized lesion in the center of the right breast. Otherwise unremarkable findings.

b T1w precontrast slice image (right breast): vague architectural distortion within the lipomatous breast area.

c IR T2w slice image (right breast): intermediate signal intensity in the center of the lesion.

d Early subtraction slice image (right breast): improved visualization of nonmasslike, spiculated enhancement. TICs unspecific, as is typical in nonmasslike lesions (not shown).

Histology: IDC (pT1 b).

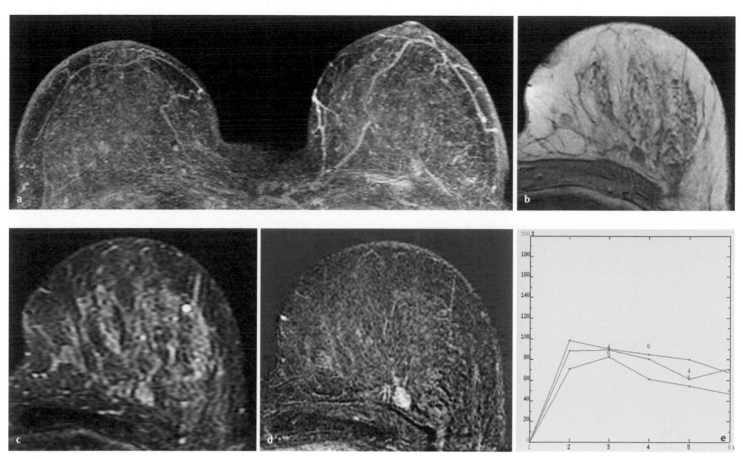

Fig. 12.3a–e Invasive ductal carcinoma (pT1b).

a Subtraction MIP: stippled enhancement pattern in both breasts. Vague, enhancing, nodular lesion near the chest wall in the left breast.

b T1w precontrast slice image (left breast): round, well-circumscribed mass with signal intensity equivalent to that of breast parenchyma.

c IR T2w slice image (left breast): intermediate signal intensity. The image gives the impression that the lesion may have internal septations.

d Early subtraction slice image (left breast): round, relatively well-circumscribed mass lesion with inhomogeneous enhancement.

e TIC: early peak with pronounced postinitial washout.

Histology: IDC (pT1b).

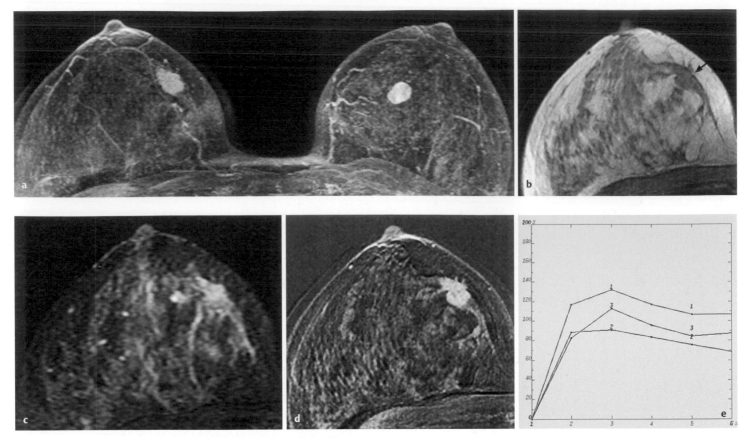

Fig. 12.4a–e Invasive ductal carcinoma (pT2) and fibroadenoma.

a Subtraction MIP: bilateral hypervascularized lesions. *Right lesion*: 12 mm, lobulated, relatively well-circumscribed lesion with inhomogeneous enhancement (carcinoma). *Left lesion*: 10 mm, oval lesion with inhomogeneous enhancement (fibroadenoma).

b T1w precontrast slice image (right breast): vague, space-occupying lesion with signal intensity equivalent to that of breast parenchyma (arrow).

c IR T2w slice image (right breast): increased signal intensity.

d Early subtraction slice image (right breast): irregular, partially ill-defined, hypervascularized lesion.

e TIC: early peak with pronounced postinitial washout.

Histology: IDC (pT1c, right breast). Fibroadenoma (left breast).

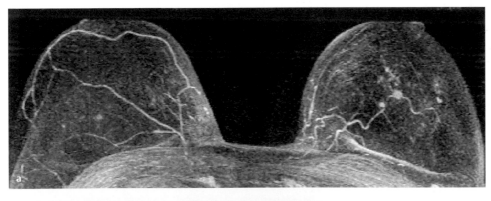

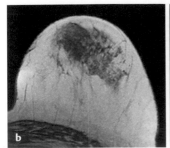
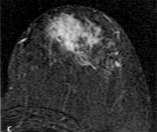
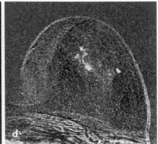

Fig. 12.5a–d Invasive ductal carcinoma with extensive intraductal component (EIC).

a Subtraction MIP: hypervascularized focus of 3 mm diameter in the center of the left breast. Adjacent linear-branching enhancement. Unremarkable findings in the right breast.

b T1w precontrast slice image (left breast): unremarkable findings.

c IR T2w slice image (left breast): unremarkable findings.

d Early subtraction slice image (left breast): Improved visualization of peritumoral ductal enhancement correlating to EIC. TICs are unspecific (not shown).

Histology: IDC (pT1a) + EIC.

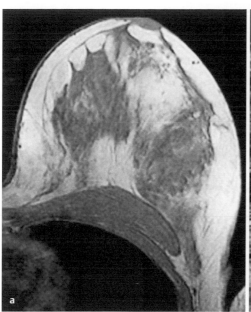
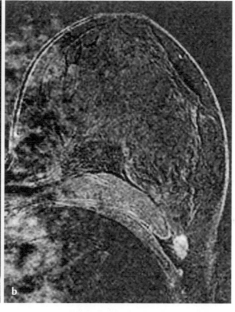

Fig. 12.6a, b   Invasive ductal carcinoma in a location that is easy to overlook.

a T1w precontrast slice image (left breast): presumptive extension of breast parenchymal body far into the axillary tail.

b Early subtraction slice image with swapped phase-encoding gradient (left breast): now discernible, oval, ill-defined lesion with accentuated enhancement in the periphery of the lesion. Dynamic examination was performed using the zebra protocol (see Chapter 3) for better assessment of the lateral breast aspects.

Histology: IDC (pT1c).

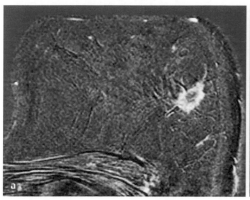
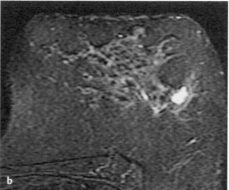

Fig. 12.7a, b   Invasive ductal carcinoma with rim-enhancement.

a Early subtraction slice image (left breast): classical breast carcinoma with ill-defined borders, rim-enhancement, and peritumoral linear extensions as an indication of concomitant EIC.

b IR T2w slice image (left breast): pronounced necrosis in tumor center with high signal intensity equivalent to that of a cyst.

Histology: IDC (pT1c).

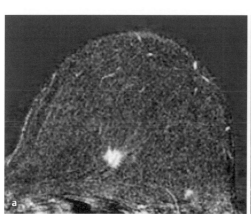
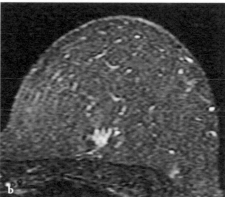

Fig. 12.8a, b   Invasive ductal carcinoma with high water content.

a Early subtraction slice image (left breast): hypervascularized, spiculated breast carcinoma.

b IR T2w slice image (left breast): high signal intensity of the entire tumor matrix.

Histology: IDC (pT1b).

Invasive Lobular Carcinoma

Synonym: infiltrating lobular carcinoma.

Invasive lobular carcinoma (ILC) is characterized histologically by a desmoplastic stromal reaction. Tumor cells are small, monomorphic, and round, and grow in a single-file ("Indian-file") or targetoid pattern encircling ducts that are dispersed throughout the fibrous matrix. Some tumors contain so-called "signet ring cells" (tumor cells with central mucoid globules) in addition to the small cells. Growth patterns are differentiated into diffuse and nodular types.

!Invasive lobular carcinomas (ILC) with a diffuse growth pattern have the greatest false-negative detection rate in all breast imaging techniques.

 MR Mammography: Invasive Lobular Carcinoma

T1-Weighted Sequence (Precontrast)

Diffuse type. When located in lipomatous areas of the breast: linear-streaky, isointense architectural distortion that respects the fat lamellae and is not space-occupying (**Figs. 12.9b, 12.10b, 12.11b, 12.12b**). No characteristic changes when located within the breast parenchyma.

Nodular type. When located in lipomatous areas of the breast: nodular, an isointense lesion (**Fig. 12.14b**). When located within breast parenchyma, often unremarkable findings (**Figs. 12.15b, 12.16b**).

T2-Weighted Sequence

Typically intermediate or slightly decreased signal intensity in comparison to the surrounding breast parenchyma (**Figs. 12.15c, 12.16c**). Occasional hyperintense zone of peritumoral edema (**Fig. 12.13c**).

T1-Weighted Sequence (Contrast Enhanced)

Diffuse type. Nonmasslike lesion that respects the fat tissue boundaries and displays a linear-streaky, sometimes "Indian-file" enhancement (**Figs. 12.9c, 12.10c, 12.11c, 12.12d**). Enhancement pattern correlates with histology and the often very discrete morphological changes seen on mammography (**Figs. 12.9a, 12.10a, 12.11a**). It is not advisable to generate TICs. The ROIs always include nontumor, lipomatous areas, producing TICs that may be misleading.

Nodular type. The nodular type of ILC displays the same features as an IDC: hypervascularized focus (**Fig. 12.14a, d**) or mass, most often with ill-defined borders (**Fig. 12.15a, d**) and rim-enhancement (**Fig. 12.16a, d**). TIC shows intermediate or rapid initial signal increase, often with postinitial plateau or washout.

Invasive lobular carcinoma: General information

Incidence:	Second most common form of invasive breast cancer (10%–15%).
Age peak:	All ages, peak between 40th and 60th years.
Grading:	*Histological grade*: well-differentiated (G1), intermediate (G2), poorly differentiated (G3).
Prognosis:	Dependent upon size, grading, N-stage, and receptor status among other factors.
Multicentricity:	>20%.
Multifocality:	10%–20%.
Coincidence:	Association with LCIS or ADH.

Findings

Clinical:	Often clinically occult.
	Tumors with large volume may cause palpable firmness.
	Nodular types may present as palpable mass.
Mammography:	*Diffuse type*: architectural distortion, localized changes in parenchymal density, structural irregularities. Rarely tumor-associated microcalcifications (<10%).
	Nodular type: may show more typical signs of malignancy. Often focal, ill-defined hyperdensity.
	Detection rate is higher when located in lipomatous breast areas than within dense parenchyma.
Ultrasonography:	*Diffuse type*: often no specific changes. Occasionally diffuse echo-alterations with multiple fine posterior acoustic shadowings.
	Nodular type: focal lesions with typical characteristics of malignancy.

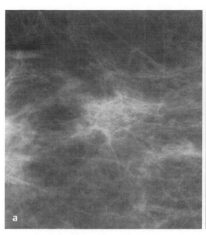
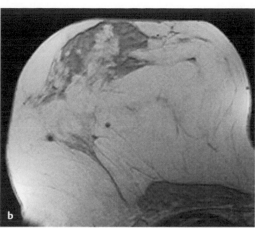
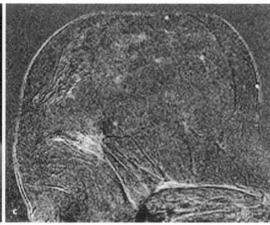

Fig. 12.9a–c   Invasive lobular carcinoma, diffuse type.
a Enlarged detail mammography image: typical nonmass density.
b T1w precontrast slice image (right breast): susceptibility artifacts due to prior surgery. Vague linear-streaky area within lipomatous breast tissue.

c Early subtraction slice image (right breast): regional, linear non-masslike enhancement.

Histology: ILC (pT1c).

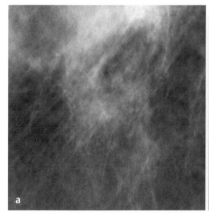
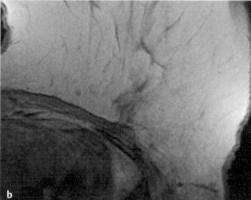
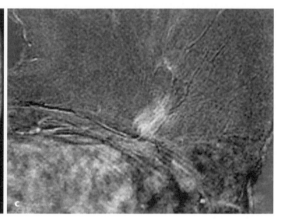

Fig. 12.10a–c   Invasive lobular carcinoma, diffuse type.
a Enlarged detail of mammography (Mx) image: localized architectural distortion (nonmasslike lesion).
b T1w precontrast slice image (left breast): linear-streaky, nonlipomatous area corresponding to mammography.

c Early subtraction slice image (left breast): Regional, linear non-masslike enhancement excluding the lipomatous areas.

Histology: ILC (pT1c).

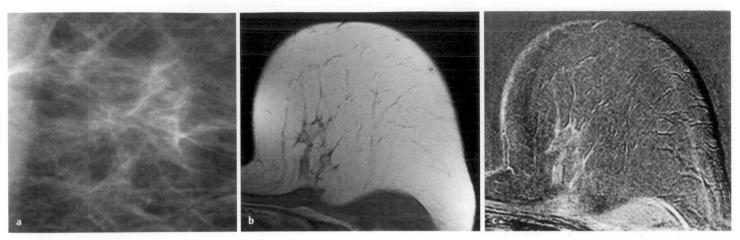

Fig. 12.11 a–c   Invasive lobular carcinoma, diffuse type.
a Enlarged detail of mammography (Mx) image: localized architectural distortion (nonmasslike lesion).
b T1w precontrast slice image (left breast): nonlipomatous, tissue streaks within lipomatous breast tissue.

c. Early subtraction slice image (left breast): linear nonmasslike enhancement ("Indian-file") excluding the lipomatous areas.

Histology: ILC (pT1c).

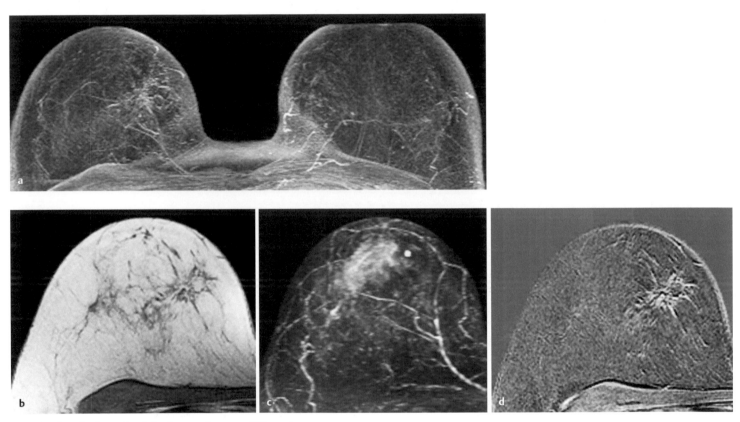

Fig. 12.12 a–d   Invasive lobular carcinoma, diffuse type.
a Subtraction MIP: reticular enhancement in the medial aspect of the right breast.
b T1w precontrast slice image (right breast): corresponding linear-branching architectural distortion within intramammary lipomatous tissue.
c IR T2w slice image (right breast): unremarkable findings in the medial aspect of the right breast.

d Early subtraction slice image (right breast): improved visualization of the nonmasslike, linear-branching enhancement which excludes the lipomatous areas. TICs are unspecific and not informative (not shown).

Histology: ILC (pT2).

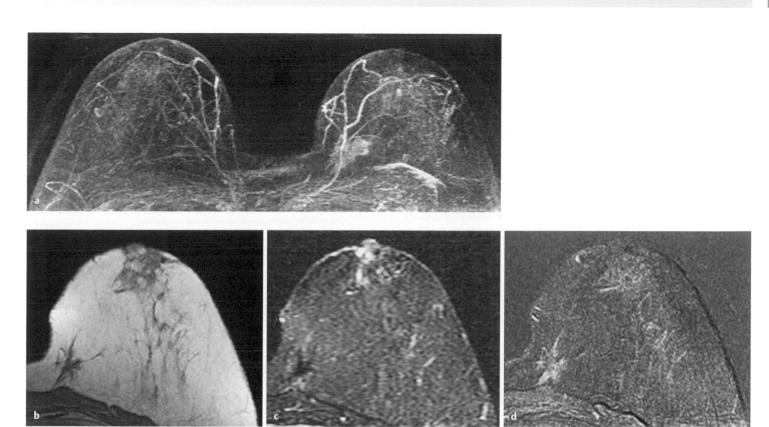

Fig. 12.13a–d Invasive lobular carcinoma, diffuse type.

a Subtraction MIP: irregular area of enhancement in the medial aspect of the left breast.

b T1w precontrast slice image (left breast): irregular shape is well-visualized within lipomatous tissue.

c IR T2w slice image (left breast): unusual signal suppression within the tumor in this fat-suppressed image. Slight peripheral edema.

d Early subtraction slice image (left breast): nonmasslike enhancement pattern within the tumor is evident. Topographical closeness to the chest wall. TICs are unspecific and not informative (not shown).

Histology: ILC (pT2).

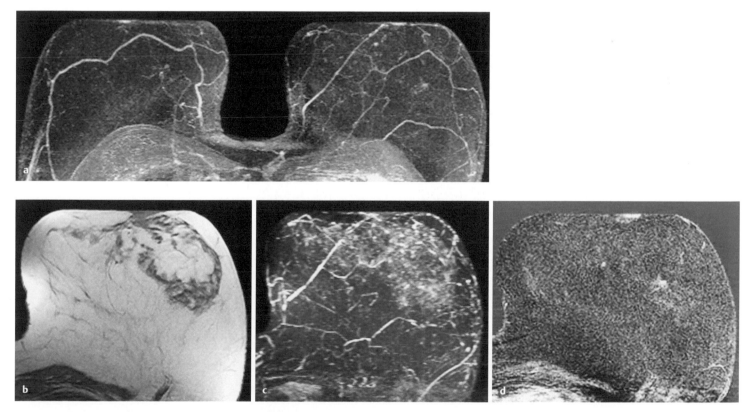

Fig. 12.14a–d Invasive lobular carcinoma, nodular type.

a Subtraction MIP: barely discernible focus in the centrolateral aspect of the left breast.

b T1w precontrast slice image (left breast): As expected, unremarkable findings.

c IR T2w slice image (left breast): Unremarkable findings.

d Early subtraction slice image (left breast): improved visualization of hypervascularized focus with fine-linear peritumoral enhancement. TICs are unspecific (not shown).

Histology: ILC (pT1a).

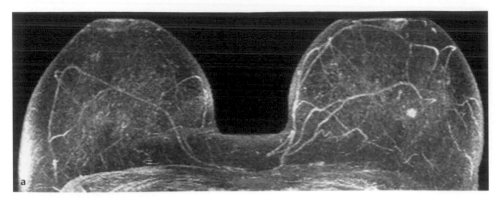

Fig. 12.15a–d Invasive lobular carcinoma, nodular type.
a Subtraction MIP: ill-defined mass lesion of 5 mm diameter in the central aspect of the left breast.
b T1w precontrast slice image (left breast): unremarkable findings.
c IR T2w slice image (left breast): no correlating tumor findings.
d Early subtraction slice image (left breast): improved visualization of the lobulated, hypervascularized mass lesion with possible internal septations. TICs are unspecific with initial increase > 100% and postinitial plateau (not shown).

Histology: ILC (pT1b).

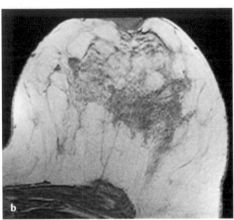
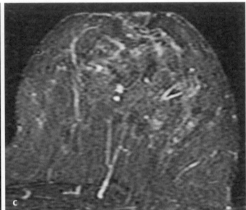
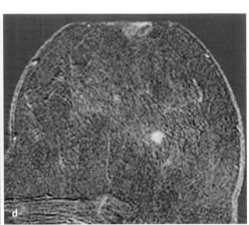

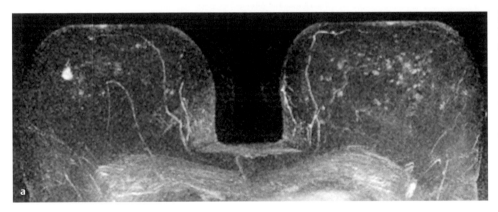

Fig. 12.16a–d Invasive lobular carcinoma, nodular type.
a Subtraction MIP: lobulated, partially ill-defined mass lesion of 7 mm diameter in the right breast. Multiple harmless foci in the left breast.
b T1w precontrast slice image (right breast): unremarkable findings.
c IR T2w slice image (right breast): unremarkable findings.
d Early subtraction slice image (right breast): improved visualization of the ill-defined borders and rim-enhancement (decreased perfusion in tumor center). TICs are unspecific with initial increase 80% and postinitial plateau (not shown).

Histology: ILC (pT1b).

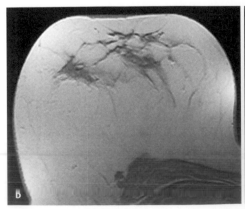
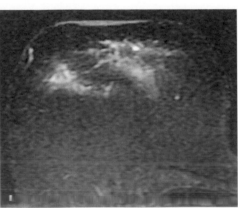
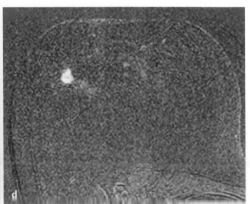

Medullary Carcinoma

The histopathological features that define the *typical form of medullary carcinoma* are a tendency for tumor cells to grow in broad sheets without distinct cell borders (syncytial growth), high nuclear grade (pleomorphic nuclei with prominent nucleoli, usually accompanied by numerous mitotic figures), well-circumscribed tumor margins, and an intense lymphoplasmacytic reaction around and within the tumor. Carcinomas that have most, but not all, of these microscopic features are referred to as *atypical medullary carcinomas*. The median size of medullary carcinomas is 2–3 cm. Lesions larger than 5 cm tend to show central tumor necrosis and calcification.

 MR Mammography: Medullary Carcinoma

T1-Weighted Sequence (Precontrast)
Round, oval, or lobulated, well-circumscribed (**Fig. 12.17b**) or partially ill-defined (**Fig. 12.18b**), isointense or hypointense mass. Difficult to detect when located within breast parenchyma.

T2-Weighted Sequence
Signal intensity is occasionally intermediate (**Fig. 12.18c**), often increased (**Fig. 12.17c**) relative to breast parenchyma. Occasional peritumoral hyperintense edematous zone (**Figs. 12.17c, 12.18c**).

T1-Weighted Sequence (Contrast Enhanced)
Enhancement typical of malignancy. Often round, oval, or lobulated mass. Boundaries are often partially well-circumscribed, but are almost always partially ill-defined (**Fig. 12.17 d**) and/or microlobulated (**Fig. 12.18 d**). Rim-enhancement is rare. TIC analysis shows an intermediate, more often a rapid initial signal increase (**Figs. 12.17e, 12.18e**). A slow initial increase is very rare. The postinitial signal course often displays a washout (**Figs. 12.17e, 12.18e**). A postinitial persistent signal increase is very rare.

Medullary carcinoma: General information

Incidence:	Rare; ~1% of all breast cancers. Often associated with *BRCA1* gene mutations.
Age peak:	All ages. Usually under 50 years, common under 35 years.
Prognosis:	*Typical form*: more favorable than that of invasive ductal carcinoma. *Atypical form*: identical with that of invasive ductal carcinoma.

Findings

Clinical:	Small tumors are clinically occult.
	Larger tumors are often well-circumscribed masses.
Mammography:	Tumors located within dense parenchyma are often mammographically occult.
	Good detection of tumors located within lipomatous breast tissue.
	Rare microcalcifications. Larger tumors appear as well-circumscribed, round or lobulated mass lesions.
	Occasionally ill-defined borders due to lymphocytic infiltrates.
Ultrasonography:	Small tumors are sonographically occult.
	Larger tumors appear round, well-circumscribed, and hypoechoic.

Because the typical appearance of a medullary breast carcinoma can make it difficult to differentiate from a benign breast mass lesion (e.g., fibroadenoma), it has a special significance in breast cancer diagnostics. Along with the mucinous carcinomas, medullary carcinomas are unlike other carcinomas in their tendency to have a high endotumoral water content (T2w signal).

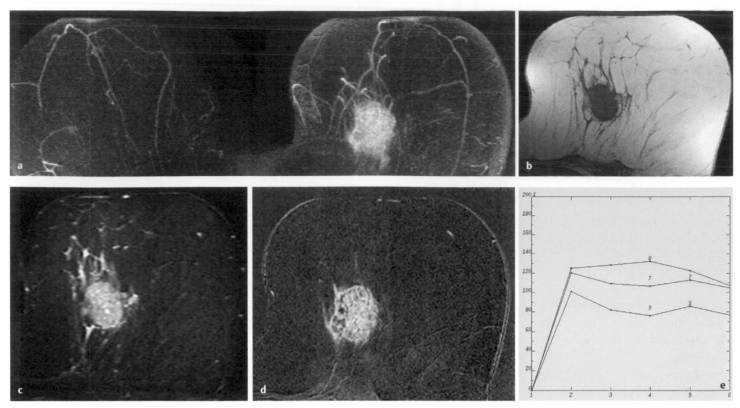

Fig. 12.17a–e   Medullary carcinoma.

a Subtraction MIP: large oval tumor in the left breast.

b T1w precontrast slice image (left breast): round, predominantly well-circumscribed mass.

c IR T2w slice image (left breast): high signal intensity of the entire lesion with punctate areas of very high signal intensity. Peritumoral edema.

d Early subtraction slice image (left breast): improved visualization of the partially ill-defined borders and very inhomogeneous enhancement.

e TIC: early peak with postinitial washout.

Histology: medullary carcinoma (pT2).

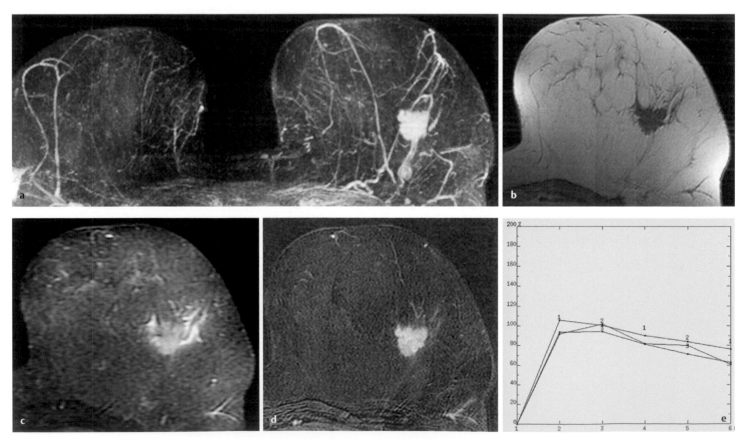

Fig. 12.18a–e   Medullary carcinoma.

a Subtraction MIP: large lobulated tumor with hypervascularized intramammary lymph node in the left breast. Unremarkable findings in the right breast.

b T1w precontrast slice image (left breast): lobulated, ill-defined mass.

c IR T2w slice image (left breast): intermediate endotumoral signal intensity. Very high peritumoral signal intensity.

d Early subtraction slice image (left breast): improved visualization of the lobulated, partially ill-defined, partially microlobulated tumor.

e TIC: early peak with postinitial washout. Typical of malignancy.

Histology: medullary carcinoma (pT2, pN1).

Mucinous Carcinoma

Synonyms: gelatinous carcinoma.

The histopathological characteristic that defines the *typical form of mucinous carcinoma* is the presence of islandlike clusters of small tumor cells floating in lakes of extracellular mucin, which makes up at least 90% of the tumor volume. Calcifications are rarely found. The *atypical or mixed variant of mucinous carcinoma* is regarded as a variant of a ductal or otherwise differentiated carcinoma with a lower proportion of mucinous secretion (75%–90% of tumor volume).

 MR Mammography: Mucinous Carcinoma

T1-Weighted Sequence (Precontrast)
Often no demarcation when located within breast parenchyma. May show discretely reduced signal intensity in comparison with parenchyma due to its high endotumoral water content (**Fig. 12.20b**). When located within lipomatous tissues, seen as a round, oval, or lobulated mass with well-circumscribed, partially ill-defined, or microlobulated borders (**Fig. 12.19a**).

T2-Weighted Sequence
Signal intensity is often increased due to the mucinous component (**Figs. 12.19b, 12.20c**).

T1-Weighted Sequence (Contrast Enhanced)
Hypervascularized round, oval (**Fig. 12.20d**), or lobulated mass (**Fig. 12.19c**). Generally well-circumscribed or microlobulated. Rim-enhancement is very rare. TIC analysis frequently shows a very strong initial signal increase (may reach values >200%). Occasionally the initial signal increase may be intermediate. The postinitial signal course usually displays a plateau. A postinitial washout is less frequent. A persistent signal increase in the post-initial phase is very rare.

Caution: Cases of mucinous carcinomas without contrast enhancement do exist (probably those with extremely high mucinous component).

Mucinous carcinoma: General information

Incidence:	Rare breast tumor (~1%–4% of all breast cancers).
Age peak:	All ages. Usually older women.
Prognosis:	*Typical form*: favorable prognosis.
	Atypical form: identical with that of invasive ductal carcinoma.

Findings

Clinical:	Small tumors are clinically occult.
	Larger tumors are often well-circumscribed masses.
Mammography:	Tumors located within dense parenchyma are often mammographically occult.
	Good detection of tumors located within lipomatous breast tissue.
	Rare microcalcifications. Larger tumors appear as well-circumscribed, round or lobulated mass lesions.
	Occasionally ill-defined or microlobulated borders.
Ultrasonography:	Small tumors are sonographically occult.
	Larger tumors are often round lesions with well-circumscribed, partially ill-defined, or microlobulated borders.
	Internal echotexture is usually hyperechoic, occasionally iso- or hypoechoic.

Mucinous carcinomas have a relatively good prognosis that depends on the degree of extracellular mucin. Along with the medullary carcinomas, mucinous carcinomas tend to have a high endotumoral water content (T2w signal).

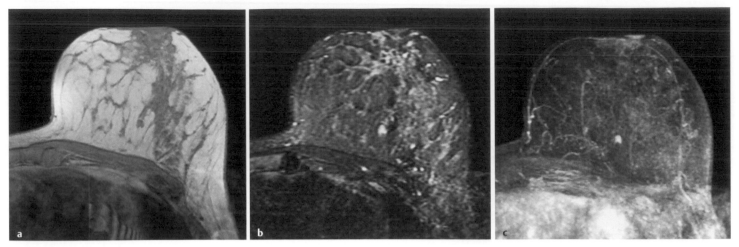

Fig. 12.19a–c Mucinous carcinoma.

a T1w precontrast slice image (left breast): lobulated, isointense mass of 4 mm diameter located within lipomatous tissue.

b IR T2w slice image (left breast): lesion displays high signal intensity.

c Early subtraction slice image (left breast): lobulated, hypervascularized tumor. TICs are unspecific (not shown).

Histology: mucinous carcinoma (pT1a).

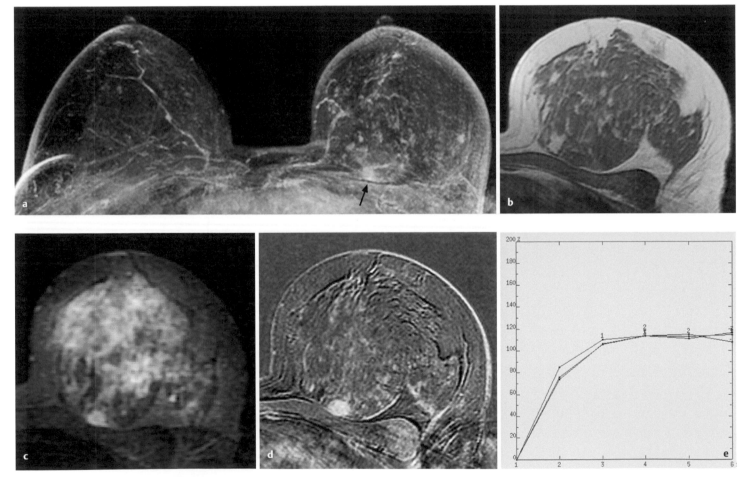

Fig. 12.20a–e Mucinous carcinoma.

a Subtraction MIP: vague hypervascularized mass lesion near the chest wall of the left breast (arrow).

b T1w precontrast slice image (left breast): with knowledge of the lesion, a vague oval mass lesion with slightly hypointense signal can be seen.

c IR T2w slice image (left breast): increased signal intensity with peripheral accentuation.

d Early subtraction slice image (left breast): oval tumor with inhomogeneous enhancement.

e TIC: Unspecific.

Histology: mucinous carcinoma (pT1c).

Invasive Papillary Carcinoma

The term *invasive papillary carcinoma* is used to describe carcinomas that have a frond-forming microscopic growth pattern. In addition, these lesions often have a cystic component. Invasive papillary carcinomas can arise in benign papillomas. *Intracystic papillary carcinomas*, which correspond to in-situ carcinomas, and *intraductal papillary carcinomas*, which are a subgroup of DCIS, must be differentiated from invasive papillary carcinomas.

 MR Mammography: Invasive Papillary Carcinoma

T1-Weighted Sequence (Precontrast)

Often no demarcation when located within breast parenchyma. When located within lipomatous breast tissue: usually a round, oval, or often lobulated (**Fig. 12.21 b**), isointense or hypointense mass lesion with well-circumscribed or predominantly well-circumscribed borders (**Fig. 12.22 b**). Location usually in the retroareolar (**Fig. 12.21 b**) or central (**Fig. 12.22 b**) region of the breast.

T2-Weighted Sequence

Intermediate (**Fig. 12.22 c**) or increased (**Fig. 12.21 c**) signal intensity.

T1-Weighted Sequence (Contrast Enhanced)

Round, oval, or often lobulated mass lesion with well-circumscribed or predominantly well-circumscribed borders (**Figs. 12.21 a, d, 12.22 a, d**). TIC analysis usually shows an intermediate or rapid initial signal increase. The postinitial signal course displays a plateau or washout (**Fig. 12.21 e, 12.22 e**). Rim-enhancement is rare.

Invasive papillary carcinoma: General information

Incidence:	Rare; <2% of all breast cancers.
Age peak:	60–65 years.
Prognosis:	5-year survival rate is 90%, better than that of invasive ductal carcinoma.

Findings	
Clinical:	Rare presentation as palpable subareolar nodule, bloody nipple discharge and/or nipple retraction.
Mammography:	Ill-defined, usually lobulated lesion. Rarely asymmetric density in the retroareolar region. Rarely associated with microcalcifications.
Ultrasonography:	Ill-defined, hypoechoic or anechoic lesion with hyperechoic wall. Central or peripheral posterior shadowing.

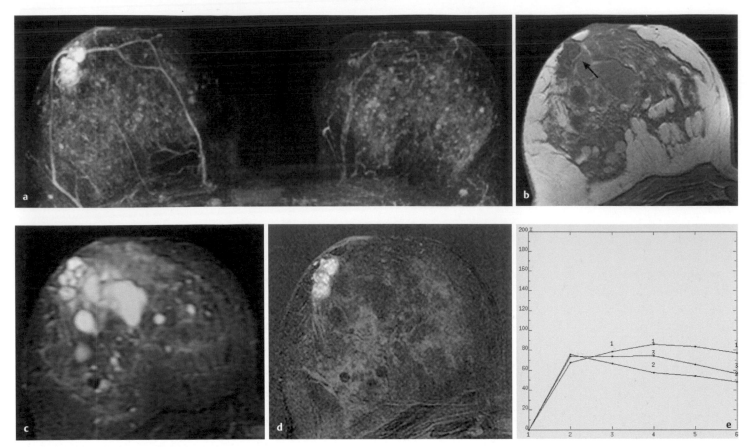

Fig. 12.21 a–e   Invasive papillary carcinoma.

a Subtraction MIP: conglomerate of several hypervascularized mass lesions in the retroareolar region of the right breast. Bilateral foci.

b T1w precontrast slice image (right breast): corresponding isointense findings in the subcutaneous fat tissue near the areola.

c IR T2w slice image (right breast): increased signal intensity of papillary tumor with internal septations. Pronounced fibrocystic changes with several macrocysts.

d Early subtraction slice image (right breast): improved visualization of the lobulated, well-circumscribed lesion with inhomogeneous enhancement and possible internal septations.

e TIC: suspicious for malignancy.

Histology: extensive papilloma with minimally invasive, unifocal carcinoma (pTmic).

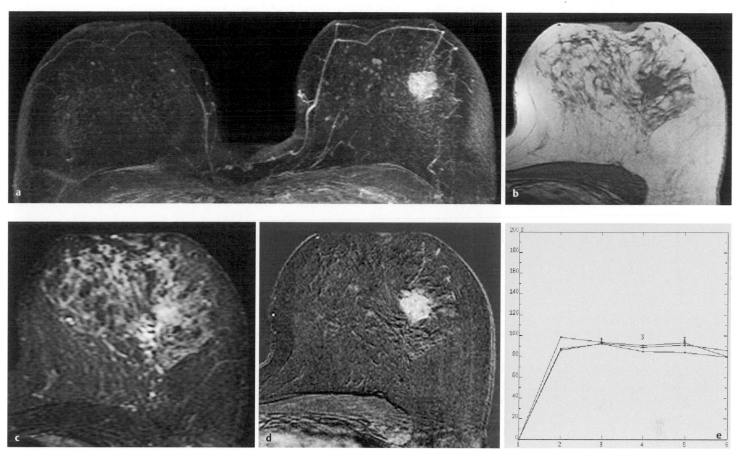

Fig. 12.22a–e Invasive papillary carcinoma.

a Subtraction MIP: large lobulated hypervascularized mass lesions in the central region of the left breast. Unremarkable findings in the right breast.

b T1w precontrast slice image (left breast): corresponding isointense, space-occupying lesion in the lipomatous breast tissue.

c IR T2w slice image (left breast): slightly increased endotumoral signal intensity.

d Early subtraction slice image (left breast): lobulated lesion with inhomogeneous enhancement.

e TIC: slight postinitial washout.

Histology: invasive papillary carcinoma (pT2).

Tubular Carcinoma

The typical *tubular carcinoma* is characterized by a proliferation of well-differentiated, often angular or branching tubular neoplastic elements resembling normal breast ductules. These are lined by a single layer of cuboid epithelium. Flat epithelial atypia is usually present. At least 90% of the tumor must have a tubular growth pattern to qualify for this diagnosis. Tubular carcinoma is accompanied by a strong fibrotic and myxoid component. Tumor margins are often stellate. Microcalcifications are found in ~50% of cases. Tumors with tubular elements constituting less than 75% are referred to as *mixed tubular carcinomas*.

! Tubular carcinomas often arise in radial scars.

MR Mammography: Tubular Carcinoma

T1-Weighted Sequence (Precontrast)
Occasionally no demarcation when located within breast parenchyma. May appear as architectural distortion. When located within lipomatous breast tissue: stellate architectural distortion with small (**Fig. 12.23b**) or large (**Fig. 12.24b**) center.

T2-Weighted Sequence
Typically intermediate (**Fig. 12.23c**) or decreased (**Fig. 12.24c**) signal intensity. Occasional hyperintense peritumoral edema.

T1-Weighted Sequence (Contrast Enhanced)
Stellate architectural distortion (**Fig. 12.23 d**) or spiculated mass (**Fig. 12.24 d**). Rim-enhancement is rare. TIC analysis is not informative. Because of the nonmasslike lesion characteristics, regions of interest (ROIs) always include nontumor, lipomatous areas producing TICs that are often unspecific.

Tubular carcinoma: General information

Incidence:	Rare; <2% of all breast cancers.
Age peak:	All ages. Peak between 40 and 50 years.
Prognosis:	Excellent for pure form.
	Less favorable when mixed with ductal carcinoma.

Findings

Clinical:	Small tumors are clinically occult.
	Larger tumors present as a palpable suspicious mass.
Mammography:	Often architectural distortion or stellate lesion with prominent spiculae, visible also when located within dense breast tissue. Microcalcifications in >50% of cases.
Ultrasonography:	Small tumors are sonographically occult.
	Larger tumors are seen as architectural distortions or ill-defined, hypoechoic lesions with posterior acoustic shadowing.

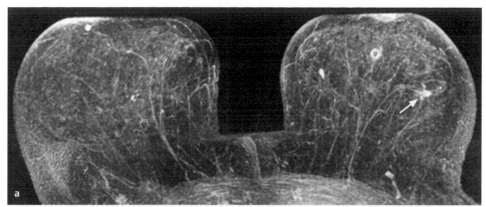
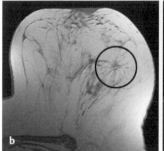
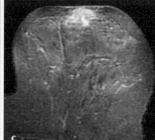
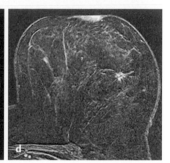

Fig. 12.23a–d Tubular carcinoma.
a Subtraction MIP: bilateral foci. Inflamed cyst in the retromamillary region of the left breast. Carcinoma in the lateral aspect of the left breast.
b T1w precontrast slice image (left breast): typical architectural distortion with lipomatous breast tissue in the lateral aspect of the left breast (circle).
c IR T2w slice image (left breast): intermediate signal intensity.
d Early subtraction slice image (left breast): improved visualization of the lesion's spiculations. TICs not informative (not shown).

Histology: tubular carcinoma (pT1b).

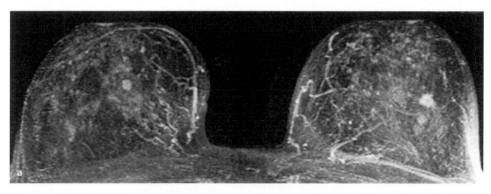
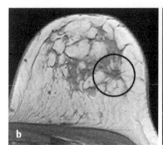
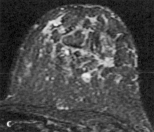
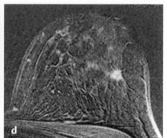

Fig. 12.24a–d Tubular carcinoma.
a Subtraction MIP: hypervascularized lesion in each breast. Carcinoma in the lateral aspect of the left breast.
b T1w precontrast slice image (left breast): typical architectural distortion with lipomatous breast tissue in the lateral aspect of the left parenchymal body (circle).
c IR T2w slice image (left breast): high signal intensity in the center of the carcinoma. No reproduction of the lesion's spiculations. Incidental cyst.
d Early subtraction slice image (left breast): spiculated mass lesion with rim-enhancement. Unspecific TICs (not shown).

Histology: tubular carcinoma (pT1c). Contralateral invasive ductal carcinoma.

Inflammatory Breast Cancer

Inflammatory breast cancer does not constitute a histological type but rather a clinical entity. Microscopically there is a diffuse infiltration of the skin and mammary tissue, usually by a poorly differentiated invasive/infiltrating ductal carcinoma (NOS). The striking clinical manifestation of inflammatory carcinoma is erythema and edema usually involving over one-third of the breast skin. In ~80% of cases, tumor cells are found within the dermal lymphatic channels.

> ! Inflammatory breast cancer is very difficult to distinguish from nonpuerperal mastitis clinically, as well as with breast imaging techniques. Skin biopsy or open surgery is, therefore, one of the first diagnostic procedures performed to make this distinction.

MR Mammography: Inflammatory Breast Cancer

T1-Weighted Sequence (Precontrast)
Asymmetric skin thickening (**Fig. 12.25b**). If intramammary tumor mass is present, it shows criteria of invasive breast cancer (**Fig. 12.25b**).

T2-Weighted Sequence
Diffuse increase in signal intensity of the entire affected breast due to lymph imbibition (**Fig. 12.25a**). Lymphatic fluid-filled interstices are seen in a single-slice image. Skin thickening (**Fig. 12.25c**).

T1-Weighted Sequence (Contrast Enhanced)
Increased contrast enhancement of thickened skin (**Fig. 12.25d**). Diffuse, often only slight enhancement of all parenchymal structures. TIC analysis is often uninformative and of little value. Occasional documentation of primary carcinoma with characteristics typical of malignancy (**Fig. 12.25d**).

Occult inflammatory breast cancer. Diffuse breast cancer with pronounced lymph imbibition but no signs of inflammation is known as *occult inflammatory breast cancer (OIBC)*. OIBC is caused by a predominantly diffuse spread of cancer cells/tumor emboli in the lymphatic vessels with little or no tumor angiogenesis.

In breast MRI, contrast enhancement of the skin is typically missing (**Fig. 12.26a, e**). Relatively slight intramammary enhancement contradicts the pronounced findings in the T2-weighted sequence (**Fig. 12.26b, d**). If an intramammary tumor mass is present, it shows criteria of invasive breast cancer (**Fig. 12.26c, e**).

Inflammatory breast cancer: General information

Incidence:	Rare (1%–2% of all mammary carcinomas).
Age peak:	40–55 years.
Bilaterality:	High (reports up to 30%).
Prognosis:	Very poor. The most aggressive form of all mammary carcinomas.

Findings	
Clinical:	Erythema, edema, hyperthermia, pain. Diffusely increased firmness. Peau d'orange (enlarged skin pores). Cancer en cuirasse.
	Often with lymph node metastases.
Mammography:	Skin thickening. Increased density of parenchyma (note asymmetry!).
	Occasionally diffuse pleomorphic microcalcifications.
	Circumscribed intramammary mass seen only in one-third of cases.
Ultrasonography:	Skin thickening, interstitial fluid collections (note asymmetry).
	Axillary lymph nodes often metastasized.

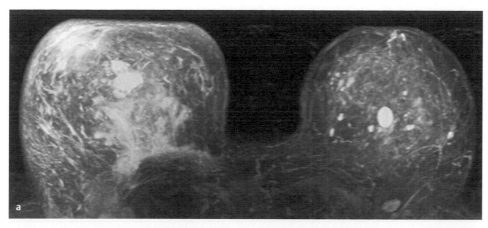
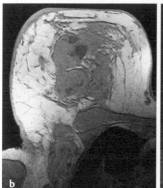
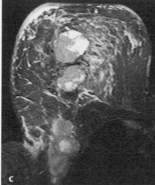
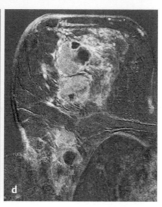

Fig. 12.25a–d   Inflammatory breast cancer.
a IR T2w MIP: pronounced inflammatory changes in the right breast—volume increase, skin thickening, and massive increase of fluid content.
b T1w precontrast slice image (right breast): skin thickening. Several tumor masses with central necrosis. Enlarged axillary lymph nodes.
c IR T2w slice image (right breast): tumor masses and lymph nodes show intermediate signal intensity. Necrotic tumor areas show high signal intensity. Skin thickening. Lymphatic fluid-filled interstices.
d Early subtraction slice image (right breast): pathological enhancement of tumor masses and lymph nodes with the exception of necrotic areas. Skin enhancement. TICs are dispensable for making diagnosis.

Histology: inflammatory breast cancer with lymph node metastases.

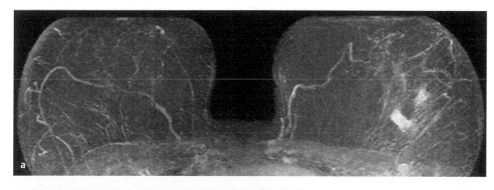
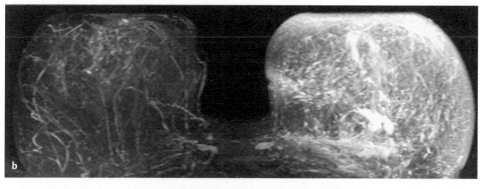
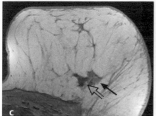
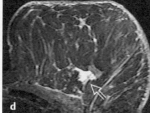
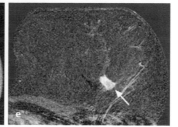

Fig. 12.26a–e   Occult inflammatory breast cancer.
a Subtraction MIP: hypervascularized carcinomas in the lateral aspect of the left breast. Discrete hypervascularization of adjacent breast tissue.
b IR T2w MIP: in contrast to the subtraction MIP, pronounced edematous changes and skin thickening in the left breast.
c T1w precontrast slice image (left breast): tumor mass (solid arrow) and fluid accumulation (open arrow). Skin thickening.
d IR T2w slice image (left breast): intermediate signal intensity of the tumor mass (ventral lesion). High signal intensity of fluid accumulation (open arrow). Skin thickening. Lymphatic fluid-filled interstices.
e Early subtraction slice image (left breast): pathological enhancement of tumor mass (white arrow) with rim-enhancement. No skin enhancement. No enhancement of retrotumoral fluid accumulation.

Diagnosis: occult inflammatory breast cancer. Biopsy of mass lesion confirmed carcinoma.

Paget Disease of the Nipple

Paget disease is considered a carcinoma in situ involving the nipple. Large, round or oval tumor cells, called *Paget cells*, are found singly or in aggregates within the epidermis of the nipple and may spread to the surrounding skin areas. In advanced stages, ulcerations—but not infiltration of the corium—can be seen. Paget disease of the nipple is typically associated with DCIS (60%) or invasive carcinoma (30%) of the breast.

 MR Mammography: Paget Disease of the Nipple

T1-Weighted Sequence (Precontrast)
Possible flattening and/or thickening of the mamillary region (**Fig. 12.27b**).

 Note: The nipples of large breasts may rest upon the ventral surface of the MRI breast coil and appear flattened (**Fig. 12.28b**).

T2-Weighted Sequence
No characteristic signal changes. Usually does not provide additional diagnostic information (**Figs. 12.27c, 12.28c**).

T1-Weighted Sequence (Contrast Enhanced)
Usually unspecific enhancement of the mamilla and mamillary region that cannot be differentiated from normal findings (**Figs. 12.27d, 12.28d**). Occasional findings indicating intramammary DCIS (**Fig. 12.28a, d**) or invasive carcinoma. TICs usually do not provide additional diagnostic information and are therefore dispensable (**Figs. 12.27e**).

Paget disease of the nipple: General information

Incidence:	Rare; ~2% of all mammary carcinomas.
Age peak:	All ages. Peak between 40 and 60 years.
Prognosis:	Usually good (depending on intramammary manifestation).
Lymph node involvement:	3%–5%.

Findings

Clinical:	Nonhealing eczematoid changes of the nipple and/or areola.
	Palpable mass in ~60% of cases.
Mammography:	Occasional flattening or thickening of nipple region, retromamillary density.
	Retroareolar microcalcifications in ~50% of cases. Occasionally findings typical of intramammary invasive cancer.
Ultrasonography:	Rarely diagnostically relevant findings.

The primary differential diagnoses of Paget disease are dermatological diseases. Confirmation of Paget disease of the nipple may be achieved by exfoliative cytology or skin biopsy.

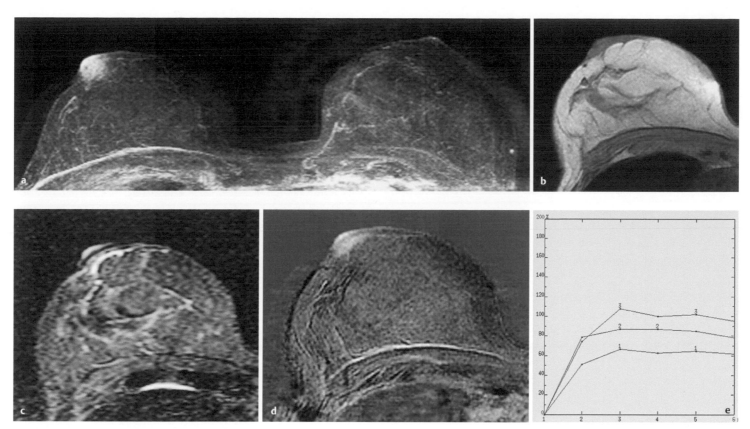

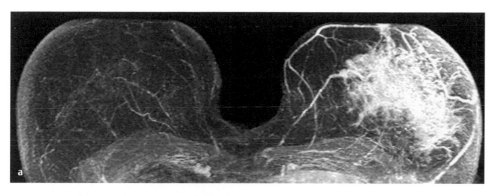

Fig. 12.27 a–e   Paget disease of the nipple.

a Subtraction MIP: asymmetric hypervascularization of the right nipple and surrounding area. Otherwise unremarkable findings.

b T1 w precontrast slice image (right breast): the right nipple appears to be laterally inclined. Otherwise no specific changes.

c IR T2 w slice image (right breast): unremarkable findings.

d Early subtraction slice image (right breast): hypervascularization of the right nipple. No pathological enhancement in the retromamillary region.

e TIC: unspecific.

Histology: Paget disease of the nipple.

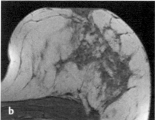
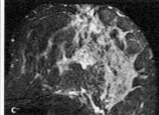
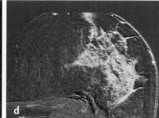

Fig. 12.28 a–d   Paget disease of the nipple.

a IR T2 w MIP: diffuse enhancement of the entire left breast, including the nipple.

b T1 w precontrast slice image (left breast): no specific changes. Nipple flattening is due to the large breast resting on the ventral surface of the MRI breast coil.

c IR T2 w slice image (left breast): no specific changes.

d Early subtraction slice image (left breast): pathological nonmasslike enhancement of all nonlipomatous breast tissues. An enhancing bridge connects the parenchymal body with the strongly enhancing nipple. TICs are unspecific and uninformative (not shown).

Histology: Paget disease of the nipple and DCIS throughout entire left breast.

Malignant Phyllodes Tumor

Synonyms: phyllodes tumor, malignant cystosarcoma phyllodes.

The phyllodes tumor is a distinctive fibroepithelial tumor that is only found within the breast. The malignant form of this tumor is characterized by its high mitotic activity (>5 mitoses/10 HPF), cellular atypia, a dominant stromal component, and a tumor growth pattern that infiltrates the surrounding tissue. The tumor stroma shows a predominantly sarcomatous differentiation. In addition, tumors may show signs of hemorrhage and ulcerations.

 MR Mammography: Malignant Phyllodes Tumor

T1-Weighted Sequence (Precontrast)
Well-circumscribed, round or lobulated, isointense lesion without pseudocapsular demarcation. Signal intensity lower than or equivalent to that of parenchyma. Occasional documentation of round, hypointense inclusions corresponding to cystic or necrotic areas.

T2-Weighted Sequence
Well-circumscribed, round or lobulated lesion with isointense to slightly hyperintense signal intensity. Occasional documentation of rounded inclusions with hyperintense signal corresponding to cystic or necrotic areas.

T1-Weighted Sequence (Contrast Enhanced)
Strong contrast enhancement within solid tumor portions. In the course of the examination, increasing demarcation of existing cystic or necrotic areas. Initial signal increase is usually 100% or more. Postinitial signal usually shows continuous increase or a plateau. When no liquid inclusions are present, differentiation from a fibroadenoma is not possible.

> **!** Breast MRI does not allow reliable differentiation between benign and malignant phyllodes tumors.

Malignant phyllodes tumor: General information

Incidence:	Rare; ~0.2% of all breast malignancies.
Age peak:	40–60 years.
Metastasis:	In 20% hematogenous. Rarely lymphogenous.

Findings

Clinical:	Rapidly growing, smooth or tuberous mass; can reach >10 cm in diameter.
	Large tumors may cause skin changes (thinning and/or livid discoloration).
Mammography:	Homogeneous, round, oval, or lobulated tumor (similar to fibroadenoma). Occasional halo sign due to compression of surrounding tissue.
	Rarely contains micro- or macrocalcifications.
Ultrasonography:	Well-circumscribed, round or lobulated lesion with posterior acoustic enhancement.
	Cystic inclusions are diagnostic substantiation.

The differential diagnosis between a phyllodes tumor and a fibroadenoma or a hamartoma is occasionally difficult. Indicative for a phyllodes tumor are the patient's age, rapid growth, and the documentation of cystic inclusions.

Sarcoma

Breast sarcomas originate in the periductal or perilobular stroma. In conformity with the manifestations of primary malignant mesenchymal tumors in other soft tissues, they are a heterogeneous histological group. The most common type is the malignant fibrous histiocytoma. Angiosarcomas are seen less frequently. In rare cases, sarcomas may occur as a consequence of radiotherapy (as fibrosarcoma, malignant fibrous histiocytoma, liposarcoma, leiomyosarcoma, chondrosarcoma, or angiosarcoma).

 MR Mammography: Sarcoma

T1-Weighted Sequence (Precontrast)
Usually well-circumscribed, isointense or hypointense lesion without pseudocapsular demarcation (**Fig. 12.29 b**).

T2-Weighted Sequence
Usually well-circumscribed, isointense or hyperintense lesion (**Fig. 12.29 c**).

T1-Weighted Sequence (Contrast Enhanced)
Well-circumscribed, round lesion with inhomogeneous contrast enhancement (**Fig. 12.29 a, d**). TIC analysis shows characteristics typical of malignancy (strong initial signal increase, postinitial plateau or washout). The general MRI impression is that of a fast-growing carcinoma (**Fig. 12.29 d**). Sarcomas display no characteristic, differentiating MRI-features.

Sarcoma: General information

Incidence:	Very rare (<1% of all malignant breast tumors).
Age peak:	All ages (mean age 30–40 years).
Prognosis:	Variable, depending on histology.
Bilaterality:	Extremely rare.

Findings

Clinical:	Painless, mobile, often fast-growing mass (at time of detection often 4–6 cm in diameter).
	Large tumors often cause skin changes (stretching, livid discoloring).
Mammography:	High density, usually well-circumscribed, occasionally lobulated mass.
	Osteosarcomas display endotumoral bony trabecular structures. Otherwise no characteristic features.
Ultrasonography:	Usually well-circumscribed, occasionally lobulated, hypoechoic mass. Otherwise no characteristic features.

Because breast sarcomas occur very rarely, they are of little clinical significance.

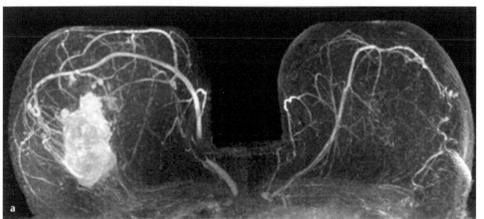

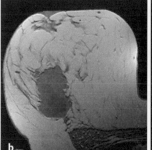
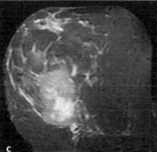
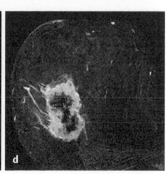

Fig. 12.29 a–d   Sarcoma of the breast.
a Subtraction MIP: large lobulated tumor in the right breast.
b T1 w precontrast slice image (right breast): lobulated, partially well-circumscribed, partially spiculated lesion; isointense lesion with hypointense inclusion.
c IR T2 w slice image (right breast): intermediate internal signal intensity of proliferating tumor areas. High signal intensity of necrotic areas.
d Early subtraction slice image (right breast): classic, pathological rim-enhancement (wide rim of proliferating tumor around necrotic tumor center).

Histology: carcinosarcoma of the breast (G4).

Triple-Negative Breast Cancer

Triple-negative breast cancer refers to any breast cancer that does not express the genes for estrogen receptor, progesterone receptor, or HER2/neu. This subtype of breast cancer is diagnosed more frequently in women with *BRCA1* mutations and those belonging to African American and Hispanic ethnic groups.

Triple-negative breast cancers often show special image characteristics and are therefore described separately in this section. Apparently due to their high cell proliferation rate, these tumors tend to display rim-enhancement more frequently than other breast cancers (**Figs. 12.30 d, 12.31 d**). This is sometimes seen as a very thin ring structure (**Fig. 12.30 e**). In addition, tumors displaying rim-enhancement also show significant (**Fig. 12.30 c**) or massive (**Fig. 12.31 c**) endotumoral T2w signal intensity increase, resulting from the liquefaction of central tumor necrosis associated with rapid tumor growth.

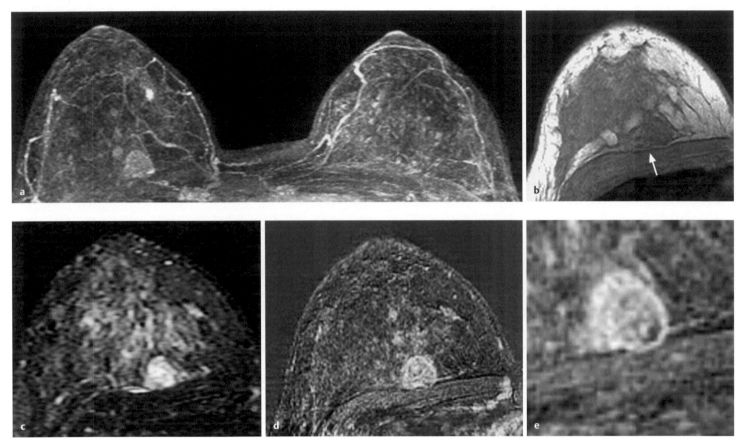

Fig. 12.30 a–e   Triple-negative breast cancer.
a Subtraction MIP: mild hypervascularization of triple-negative carcinoma near the chest wall of the right breast. Incidental finding: strongly hypervascularized fibroadenoma in the medial aspect of the right breast.
b T1w precontrast slice image (right breast): mass lesion isointense to normal tissue (arrow).
c IR T2w slice image (right breast): high endotumoral signal intensity (water content).

d Early subtraction slice image (right breast): rim-enhancement with inhomogeneous internal enhancement pattern.
e Zoomed subtraction slice image: improved visualization of thin rim-enhancement in the peripheral zone with increased proliferation.

Histology: invasive ductal carcinoma, G3, triple-negative.

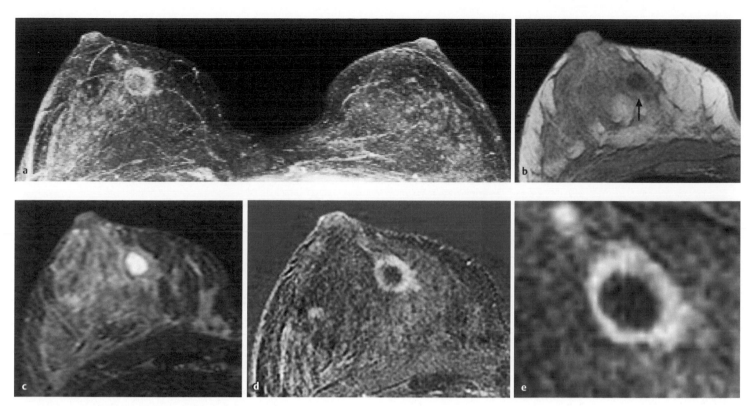

Fig. 12.31 a–e   Triple-negative breast cancer.

a Subtraction MIP: rim-enhancement of hypervascularized tumor in the medial aspect of the right breast. Additional signs indicating an EIC toward the nipple.

b T1w precontrast slice image (right breast): isointense mass lesion with hypointense center (arrow).

c IR T2w slice image (right breast): high, water-equivalent endotumoral signal intensity corresponding to the area of tumor necrosis.

d Early subtraction slice image (right breast): broad rim-enhancement without any central enhancement.

e Zoomed subtraction slice image: improved visualization of broad rim-enhancement in the peripheral zone of increased proliferation with relatively smooth demarcation from central necrosis.

Histology: invasive ductal carcinoma, G3, triple-negative.

Breast Carcinomas during Pregnancy and/or the Lactational Period

During pregnancy and the following lactational period, the female breast is subject to strong hormonal stimulation. When carcinomas of the breast develop during this period, they usually show a significantly increased proliferation rate (**Fig. 12.33**). Furthermore, this constellation is usually encountered in younger women who do not normally (yet) take part in a routine early detection program. As a consequence, these tumors are often very large at the time of detection (**Fig. 12.32**). In addition, the informative value of breast imaging during pregnancy and the lactational period is often very limited due to the density of parenchymal tissues and maximal hormonal stimulation. Of all imaging modalities, breast MRI usually offers the best estimation of a tumor's actual dimensions (**Fig. 12.34**).

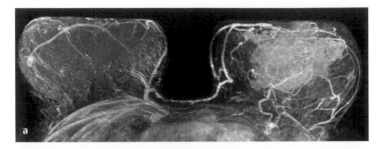
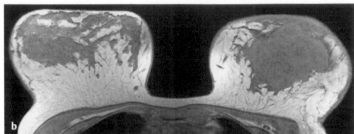
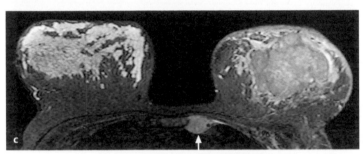
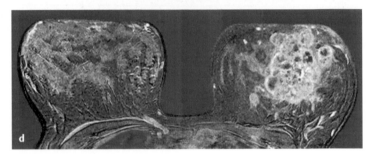

Fig. 12.32 a–d   Breast cancer in early pregnancy.
a Subtraction MIP: widespread carcinoma of the entire left breast.
b T1w precontrast slice image (left breast): enormous mass lesion isointense to normal tissue.
c IR T2w slice image (left breast): intermediate endotumoral signal intensity (water content). Enlarged internal mammaria lymph node (arrow) as a reliable sign of lymphogenous spread.

d Early subtraction slice image (left breast): multiple areas with rim-enhancement in tumor conglomerate.

Histology was verified before neoadjuvant chemotherapy.

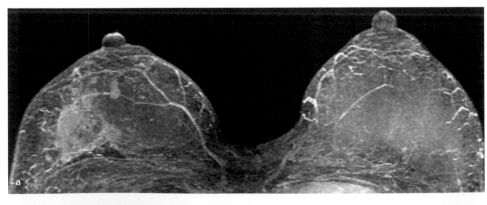
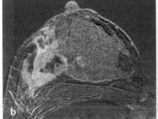
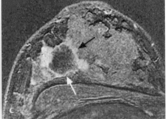
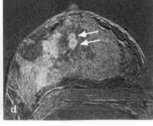

Fig. 12.33 a–d   Breast cancer during the lactational period.
a Subtraction MIP: normal homogeneous enhancement of the left breast. Primary enhancement of the extensive carcinoma in the lateral and central aspects of the right breast with steal phenomenon (lower enhancement of the normal right breast parenchyma in comparison with the left breast).
b Representative early subtraction slice image (right breast): signs of strongly increased proliferation.
c Representative early subtraction slice image (right breast): thin rim-enhancement (arrows).
d Representative early subtraction slice image (right breast): multiple tumor manifestations with typical n-enhancement despite small individual tumor sizes.

Histology was verified before neoadjuvant chemotherapy.

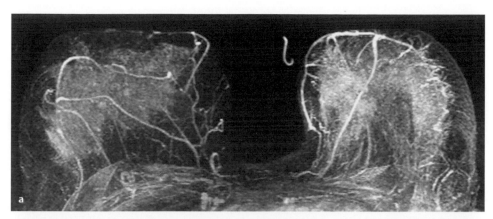

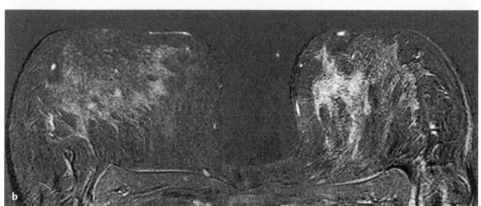

Fig. 12.34a, b Breast cancer during the lactational period.

a Subtraction MIP: strong early bilateral enhancement with asymmetry on the left side.

b Representative early subtraction slice image: stronger enhancement in the medial aspect of the left breast. Histological verification of breast cancer in this area.

Study Results

Breast MRI and invasive breast cancer. Invasive ductal carcinomas are the best-studied breast cancers in breast MRI. Results from different working groups have concurred for many years and document a sensitivity for this imaging method between 80% and 90% (**Table 12.1**). These results are even better and reach a sensitivity of >95% when using high-resolution MRI techniques and performing high-quality breast MRI examinations (**Table 12.1**). Poorer sensitivities reported in older studies are due to technical and methodical insufficiencies. In summary, breast MRI is the most sensitive method for the detection of invasive carcinomas.

Breast MRI exhibits an extremely high sensitivity (>95%) for the two most common forms of invasive breast cancer (IDC and ILC). X-ray mammography (Mx) and breast ultrasound (US) show a relatively good, albeit inferior, sensitivity for the detection of the usually nodular forms of IDC. The discrepancy between the sensitivity of these imaging methods is, however, much higher for the detection of ILC (**Table 12.2**). This is due to the difficulties encountered in the detection of nonmasslike lesions, the usual image correlate of ILC, in Mx and US.

The high diagnostic significance of breast MRI is especially obvious in the detection of small breast cancers up to a maximum of 10 mm in diameter (early detection). The sensitivity of the other imaging techniques in these cases is significantly inferior to that of breast MRI (**Table 12.3**).

! The excellent sensitivity of breast MRI in the detection of invasive breast carcinomas can only be achieved when MRI is performed in HR technique and with effective breast compression.

Table 12.1 Sensitivities of breast imaging techniques for the detection of invasive breast cancers

Author	Year	Cohort	Invasive breast cancers			
			Palpation	Mx	MRI	US
Kriege et al.[a]	2004	1909	17.9%	33.3%	79.5%	n.a.
Sardanelli	2004	99[b]	n.a.	72%	89%	n.a.
Fischer	2008	3750[a,c]	n.a.	72%	98%	61%

Mx: x-ray mammography. US: ultrasonography. n.a.: not applicable.
[a] High-risk cohort, average age 40 years.
[b] Mastectomy specimens with breast carcinomas.
[c] Early detection program, asymptomatic women, average age 53.7 years.

Table 12.2 Sensitivities of breast imaging techniques for the detection of IDC and ILC

Author	Year	Cohort	IDC			ILC		
			Mx	MRI	US	Mx	MRI	US
Berg et al.	2004	111	89%	95%	94%	34%	96%	86%

IDC: invasive ductal carcinoma. ILC: invasive lobular carcinoma. Mx: x-ray mammography. US: ultrasonography.

Table 12.3 Sensitivities of breast imaging techniques for the detection of small invasive breast cancers (diameter up to 10 mm, pT1a and pT1b)

Author	Year	Cohort	Invasive breast cancers			
			Palpation	Mx	MRI	US
Fischer et al.	2009	84[a]	16.5%	50.0%	94.4%	53.7%

Mx: x-ray mammography. US: ultrasonography.
[a] Carcinomas with histological stage pT1a and pT1b.

13 Lymph Node Diagnostics

Lymphogenous spread of breast cancer is most commonly to the axillary lymph nodes. Rarely, breast cancer may also spread to the internal mammary lymph nodes or, even more rarely, to intra-parenchymal lymph nodes.

> ! Breast imaging does not usually allow a reliable evaluation of metastatic tumor spread to local and regional lymph nodes.

 MR Mammography: Lymph Nodes

T1-Weighted Sequence (Precontrast)
Good demarcation when in typical locations in subcutaneous fat tissue. Lobulated (**Fig. 13.1 a**), oval (**Fig. 13.1 b**), or bean-shaped (**Fig. 13.1 c**), well-circumscribed, hypointense mass lesion. Lesions often display a central hyperintense area (fatty hilus) (**Fig. 13.1**). Rarely located within parenchyma, where the detection rate is reduced.

T2-Weighted Sequence
Often a hyperintense mass (**Fig. 13.2**). When using a fat-suppressed sequence (e.g., IR sequence), a central signal-free zone is the correlate of the lipomatous lymph node hilus (**Fig. 13.7 b**).

T1-Weighted Sequence (Contrast Enhanced)
Occasionally no or very little contrast enhancement within normal lymph nodes. Often reactive-inflammatory changes with increased peripheral perfusion (**Figs. 13.4 c**, **13.5 c**, **13.6 c**). No perfusion of lymph node hilus (**Fig. 13.5 c**). TIC usually shows intermediate or rapid initial signal increase and postinitial plateau or washout (**Fig. 13.3 d**).

Note: Lymph nodes with inflammatory changes and a fatty hilus may show findings resembling rim-enhancement (**Fig. 13.3 b, c**).

> ! The size of axillary lymph nodes is reliably well visualized in the T1w and T2w images. Images after contrast administration are often of limited informative value in these areas due to overlapping of phase-encoding gradients.

Lymph node locations. Axillary lymph nodes typically lie dorsal or lateral to the pectoral muscle (**Fig. 13.4**). Occasionally they lie in the prepectoral area (**Fig. 13.3**) or in the subcutaneous fat tissue lateral to the nipple (**Fig. 13.5**). Intramammary lymph nodes are typically found within the breast parenchyma (**Figs. 13.6, 13.10, 13.11**). Parasternal lymph nodes lie within the thorax along the internal mammary vessels (**Figs. 13.12, 13.13**).

> ! The detection of a fatty hilus within a mass is almost always confirmation of a lymph node. It is not, however, proof that the lymph node is free of metastatic tumor spread (**Fig. 13.7**).

Lymph node size and morphology. The average diameter of typical, normal axillary lymph nodes is 5–10 mm. Lymph nodes with reactive-inflammatory changes, however, can easily reach diameters of 15–20 mm. Displacement or complete disappearance of a lymph nodes fatty hilus can be an indication of metastatic spread. A lymph node size over 15–20 mm (**Fig. 13.9**), or disappearance of the typical bean shape with an increasingly rounded shape (**Figs. 13.8, 13.9**) are indications of possible metastatic spread. The threshold values for parasternal lymph nodes is lower (**Figs. 13.14, 13.15**).

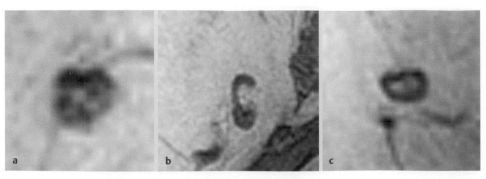

Fig. 13.1 a–c Normal lymph nodes. Normal-sized lymph nodes in T1w precontrast images showing typical increased signal in the node center due to fatty hilus.
a Round shape with lobulated borders.
b Oval shape.
c Bean shape.

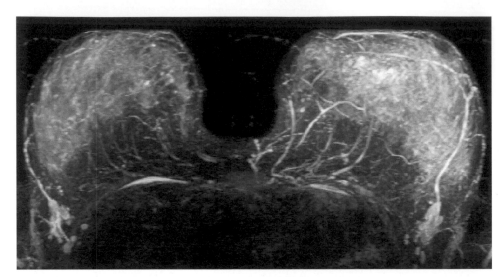

Fig. 13.2 Normal lymph node. Normal-sized axillary lymph nodes in fat-suppressed IR T2w MIP.

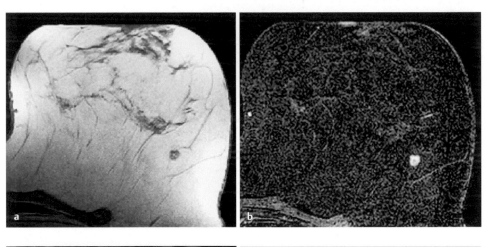

Fig. 13.3 a–d Lymph node with "rim-enhancement."
a T1w precontrast slice image (left breast): normal-sized, lobulated lymph node with central fatty hilus.
b Early subtraction slice image (left breast): rim-enhancement is seen due to missing perfusion in the central fatty hilus.
c Zoom
d TIC: typical of malignancy with rapid initial signal increase and postinitial washout.

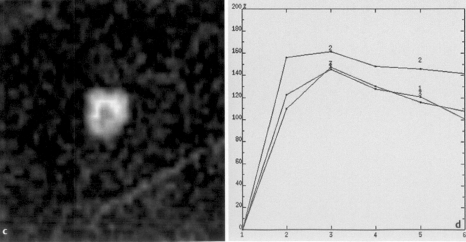

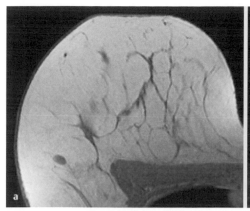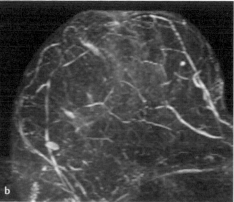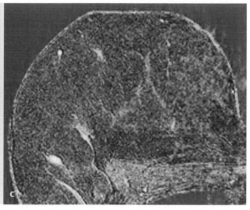

Fig. 13.4a–c Axillary lymph node.

a T1w precontrast slice image (right breast): axillary lymph node in typical location lateral to the pectoral muscle.

b IR T2w slice image (right breast): increased signal intensity.

c Early subtraction slice image (right breast): increased vascularization.

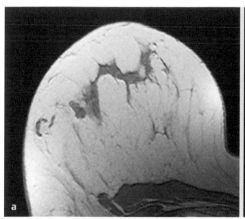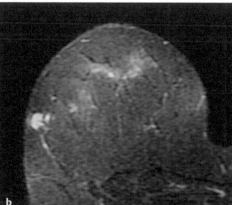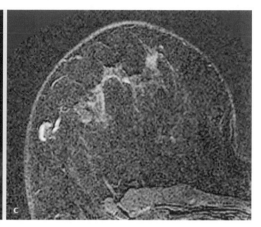

Fig. 13.5a–c Axillary lymph node.

a T1w precontrast slice image (right breast): axillary lymph node located in subcutaneous fat.

b IR T2w slice image (right breast): increased signal intensity.

c Early subtraction slice image (right breast): increased peripheral vascularization.

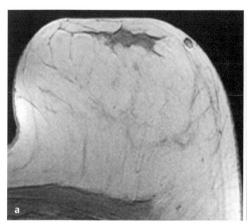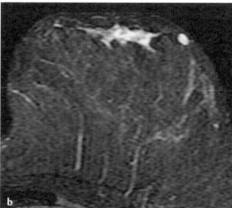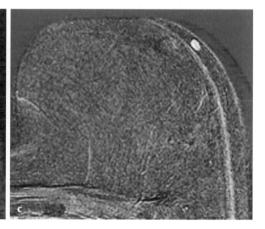

Fig. 13.6a–c Intramammary lymph node.

a T1w precontrast slice image (left breast): lymph node with more atypical location in ventral subcutaneous fat.

b IR T2w slice image (left breast): increased signal intensity.

c Early subtraction slice image (left breast): increased vascularization.

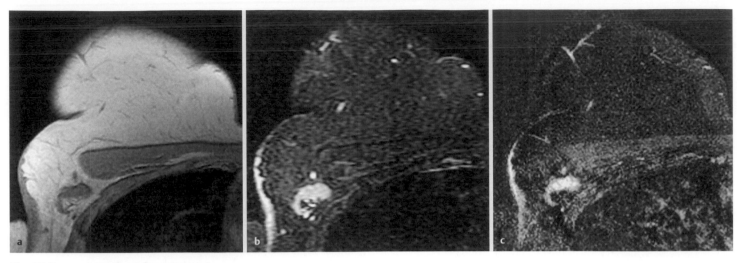

Fig. 13.7a–c   Lymph node metastasis.
a T1w precontrast slice image (right breast): axillary lymph node with borderline size and fat-equivalent signal intensity in hilus area.
b IR T2w slice image (right breast): increased parenchymal signal intensity.

c Early subtraction slice image (right breast): increased vascularization of the parenchymal zone.

Histology: lymph node metastasis of breast carcinoma.

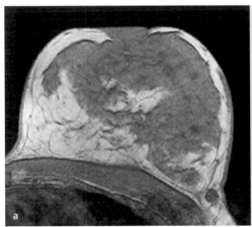
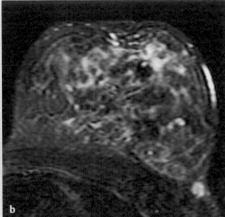

Fig. 13.8a, b   Suspicious axillary lymph node.
a T1w precontrast slice image (left breast): axillary lymph node with borderline size and conspicuous round shape.
b IR T2w slice image (left breast).

Imaging is suspicious for, but not proof of, lymph node metastasis.

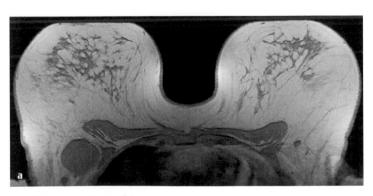
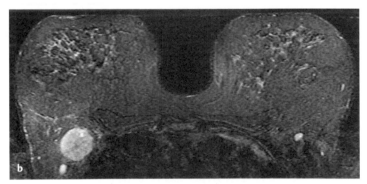

Fig. 13.9a, b   Typical lymph node metastasis.
a T1w precontrast slice image: pathologically enlarged, round lymph node in the right axilla. Typical finding indicating metastatic spread of known breast carcinoma.

b IR T2w slice image: right axillary lymph node metastasis. Normal left-sided lymph node.

Cytologically proven lymph node metastasis.

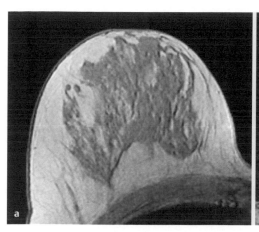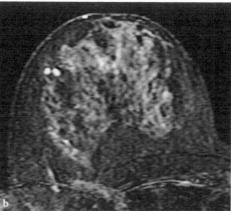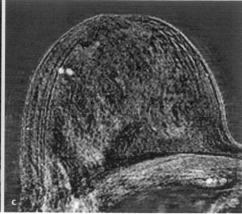

Fig. 13.10a–c Intramammary lymph node.

a T1w precontrast slice image (right breast): inhomogeneously dense breast parenchyma. Two small round masslike lesions in the lateral aspect correlate with intramammary lymph node.

b IR T2w slice image (right breast): increased signal intensity.
c Early subtraction slice image (right breast): increased vascularization.

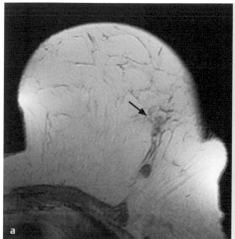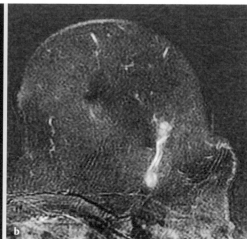

Fig. 13.11 a, b Intramammary lymph node metastasis.

a T1w precontrast slice image (left breast): breast carcinoma (arrow) with visible lymph channels and intramammary lymph node of borderline size.

b Early subtraction slice image (left breast): enhancement of carcinoma, lymph channels and intramammary lymph node.

Histology: intramammary lymph node metastasis (pN1).

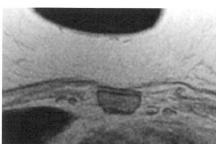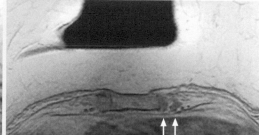

Fig. 13.12 Normal parasternal lymph nodes. Normal-sized intrathoracic, parasternal lymph nodes in T1w precontrast image.

Fig. 13.13 Parasternal lymph nodes, with reactive hyperplasia on the left. Right-sided intrathoracic, parasternal lymph nodes in T1w precontrast image are of normal size. Left-sided parasternal lymph nodes show volume increase after radiotherapy of the left breast (arrows).

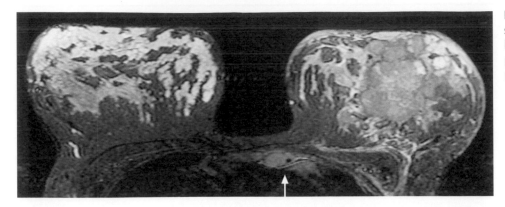

Fig. 13.14 Parasternal lymph node metastasis. Extensive breast carcinoma of the left breast with pathological enlargement of left parasternal lymph node (arrow) in fat-suppressed IR T2w slice image.

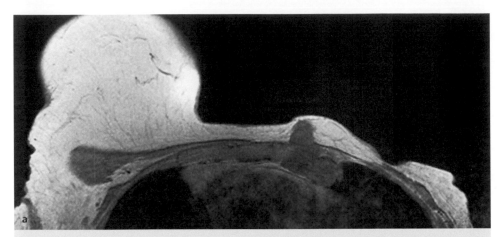

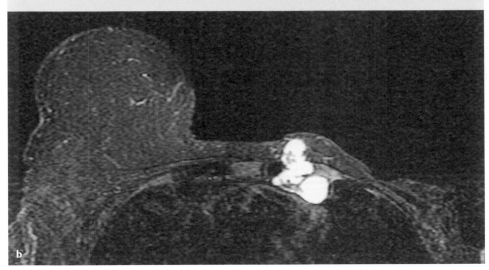

Fig. 13.15a, b Late parasternal lymph node metastasis. Cystic-solid, intra- and extrathoracic, parasternal tumor conglomerate along the internal mammary vessels as the imaging correlate of a late lymph node recurrence after mastectomy for breast cancer 18 years earlier.
a T1w precontrast slice image.
b IR T2w slice image.

14 Autologous and Prosthetic Breast Reconstruction

In general, breast plastic surgery techniques are performed for breast size reduction (**Fig. 14.1**), breast augmentation, and breast reconstruction. Reconstruction of the female breast can be per- formed using autologous tissue or prosthetic material, both of which are discussed here separately.

Diagnostic MRI after Autologous Breast Reconstruction

Breast MRI images after flap reconstruction are dependent upon the technique and type of donor tissue used. The most commonly used techniques are the *latissimus dorsi myocutaneous flap tech- nique* (**Fig. 14.2**) and the *thoracoepigastric flap technique*, which typically leave the donor tissue connected to the original blood supply (pedicled flap). The pedicle can either be ipsilateral to the reconstructed breast, with the pedicle leading to the recon- structed area from the caudal aspect (**Fig. 14.4**), or contralateral to the reconstructed breast, with the pedicle leading to the re- constructed area from the mediocaudal aspect. The most com- monly used technique for autologous breast reconstruction is the TRAM (transverse rectus abdominis myocutaneous) flap tech- nique (**Fig. 14.3**). In addition, there are other flaps that can be used for breast reconstruction (e.g., contralateral superior rectus flap, vertical rectus flap, gluteal flaps).

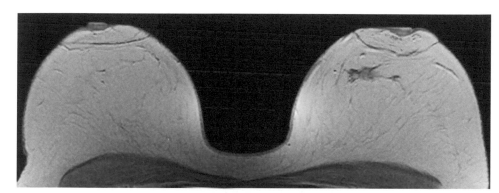

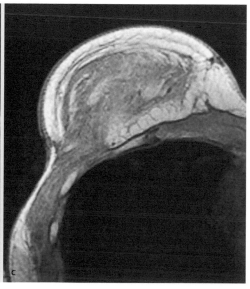

Fig. 14.1 Reduction mammaplasty with periareolar incision. T1w precontrast image shows retromamillary scar after periareolar incision.

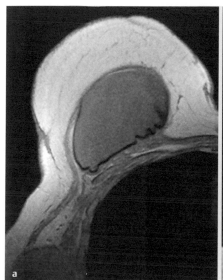
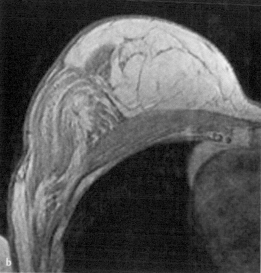

Fig. 14.2a–c Different forms of latissimus dorsi flaps.
a T1w precontrast slice image: latissimus dorsi flap combined with breast implant.
b T1w precontrast slice image: latissimus dorsi flap for reconstruction of lateral breast aspect.

c T1w precontrast slice image: latissimus dorsi flap for reconstruction of entire breast.

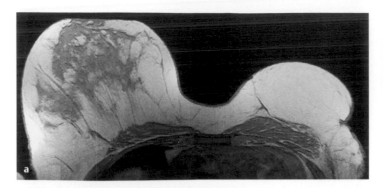

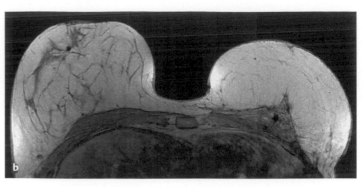

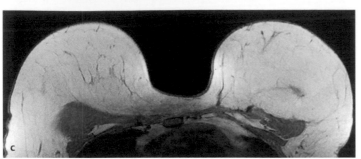

Fig. 14.3 a–c   TRAM flaps.
a T1w precontrast slice image: predominantly lipomatous flap.
b T1w precontrast slice image: TRAM flap with pedicle near the thoracic wall.
c T1w precontrast slice image: fasciocutaneous TRAM flap.

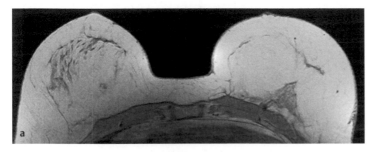

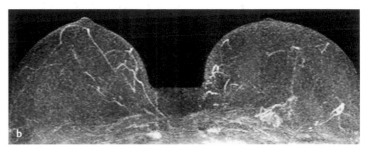

Fig. 14.4 a, b   TRAM flap pedicle.
a T1w precontrast slice image: typical TRAM flap for reconstruction of the left breast with pedicle near the thoracic wall.

b Subtraction MIP.

Diagnostic MRI of Breast Prostheses

Examinations performed for the purpose of detecting and evaluating complications of prostheses are fundamentally different from those performed to rule out malignancy (**Fig. 14.5**). First, no dynamic study is performed in such an examination, dispensing with the need for intravenous administration of contrast material. Second, special sequences are employed to selectively evaluate the different prosthesis components (e.g., silicone, water).

Orientation. In contrast to the dynamic breast MRI examination, it is obligatory in the examination of a woman with breast prostheses to use several orientations (**Fig. 14.6**). In addition to the customary axial slice orientation, images with sagittal orientation have proven advantageous for the detection of extramammary silicone accumulations, especially cranially and caudally to the

prosthesis, as well as prosthesis deformations in the craniocaudal direction. Thin slices (2 mm) should be attained to detect subtle changes (see gel bleeding, p. 207).

IR sequences. The relative resonant frequencies of fat and silicone differ only slightly. Silicone has a resonant frequency ~100 Hz lower than that of fat, and ~320 Hz lower than that of water (**Fig. 14.7c, e, g**). The most effective sequences for differentiating the different fluid components of a prosthesis are the inversion recovery (IR) sequences with fat suppression (**Fig. 14.7b, d, f**). Using such IR sequences with additional suppression of the water signal allows the signal-intense depiction of silicone, while suppressing the signal of the saline component and the surrounding fat tissue (**Fig. 14.7f**). On the other hand, IR sequences performed with the additional suppression of the silicone signal allow the

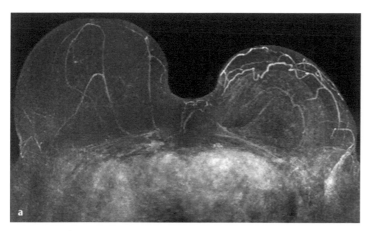

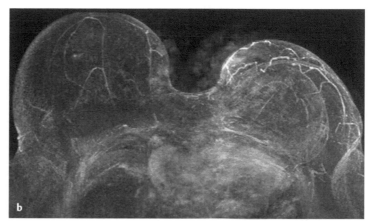

Fig. 14.5a, b   Diagnostic MRI in patient with breast prosthesis: with and without swapped phase-encoding gradient.
a Subtraction MIP with mediolateral phase-encoding gradient.   **b** Subtraction MIP with ventrodorsal phase-encoding gradient.

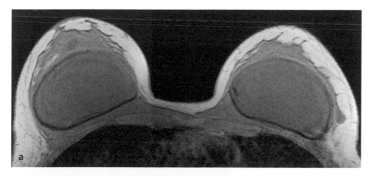

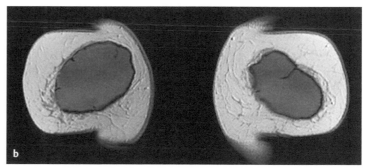

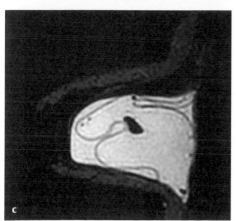

Fig. 14.6a–c   Diagnostic MRI in patients with breast prosthesis: different orientations.
a Axial orientation.
b Coronal orientation.
c Sagittal orientation.

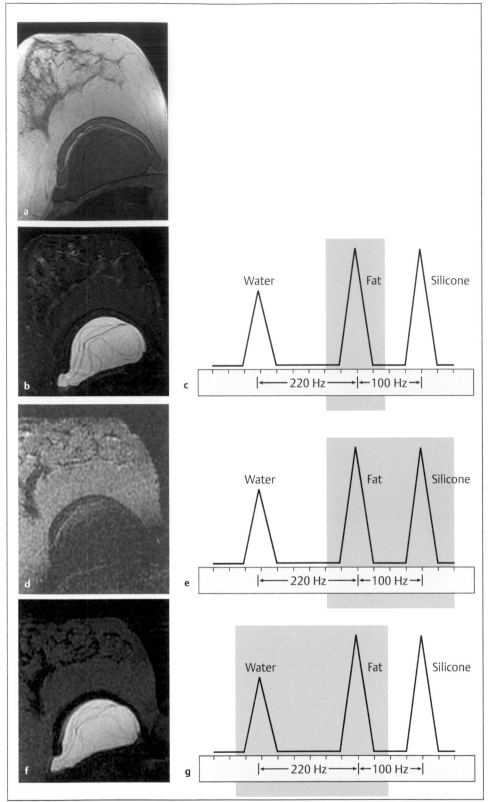

Fig. 14.7a–g Special silicone-specific sequences for diagnostic MRI examination of breast prostheses.
a Standard MRI with usual T1w precontrast images.
b IR T2w examination with signal-intense depiction of water and silicone, and suppression of the fat signal. Signal-intense areas within prosthesis and parenchyma.
c Schematic diagram of fat suppression.
d Silicone-suppressed IR examination with fat suppression.
e Schematic diagram of fat and silicone suppression.
f Water-suppressed IR examination with fat suppression. Only silicone is depicted with high signal intensity.
g Schematic diagram of fat and water suppression.

selective depiction of the saline component. In this way it is possible to image both lumina of a double-lumen prosthetic implant separately (silicone/saline). In addition, fluid accumulations between the prosthesis shell and the capsule of single-lumen implants can also be more easily detected using such protocols.

SE sequences. Other measurement sequences used for the imaging of breast prostheses include fast SE sequences, with and without water-signal suppression. These sequences, however, do not allow such selective imaging of the prosthesis silicone component as can be achieved with the IR sequences described above.

Normal Findings

Position. Breast prostheses can be surgically implanted ventral to the pectoralis major muscle (**prepectoral/subglandular position, Fig. 14.8**), or dorsal to it (**subpectoral position, Fig. 14.9**).

Shape. A breast implant is typically oval in shape, or rarely round. Deformation of the surface is not a pathological finding as long as the outer shell is intact. The outer surface of the implant shell is smooth or textured. It is usually made of silicone elastomers and there is typically a reactive formation of a thin surrounding fibrous capsule after surgical implantation. Silicone found outside this capsule is pathological.

Because of the limited scope of this atlas, it is not possible to give detailed information on the great variety of implants available on the market; for such information the reader is referred to specialist literature on the subject. The following discourse is therefore confined to the materials most often used: saline and silicone.

> **!** The prosthesis **shell** is the silicone elastomer casing surrounding the prosthesis contents (a part of the prosthesis). The shell must be differentiated from the collagen tissue **capsule** (scar tissue) that is formed around the breast implant as a reactive process after implantation.

Single- and double-lumen prostheses. When evaluating the internal structures of an implant, it is necessary to differentiate between single-lumen and double-lumen implants. The **single-lumen** prosthesis consists of a single chamber typically filled with a viscous silicone gel (**Fig. 14.10a**) or (increasingly) a saline solution. The **double-lumen** prosthesis consists of an inner chamber typically filled with a viscous silicone gel, and an outer chamber containing saline (**Fig. 14.10b**). A modification of this prosthesis in which the inner chamber contains saline and the outer chamber contains silicone is referred to as a "reverse double-lumen."

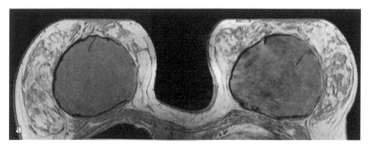

Fig. 14.8a, b   Prepectoral/subglandular prostheses.
a T1w precontrast slice image: prostheses implanted ventral to the pectoral muscle.

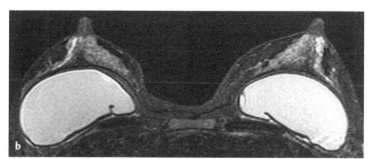

b IR T2w MIP.

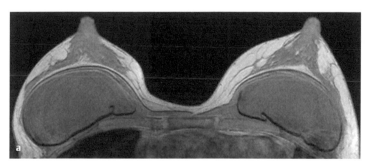

Fig. 14.9a, b   Subpectoral prostheses.
a T1w precontrast slice image: prostheses implanted dorsal to the pectoral muscle.

b IR T2w slice image.

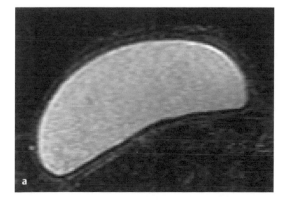

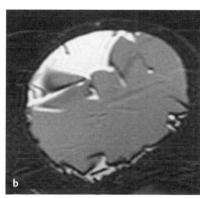

Fig. 14.10a, b   Single- and double-lumen prostheses.
a IR T2w slice image: homogeneous internal signal within prosthesis.
b IR T2w slice image: the silicone inner chamber and saline outer chamber are easily differentiated in a double-lumen prosthesis.

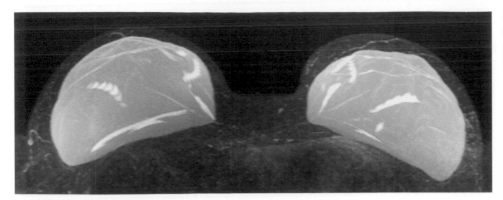

Fig. 14.11   Radial folds. IR T2w MIP shows elastomer shell folds originating in the periphery of the implant. This is a normal finding in breast implant imaging.

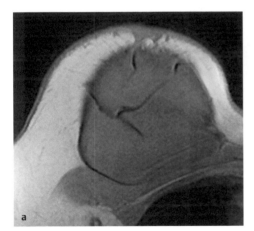
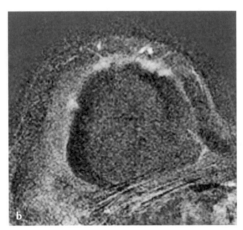

Fig. 14.12 a, b   Prosthesis rotation (dislocation). Right prosthesis shows atypical shape in axial image. Normal left prosthesis.
a IR T2w slice image.   **b** IR T2w MIP.

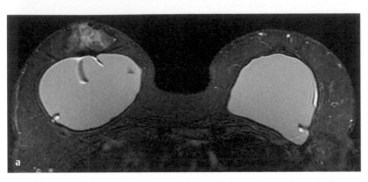

Fig. 14.13 a, b   Capsulitis.
a T1w precontrast slice image (right breast): subglandular prosthesis.
b Subtraction slice image (right breast): periprosthetic enhancement of the ventral aspect of the prosthesis circumference.

Folds. Folds of the intact silicone shell into the lumen of the prosthesis (*radial folds*) are commonly seen. They are often only 1–2 cm long and originate at the fibrous capsule, ending blindly in the silicone gel (**Fig. 14.11**). They represent a normal finding as long as they exhibit a connection to the implant shell.

Complications

Displacement. Breast implant displacement is the migration of the implant out of the original position at any time after surgery (**Fig. 14.12**). As long as the implant carrier is satisfied with the cosmetic result, it is of no clinical significance.

Capsulitis

Capsulitis is an inflammatory defense reaction of the body (in the outer capsule) to the foreign material of the breast implant (**Fig. 14.13**).

Capsular Contracture

The formation of a tough fibrous capsule (scar tissue) around the breast prosthesis may lead to painful hardening and deformation (contracture) of the implant. Extensive periprosthetic calcifications are often associated with this complication.

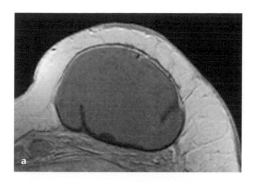
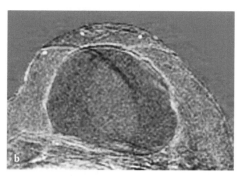

Fig. 14.14a, b Capsular contracture.
a T1w precontrast slice image (left breast): the ventral aspect of the prosthesis capsule is seen as a thin, low-signal-intensity structure.
b Subtraction slice image (left breast): a thin line of enhancement around entire prosthesis.

Clinical symptoms: painful hardening of the left prosthesis.

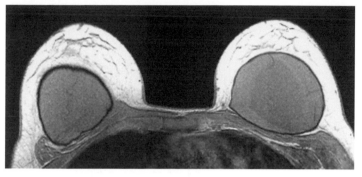

Fig. 14.15 Capsular contracture/fibrosis. T1w slice image shows asymmetric, greater capsule fibrosis around the right prosthesis due to periprosthetic calcifications. Clinical symptoms: painful hardening of right prosthesis.

Classification of capsular contracture (according to Baker)
- Grade I: Soft breast. Normal shape.
- Grade II: Firm breast. Normal shape.
- Grade III: Firm breast. Visible breast deformation.
- Grade IV: Hard, painful breast. Marked spherical deformation of the breast.

 Formation of a soft, nonpalpable periprosthetic capsule is a normal finding. Formation of a hard, thick fibrous capsule is pathological.

MR Mammography: Capsular Contracture

Occasionally there are no conspicuous image findings (**Fig. 14.14a**). Sometimes the periprosthetic capsule appears thickened and may show calcifications, occasionally demonstrating an increased contrast enhancement as the expression of a granulomatous inflammatory process (**Fig. 14.14b**). Signal-free

Capsular contracture: General information

Incidence:	Up to 20% of all prostheses.
Significance:	Pain. Dissatisfaction with cosmetic results.
Consequences:	Depending upon the degree of pain and/or dissatisfaction, surgical removal of the scar tissue and prosthesis, with or without placement of a new implant.

capsule thickening or plaques correspond to macrocalcifications (**Fig. 14.15**). Tightening of the capsular scar tissue around the implant with deformation and acquisition of a spherical configuration is possible (**Fig. 14.14**).

 Capsular contracture is a clinical diagnosis. Breast MRI is of little additional diagnostic value.

Silicone Gel Bleeding

Microscopic leakage of silicone out of the prosthesis through an intact implant shell. As a consequence, silicone accumulates between the fibrous capsule and the implant shell, i.e., within the radial folds (**Fig. 14.16**). The fibrous capsule is intact.

MR Mammography: Silicone Gel Bleeding

Accumulation of silicone is seen within the radial folds. This is most clearly visible at the keyhole-shaped terminal bend of the fold ("teardrop sign") (**Fig. 14.16**). It is often difficult to detect the accumulation of silicone between the implant shell and the capsule.

Silicone gel bleeding: General information

Incidence:	No available data. Diagnosis is only possible using high-resolution technique.
Significance:	Sign of material fatigue. Preliminary stage of implant shell recession.
Consequences:	None. Follow-up examinations.

Implant Shell Recession

With greater silicone leakage out of the prosthesis there is an increasing accumulation of silicone between the capsule and the implant shell, increasing the distance between them. The fibrous capsule is intact.

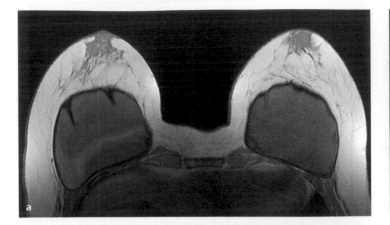

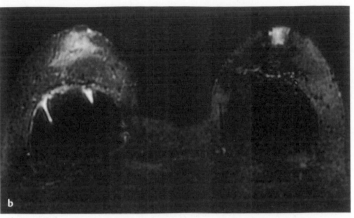

Fig. 14.16a–c Silicone gel bleeding.
a T1w precontrast slice image: bilateral subglandular prostheses.
b IR T2w, water-sensitive slice image: signal-intense depiction of saline within the radial folds of the right prosthesis. No saline-signal in the radial folds of the left prosthesis.
c IR T2w, silicone-sensitive slice image: signal-intense depiction of extruded silicone within the radial folds of the left prosthesis as an indication of gel bleeding. No silicone signal is detected within the radial folds in the right prosthesis

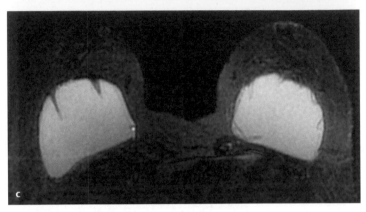

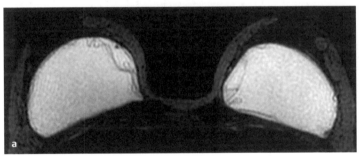

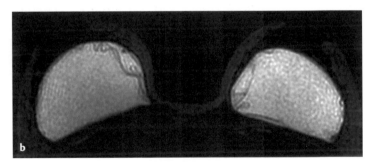

Fig. 14.17a, b Implant shell recession. Both implant shells have receded from the fibrous capsule in the medial aspects of the prostheses, indicating localized silicone extrusion into the subcapsular space. Implant shells are intact.
a IR T2w, silicone-sensitive slice image: suppressed water signal and wide window.
b IR T2w, silicone-sensitive slice image: suppressed water signal and narrow window.

 MR Mammography: Implant Shell Recession

The implant shell appears constricted by a visible amount of silicone between implant shell and capsule (**Fig. 14.17**).

Implant shell recession: General information

Incidence:	No available data.
Significance:	Sign of material fatigue. Preliminary stage of intracapsular rupture.
Consequences:	None. Follow-up examinations.

Intracapsular Rupture

The implant shell is damaged; it typically collapses and floats within the silicone gel. Leaked silicone lies outside the prosthesis but inside the intact fibrous capsule. Intracapsular ruptures occur in both single-lumen and double-lumen prostheses.

Note: The term "intracapsular rupture" is not equivalent to a rupture of the inner of the two shells in a double-lumen prosthesis.

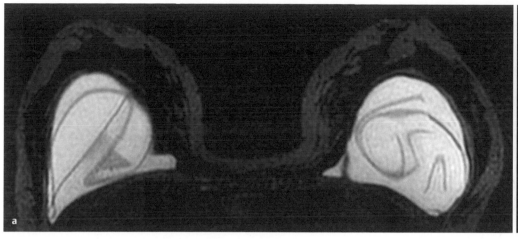
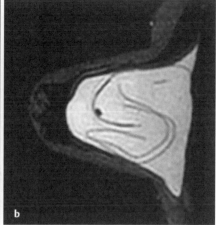

Fig. 14.18a, b Intracapsular rupture: linguine sign.
a IR T2w, silicone-sensitive slice image (axial view): depiction of free-floating, winding, torn and collapsed elastomer shells of both prostheses.

b IR T2w, silicone-sensitive slice image (sagittal view).

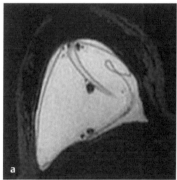
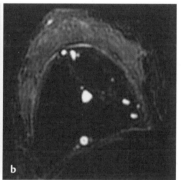

Fig. 14.19a, b Implant shell recession: salad oil sign.
a IR T2w, silicone-sensitive slice image: depiction of receded elastomer prosthesis shell and signal-free areas within silicone gel.
b "Negative image" in the water-sensitive, silicone-suppressed sequence. Droplets now appear signal-intense. This is not a reliable indication of an intracapsular rupture when the linguine sign is missing.

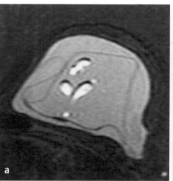
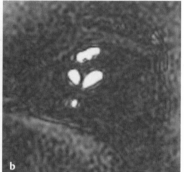

Fig. 14.20a, b Intracapsular rupture: linguine sign and salad oil sign.
a IR T2w water-sensitive slice image: depiction of incipient linguine sign and large signal-intense droplets within silicone gel.
b IR T2w water-sensitive slice image with silicone suppression: droplets still appear signal-intense while the silicone signal is completely suppressed.

MR Mammography: Intracapsular Rupture

Multiple curvilinear low-signal-intensity lines (corresponding to the collapsed prosthesis shell) are seen within the silicone-filled fibrous capsule ("linguine sign"). This is the most reliable sign of an intracapsular rupture when silicone is not demonstrated outside the fibrous capsule (**Fig. 14.18**). A less reliable sign of an intracapsular rupture is the demonstration of saline droplets within the silicone compartment ("salad-oil-sign," **Fig. 14.19**). It can only be used as a diagnostic criterion indicating an intracapsular rupture in combination with the linguine sign (**Fig. 14.20**).

 A collapsed prosthesis shell (intracapsular rupture) and a radial fold (normal finding) may be difficult to differentiate.
Tip: Radial folds run from the periphery to the center. A collapsed prosthesis shell often runs parallel to the capsule.

Intracapsular rupture: General information

Incidence:	Approx. 80%–90% of all prostheses rupture. A typical complication ~15–20 years after implantation.
Significance:	Sign of material fatigue. Additional risk of extracapsular rupture.
Consequences:	None. Follow-up examinations.

Extracapsular Rupture

Rupture of both the implant shell and the fibrous capsule with macroscopic extrusion of silicone into the surrounding tissues.

Extracapsular rupture: General information

Incidence:	Approx. 10%–20% of all prostheses rupture. A typical complication ~15–20 years after implantation.
Consequences:	Removal or replacement of prosthesis

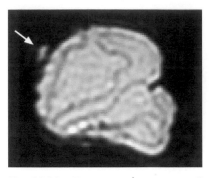

Fig. 14.21 Extracapsular rupture. Depiction of radial folds and a small "polyplike" area of silicone gel (arrow) that has leaked through the fibrous capsule in the silicone-sensitive T2w sequence (partial image). Additional linguine sign.

 MR Mammography: Extracapsular Rupture

Detection of signal-intense silicone in the periprosthetic tissues (**Fig. 14.21**). Typically, free silicone is seen near the cranial aspect of the implant. Signs of an intracapsular rupture are obligatory. Other than silicone, there are no signal-intense intramammary structures. In the silicone-suppressed IR sequence there is complete signal loss of those signal-intense structures seen in the silicone-sensitive IR sequence (**Fig. 14.22c**).

! An extracapsular rupture always presupposes an intracapsular rupture.

Complete Prosthesis Rupture

The ruptured prosthesis collapses due to subtotal/total loss of lumen contents (**Fig. 14.23**).

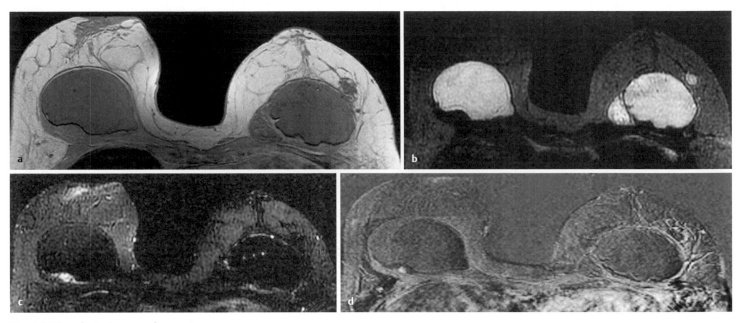

Fig. 14.22a–d Extracapsular rupture.
a T1w precontrast slice image: unspecific space-occupying lesions medially and laterally of the left prosthesis.
b IR T2w silicone-sensitive slice image: both lesions appear signal-intense.

c IR T2w water-sensitive slice image with silicone suppression: complete signal suppression within both periprosthetic lesions is a reliable indication that these contain silicone gel.
d Subtraction slice image: no reactive enhancement is an indication that the extracapsular silicone areas are not a recent development.

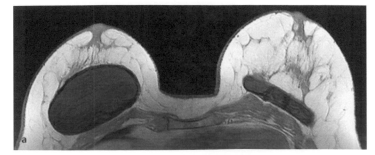

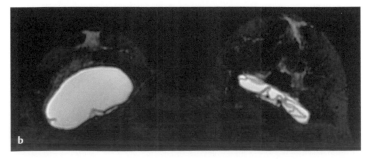

Fig. 14.23a, b Complete prosthesis rupture.
a T1w precontrast slice image: ruptured left saline prosthesis has collapsed with subtotal leakage of the internal saline solution.

b IR T2w water-sensitive slice image: normal right prosthesis.

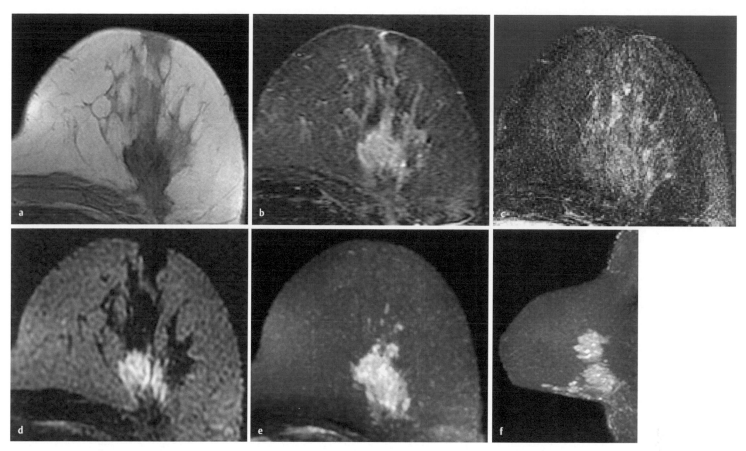

Fig. 14.24a–f   Siliconoma. Silicone can be seen in the caudal aspect of the breast after rupture of a silicone implant during surgical removal.
a   T1w precontrast slice image (left breast).
b   IR T2w water-sensitive slice image without silicone suppression.
c   Subtraction slice image: no significant reactive hyperemia.
d   IR T2w silicone-sensitive slice image with water and fat suppression: excellent depiction of intramammary silicone.
e   IR T2w silicone-sensitive MIP with water and fat suppression ("silicone MIP," axial orientation): excellent depiction of intramammary silicone.
f   "Silicone MIP" in sagittal orientation.

Free Silicone and Silicone Granuloma (Siliconoma)

Silicone collects within the breast parenchyma with a concomitant granulomatous component, equivalent to a foreign body granuloma. This develops after direct silicone injection into breast tissue (**Figs. 14.25**, **14.26**) or incomplete removal of a defective silicone prosthesis (**Fig. 14.24**).

 MR Mammography: Free Silicone and Siliconoma

Free silicone and siliconoma: General information

Incidence:	May develop after any extracapsular rupture with silicone leakage, occasionally after removal of a defective prosthesis with remaining intramammary silicone, or after direct silicone injection into the breast (very rare).
Significance:	Risk of distant intracorporeal silicone spread and antibody development.
Consequences:	Siliconoma excision.

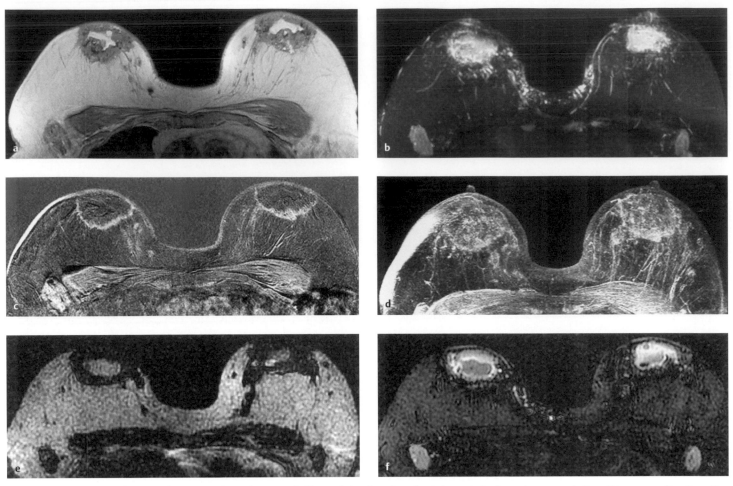

Fig. 14.25 a–f Free silicone. The patient has a history of silicone injections into both breasts for breast augmentation 25 years earlier. Reactive inflammatory changes (chronic granulomatous inflammation).

a T1w precontrast slice image: ringlike silicone deposits in the retroareolar regions of both breasts.

b IR T2w water-sensitive MIP without silicone suppression: reactive edema in these areas.

c Subtraction slice image: reactive marginal hyperemia at the borders of the silicone deposits.

d Subtraction MIP: reactive marginal hyperemia at the borders of the silicone deposits.

e IR T2w water-sensitive slice image with silicone suppression: exact depiction of intramammary silicone as signal-free retroareolar zones.

f IR T2w silicone-sensitive slice image: silicone deposits depicted as hyperintense zones. Additional depiction of bilateral pathologically enlarged axillary lymph nodes with silicone-equivalent signal intensity.

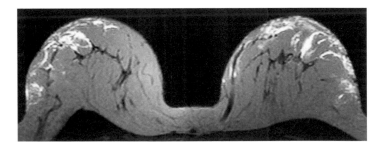

Fig. 14.26 Free silicone. The patient has a history of silicone injections into the subcutaneous tissues of both breasts for breast augmentation 20 years earlier. The T2w silicone-sensitive image shows silicone distribution in the peripheral breast aspects (image courtesy of Daniela Wruk, MD, Switzerland).

15 Breast MRI in Men

Gynecomastia

The term *gynecomastia* goes back to Galen (129–200 CE). It describes a benign, usually reversible, unilateral or bilateral enlargement of the male breast. Gynecomastia is due to an increase in breast stroma and, to a lesser extent, to ductal proliferation. It is classified into several different categories and may be a normal physiological phenomenon or a pathological finding associated with an underlying disease.

Neonatal gynecomastia, pubertal gynecomastia, senescent gynecomastia. These forms of gynecomastia represent physiological conditions due to the status with respect to the appropriate hormones. Breast imaging techniques play no role in the diagnostic work-up.

Pathological gynecomastia. Pathological gynecomastia of the adult male develops under the influence of excess estrogen or decreased androgen hormones. In addition, many drugs with an "estrogen-effect" have been found to cause gynecomastia. The following causes deserve special attention:
- Estrogen therapy
- Estrogen- or human chorionic gonadotropin-secreting testicular or adrenal tumors
- Paraneoplastic syndrome
- Cirrhosis of the liver
- Anorchism, castration, hypogonadism, Klinefelter syndrome
- Hyperthyroidism
- Treatment with spironolactone, cimetidine, or verapamil
- Marijuana use

 MR Mammography

In the T1-weighted precontrast sequence, MR mammography shows a retromamillary area with a low signal-intensity (**Fig. 15.1c** and **Fig. 15.2b**). After CM administration this area usually shows no to moderate contrast enhancement (**Figs. 15.1a, e, 15.2a, c**). The water signal of the parenchymal area is normally somewhat increased (**Fig. 15.1b, d**). If strong or suspicious contrast enhancement is found, biopsy must be performed to exclude malignancy.

> *! Gynecomastia can occur unilaterally or bilaterally.

Pseudogynecomastia (lipomastia). The enlarged breast in pseudogynecomastia is solely due to excessive adipose tissue (obesity) without evidence of parenchyma (**Fig. 15.3**). Corresponding findings in breast MRI rule out true gynecomastia (**Fig. 15.4**).

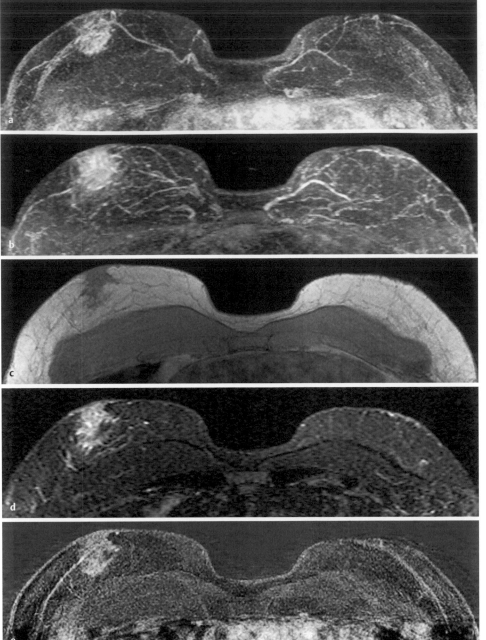

Fig. 15.1 a–e Unilateral gynecomastia.
a Subtraction MIP: localized area with increased enhancement in the right breast.
b IR T2w MIP: corresponding area with increased water content of nonlipomatous tissues.
c Representative T1w precontrast slice image.
d Representative T2w slice image.
e Representative subtraction slice image.

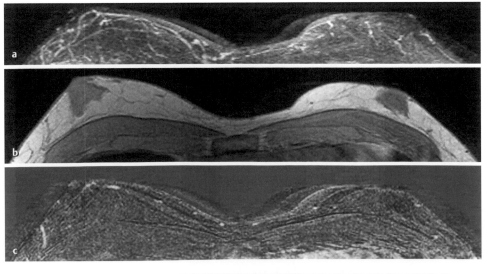

Fig. 15.2 a–c Bilateral gynecomastia.
a Subtraction MIP: no enhancement.
b T1w precontrast slice image: nonlipomatous, triangularly-shaped body of parenchyma in the retromamillary region of both breasts.
c Corresponding subtraction slice image shows no enhancement.

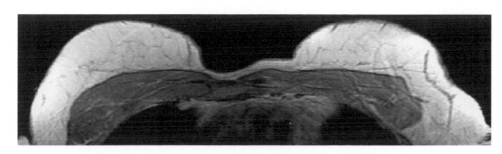

Fig. 15.3   Pseudogynecomastia. Representative T1w precontrast slice image shows bilateral breast enlargement due to an increase in lipomatous tissue volume. No evidence of parenchymal tissues.

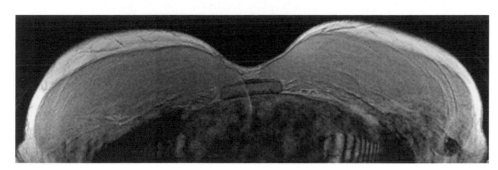

Fig. 15.4   Body builder. Representative T1w precontrast slice image shows bilateral breast enlargement due to an extreme increase in pectoral muscle volume. No evidence of parenchymal tissues.

Male Breast Cancer

Histology. Contrary to earlier opinion, there is no significant difference between the histology of male and female breast carcinomas. However, since tubular structures are not usually found in the male breast, there are only rare reports of invasive lobular carcinomas in males. All other histological types of breast cancer (NOS, medullary, papillary, colloid, and Paget disease) have been reported in men, although the majority of tumors are infiltrating ductal carcinomas (**Fig. 15.5**).

Epidemiology. Breast cancer in males is a rare disease, representing less than 1% of all breast cancers. The incidence of male breast cancer increases with age and shows a peak between the 50th and 70th years of life (incidence: 0.1/100 000 for 35-year-olds; 11/100 000 for 85-year-olds).

Only 0.3 men per 100 000 die of breast cancer. For comparison, 23.9 women per 100 000 die of breast cancer

Risk factors. Risk factors implicated in the increased incidence of male breast cancer include a history of undescended testicles,

orchitis, infertility, hypercholesterolemia, exogenous estrogen administration, and radiation exposure (latent period 12–35 years). Approximately 30% of men with breast cancer have a family history of the disease in female or male family members. It should be noted that men can be carriers of *BRCA* mutations and can pass the defective gene on to their daughters without having breast cancer themselves. Women with a family history of breast cancer in a younger male relative are considered to be at high risk for the development of breast cancer.

Diagnostics. Mammography and percutaneous biopsy are the primary diagnostic procedures performed when breast cancer is suspected in a man. Gynecomastia, which itself is not a risk factor for the development of breast cancer, must be considered as a differential diagnosis.

! Breast MRI findings associated with breast cancer in males and females show the same characteristics of malignancy.

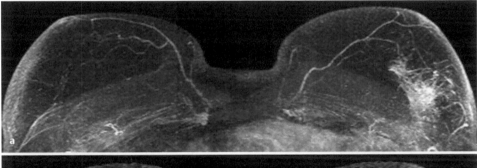

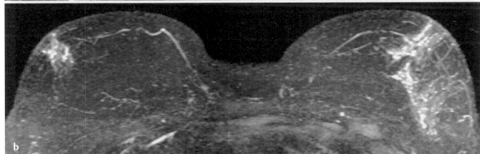

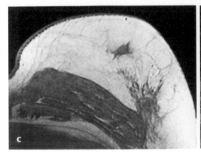
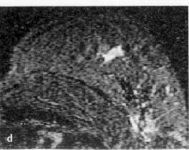
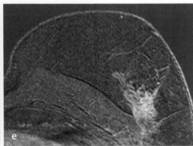
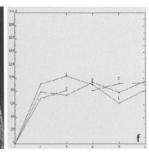

Fig. 15.5a–f   Male breast cancer.
a Subtraction MIP: regional area of enhancement in the lateral aspect of the left breast
b IR T2w MIP: partially increased signal intensity of enhancing area and retromamillary parenchyma (gynecomastia).
c T1w precontrast slice image (left breast): irregularly shaped mass-lesion in the lateral aspect (carcinoma). Smaller, ventrally located parenchymal area not associated with primary tumor.
d IR T2w slice image (left breast): inhomogeneously increased signal intensity within tumor. Increased signal intensity within parenchymal area.
e Subtraction slice image (left breast): diffuse enhancement within carcinoma. No enhancement within parenchymal area.
f TIC: rapid initial signal increase and postinitial plateau.
Histology: invasive ductal breast carcinoma.

16 MRI-Guided Interventions

Special Considerations in MRI-Guided Interventions

Equipment and procedures used for MRI-guided interventions must accommodate the special conditions encountered during an MRI scan. This applies especially to the extremely strong magnetic field, and to the short time slot of only a few minutes during which the hypervascularized target is visible. The materials used (needles, wires, clips, and coils) must therefore have favorable ferromagnetic characteristics so that they are easily identified within the breast but do not cause susceptibility artifacts that will interfere with image acquisition and target identification. In addition, measurement sequences that show as little vulnerability as possible to signal extinction due to susceptibility artifacts must be chosen for MRI-guided interventions.

MRI-Compatible Surface Coils for Breast Interventions

First attempts at MRI-guided preoperative localization were made in the 1990s using the so-called "free-hand" technique. For this, cutaneous markers were placed on the skin for better orientation and the position of the lesion was estimated. Because this method is relatively inexact, it was quickly abandoned. Later, dedicated puncture devices for interventions in the supine, oblique, or sitting body positions, depending on the particular work group, were developed using appropriate breast surface coils. These systems were used primarily for MRI-guided preoperative localizations, and increasingly also for large-core and vacuum-assisted biopsies, mostly with a lateral approach. The

decisive breakthrough for the routine and reliable performance of percutaneous MRI-guided biopsies occurred with the development of **open breast surface coils** into which dedicated targeting devices can be integrated.

Nowadays MRI-guided breast interventions are performed using open surface coils that allow access to the breast and integration of a dedicated puncture device. Open surface coils that also allow the integration of compression paddles for diagnostic examinations are available from various companies (**Fig. 16.1**). Two systems are usually used to calculate and mark the appropriate puncture coordinates, as well as to guide the puncture needle:

- The *post-and-pillar targeting equipment* (**Fig. 16.2**), allowing continuous adjustment of the *x*- and *y*-axes
- The *biopsy and localization grid* (**Fig. 16.3**), a grid system with flexible positioning of insertable guide blocks

Computer-Aided Calculation of Puncture Coordinates

Several different companies offer software for the calculation of the appropriate puncture coordinates in the *x*-, *y*-, and *z*-axes for MRI-guided breast interventions. In principle, the coordinate data are calculated in relation to an arbitrarily chosen zero-point, from which the distance to the target lesion is calculated in the three spatial planes. Currently available systems include *SureLoc* from Confirma Europe Corp., *DynaLOC* from Invivo Corp., and *MICS MIA* from Machnet B.V.

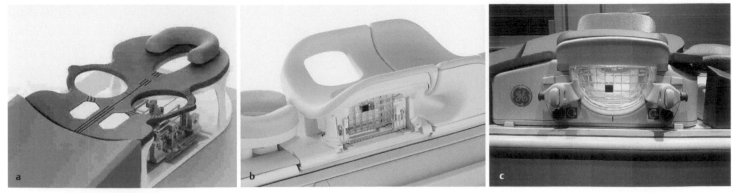

Fig. 16.1   Equipment. Different models of open breast surface coils with integrated puncture devices for MRI-guided breast interventions.

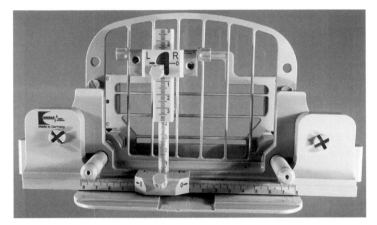

Fig. 16.2   Post-and-pillar targeting equipment for MRI-guided breast interventions. NORAS Co. breast biopsy unit with compression grid. Continuous adjustment of the *x*- and *y*-axes is possible by sliding the telescopic post-and-pillar system. Compatible with all customary open surface coils.

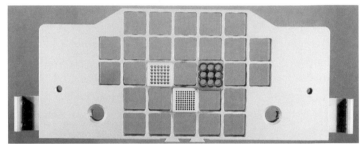

Fig. 16.3   Biopsy and localization grid for MRI-guided breast interventions. NORAS Co. breast biopsy unit with compression grid with chambers for the insertion of perforated guide blocks with various puncture opening sizes. Compatible with all customary open surface coils.

Diagnostic MRI-Guided Vacuum-Assisted Biopsy

Indications and Objectives

Conspicuous breast findings that fall into the BI-RADS category 4 or 5 should be verified histologically. This is preferably achieved by a percutaneous biopsy. In exceptional cases, however, primary open surgery may be an option. If a suspicious finding has a clear sonographic correlate, then ultrasound-guided percutaneous biopsy is the method of choice. If a suspicious finding has a mammographic correlate and no clear sonographic correlate (e.g., microcalcifications), then a stereotactic percutaneous vacuum-assisted biopsy is usually performed. Findings detected solely on breast MRI should be histologically verified by MRI-guided vacuum-assisted biopsy.

> **Good Practice Recommendations***
>
> Image-guided biopsies should be undertaken to obtain tissue samples from abnormalities found in the MRI BI-RADS categories 4 and 5 for histopathological verification and therapy planning.
> * European S 3 Guidelines: Early Breast Cancer Detection (Level of Evidence B).

A major purpose of the primary performance of percutaneous breast biopsy of findings suspicious for malignancy is to reduce the number of unnecessary open biopsies (diagnostic excisions). In cases when a benign histological result is attained (without uncertain biological potential), open biopsy can be avoided and a follow-up imaging examination in 6 months is initiated. When malignancy is confirmed, it is possible to offer appropriate patient information about the necessary therapeutic consequences. In addition, surgery is planned taking oncological aspects into consideration. In this context, it is also possible to arrange for sentinel lymph node biopsy (SLNB).

> **Good Practice Recommendations***
>
> When image-guided percutaneous biopsy yields a benign histopathological result, a short-term follow-up examination (6 months) using the corresponding imaging modality should be initiated.
> * European S 3 Guidelines: Early Breast Cancer Detection (Grade of Recommendation A).

> **Recommendations:**
>
> Equipment for MRI-Guided Vacuum-Assisted Interventions*
> * MRI system of at least 1.0 T
> * Open surface coil allowing access to the breast
> * MRI-compatible localization device
> * MRI-compatible biopsy device: vacuum-assisted biopsy (method of choice) or large-core biopsy (when justified)
> *German Radiological Society Breast Diagnostics Working Group (2007).

Biopsy Equipment

In accordance with good practice recommendations, MRI-guided biopsies should preferably be performed as vacuum-assisted biopsies using coaxial technique. Fine-needle biopsies are obsolete. Large-core biopsies should only be performed in justified exceptions.

Depending upon needle size, 6–12 tissue samples are obtained during a *vacuum-assisted biopsy*. The average volume of the samples obtained is ~1 cm^3. Several MRI-compatible vacuum-assisted biopsy systems are currently available. These differ only slightly from one another (**Fig. 16.4**).

> **Good Practice Recommendations***
>
> MRI-guided biopsies should be performed using vacuum-assisted technique.
> *European S 3 Guidelines: Early Breast Cancer Detection, Level of Evidence 3a, evidence report 2007 (Grade of Recommendation B).

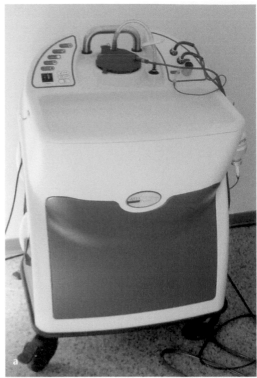

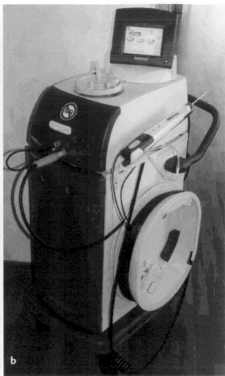

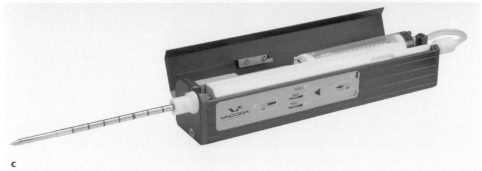

Fig. 16.4a–c MRI-compatible vacuum-assisted biopsy systems.
a ATEC breast biopsy system (Suros Surgical Systems, Inc., Indianapolis, IN, USA).
b Mammotome biopsy system (Ethicon Endo-Surgery, Cincinnati, OH, USA).
c Vacora VAB system (Bard Biopsy Systems, Tempe, AR, USA).

Procedure

MRI-Guided Percutaneous Biopsy*

- Contrast-enhanced breast MRI is performed with the localization equipment positioned on the affected side. An external marker (e.g., oil-containing) is placed at the estimated puncture site.
- If the target lesion is not or is only questionably reproduced, then the intervention should be discontinued and a short-term follow-up examination in 6 months recommended.
- If the target lesion is clearly identified, then the puncture coordinates (x-, y-, and z-axes) are calculated. The external marker is moved to the calculated puncture site and an MRI check is performed without additional contrast administration.
- If the marker position is incorrect, a new calculation is done and the marker position is corrected. If the marker position is correct, the skin is disinfected and local anesthesia is administered (if necessary, skin nick incision). The coaxial introduction needle is positioned (e.g., using the metal puncture stylet) to the appropriate depth (z-axis). The correct depth in relation to the lesion depends on the vacuum-assisted biopsy system being used.
- The puncture stylet is replaced by an MRI-compatible mandrin and the position of the coaxial introduction needle is checked by performing a T1w MRI series without contrast. If the position is incorrect, a new calculation is performed and the needle is repositioned and rechecked. If the position is correct, the MRI-compatible mandrin is removed and replaced with the vacuum-assisted biopsy needle.
- Contiguous tissue cylinders are then harvested using the vacuum-assisted biopsy needle by rotating the biopsy notch. It is recommended to obtain ≥ 12 tissue cylinders, which is the equivalent of one complete rotation around the position "clock" (1-o'clock to 12-o'clock positions). When appropriate, an additional MRI check can be performed before ending the intervention to confirm the representative position of the biopsy cavity or to redirect further sampling.
- Final documentation of representative tissue sampling (target size is reduced, target is no longer detected, the biopsy cavity position is correct) in postinterventional MRI check (when indicated with contrast administration, e.g., mass lesions). If necessary, further sampling should be performed.

- Optional placement of a marker coil/clip in the biopsy cavity through the coaxial introduction cannula. MRI documentation (without contrast) of intramammary coil position.
- Removal of the coaxial introduction needle. Compression and cooling of puncture channel. Compression bandage.
- Optional performance of postbiopsy mammograms in CC and ML projections for the topographic localization of the biopsy cavity, or to document the coil position in case surgery is indicated.
- *Report:*
  - Was the target finding reproducible? (yes/no)
  - Position of target finding (quadrant, clock time position, distance from the skin)
  - Vacuum needle caliber (e.g., 11G, 9G)
  - Number of tissue cylinders primarily harvested (if applicable, number harvested secondarily)
  - Documentation of relevant complications
- *Documentation:*
  - MRI subtraction image of target finding (**Figs. 16.5a, 16.6a, 16.7a**)
  - MRI prefire image documentation of coaxial introduction needle position (**Fig. 16.7b**)
  - MRI image documentation of biopsy cavity or of vacuum-assisted biopsy needle position after biopsy (**Figs. 16.5b, 16.6b**)
  - Optional: MRI check with additional contrast administration
  - Optional: Mammography in CC and ML projections
- *Quality criteria:*
  - Complete or partial removal of target lesion to be histologically verified by MRI-guided percutaneous biopsy
  - Compatibility of histology and target lesion MRI image
- Postbiopsy procedure depending on the reported category B pathology (**Table 16.1**):
  - B1 or B2: Short-term MRI follow-up in 6 months (in special cases earlier)
  - B3 or B4: Interdisciplinary conference to decide on the course of action (e.g., MRI follow-up, rebiopsy, surgery)
  - B5a or B5b: Initiation of appropriate therapy

*Recommendations of the German Radiological Society Breast Diagnostics Working Group 2007.

Table 16.1 Five-category classification system for pathological findings of minimally invasive breast biopsies

Category	Definition
B1	Normal tissue/unsatisfactory biopsy
B2	Benign lesion
B3	Lesion of uncertain malignant potential
B4	Lesion suspicious for malignancy
B5a	DCIS
B5b	Invasive carcinoma
B5c	Invasion not assessable
B5d	Other malignant lesion

Postbiopsy MRI Check That Tissue Samples Are Representative

After preoperative US-guided or stereotactic localization, correct and complete excision of the localized lesion can be confirmed in the perioperative ultrasound examination or radiography (microcalcifications) of the excised tissue. Perioperative confirmation that a lesion seen only on breast MRI has been completely excised is not possible as the pathological tumor hypervascularization cannot be imaged in the excised tissue. It is therefore all the more important to routinely evaluate whether histology and the MRI lesion image are compatible, and to perform a breast MRI follow-up examination 6 months after biopsy for all benign histological results (B1 and B2 lesions).

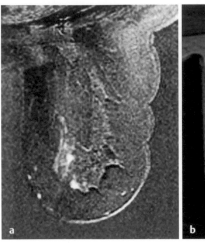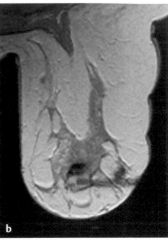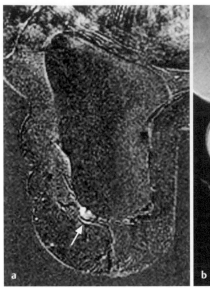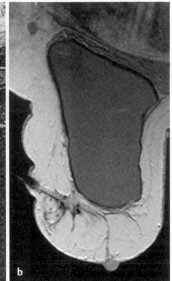

Fig. 16.5a, b   MRI-guided vacuum-assisted biopsy of suspicious focus.
a Subtraction slice image: clear identification of suspicious focus seen in diagnostic breast MRI examination.
b T1w postbiopsy image: the corresponding position of the resection cavity is documentation of representative sampling.

Histology: LIN (B3 lesion).

Fig. 16.6a, b   MRI-guided vacuum-assisted biopsy of a mass lesion near a breast prosthesis.
a Subtraction slice image: clear identification of a hypervascularized mass lesion near a prosthesis (arrow).
b T1w postbiopsy image: an angulated access path was chosen so as not to damage the prosthesis. The corresponding position of the resection cavity is documentation of representative sampling.

Histology: invasive tubular breast carcinoma (B5b lesion).

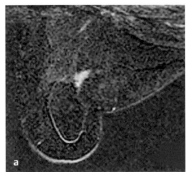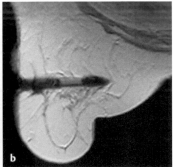

Fig. 16.7a, b   MRI-guided vacuum-assisted biopsy of a nonmass-like lesion.
a Subtraction slice image: clear identification of triangular nonmass-like lesion.
b T1w biopsy image: the biopsy needle is in place with the notch opening in the correct position.

Histology: radial scar (B3 lesion).

Checklist

MRI-Guided Vacuum-Assisted Biopsy

- Establish the indication.
- Confirm that there is no correlative finding on mammography and/or (second-look) ultrasonography.
- Obtain informed consent (in advance).
- Position the patient properly and comfortably in an open breast surface coil with biopsy option.
- Choose the appropriate puncture equipment (grid, post-and-pillar).
- Position external markers at the estimated target position (arbitrary zero-point).
- Carry out the dynamic MR mammography examination with image subtraction.
- Identify the target.
- Calculate appropriate x-, y-, and z-coordinates.
- Move the external markers to the appropriate puncture site and perform an MRI check.

- Disinfect the breast skin and administer local anesthesia; if necessary make a nick incision.
- Introduce the coaxial introduction needle.
- Perform an MRI check of the needle position in relation to the target lesion and correct the position if necessary.
- Demonstrate biopsy sounds.
- Obtain tissue samples: at least 12 tissue cylinders with 11G needle, or volume equivalent.
- Perform an MRI check of biopsy cavity position in relation to the target lesion (possibly with additional contrast administration).
- If necessary, harvest additional tissue samples.
- Consider placing a marker coil/clip.
- Remove the coaxial introduction needle.
- Release the breast from the puncture device while applying compression to the puncture site. Move the patient to a reclining chair, apply compression, and cool.
- Obtain the final mammograms in two orthogonal planes.

Table 16.2 Study results for MRI-guided vacuum-assisted breast biopsies

Parameter	Schrading, Kuhl	Libermann	Viehweg	Orel	Lehmann	Perlet	Women's Health Center Göttingen
Year	2007	2005	2007	2006	2005	2006	2008
Number of patients	200	106	39	75	28	538	365
Number of biopsies	316	112	53[a]	85	38	538	389
Gauge	10,9	9	11	9	9	11	10,9
Number of tissue samples	n.a.	~12	>20	n.a.	n.a.	20	~15
Malignant	43%	25%	26%	61%	37%	27%	27%
Borderline	5%	20%	4%	21%	5%	3%	13%
Benign	52%	55%	70%	18%	58%	70%	60%
Accuracy	99%	97%	100%	98%	100%	96%	99%
No lesion reproduction	n.a.	12%	12%	n.a.	n.a.	16%	6.8%
Time expenditure (11G)	n.a.	n.a.	60 minutes	n.a.	n.a.	70 minutes	n.a.
Time expenditure (10G)	62 minutes	n.a.	n.a.	n.a.	n.a.	n.a.	46 minutes
Time expenditure (9G)	34 minutes	33 minutes	n.a.	30–60 minutes	n.a.	38 minutes	39 minutes
Complications	3%	5.3%	n.a.	0%[b]	0%	<1%	<1%

n.a.: not applicable.
[a] Including eight preoperative wire localizations.
[b] "No major complications."

Results. Several working groups have evaluated the results of MRI-guided vacuum-assisted breast biopsies in large patient cohorts (**Table 16.2**). The data show that this is a safe, reliable, and time-efficient procedure when performed in specialized medical centers. Results for MRI-guided vacuum-assisted breast biopsies are comparable to those for stereotactic vacuum-assisted biopsies of ambiguous microcalcifications.

Therapeutic MRI-Guided Vacuum-Assisted Biopsy

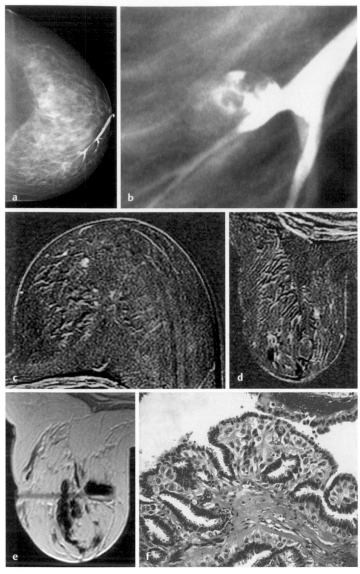

MRI-guided vacuum-assisted biopsy can be performed as a therapeutic procedure for small borderline lesions. This is especially true for papillomas. Because of their increased potential for malignant transformation, it is recommended that borderline lesions be excised. As an alternative to open surgery, vacuum-assisted biopsy is a reliable method for the complete removal of small lesions (≤ 10 mm diameter) and can be done as an outpatient procedure (**Fig. 16.8**).

Fig. 16.8a–f   MRI-compatible vacuum-assisted excision of breast papilloma.

a Galactography: localized contrast-filling defect within breast duct in patient with bloody discharge.

b Galactography (zoomed partial image).

c MRI subtraction image: corresponding hypervascularized lesion.

d Subtraction slice image before intervention: clear identification of the hypervascularized lesion seen in diagnostic breast MRI examination.

e T1w postbiopsy image: corresponding position of the resection cavity is documentation of representative sampling.

f Histology specimen: intraductal papilloma. No further pathological secretion during follow-up period.

MRI-Guided Localization

Indications and Objectives

MRI-guided localizations are indicated in cases when the MRI lesion to be excised cannot be clinically palpated or detected by ultrasound or mammography. In this context we distinguish **direct localization**, with placement of one localization wire within or near the target lesion, and **target volume localization**, in which several localization wires are placed at the surgically relevant target lesion borders.

The aim of a preoperative MRI-guided localization is to aid the surgeon in completely excising the target tissue while limiting the excision volume to the necessary extent. In addition, the preoperative markers also aid the pathologist in examining the tissue sample more selectively.

Localization Equipment

Various MRI-compatible localization needles are available for the MRI-guided preoperative localization of suspicious lesions. In terms of wire configuration, they do not differ from localization wires used for stereotactic and ultrasound-guided localizations. Generally, however, they can be categorized into manually retractable wires (whose position can be corrected, **Fig. 16.9**) and nonretractable wires (which must usually be removed surgically after placement, **Figs. 16.10, 16.11**). Another possibility for the preoperative localization of a MRI breast lesion is the placement of a skin marker. This is acceptable provided that the lesion has a close topographic relation to a clearly reproducible skin structure (e.g., nipple). In addition, MRI-compatible clips and coils are available for marking carcinoma borders prior to neoadjuvant chemotherapy or when the localization procedure is performed at an institution distant from that where the surgical procedure is performed (**Fig. 16.12**). Recent developments include combining metal clips with a special sponge detectable by ultrasound (**Figs. 16.12h, 16.13**).

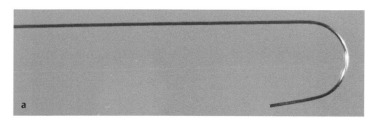

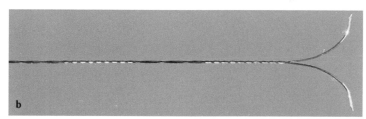

Fig. 16.9a, b   Manually retractable localization wires.
a Homer Mammalok J-wire (Mitek, Westwood, MA, USA).

b Double-tipped wire (Bard Biopsy Systems, Tempe, AZ, USA).

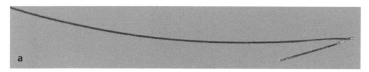

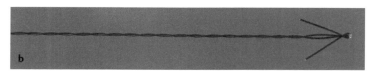

Fig. 16.10a, b   Nonretractable localization wires. These require surgical removal after placement.
a Single-hook wire (Invivo Corp., Orlando, FL, USA).

b Double-hook wire (Invivo Corp., Orlando, FL, USA).

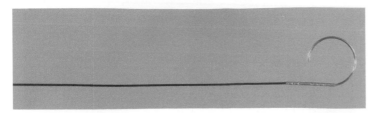

Fig. 16.11 Localization coil with attached thread. "Ariadne localization coil" (RepoLoc, Bard Biopsy Systems, Tempe, AZ, USA). A combination of metal coil with attached guiding thread.

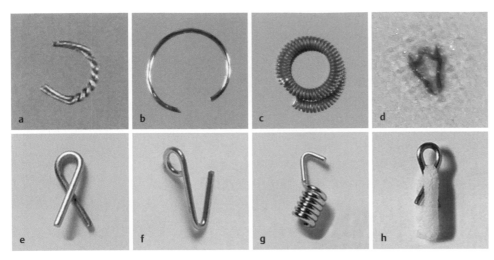

Fig. 16.12a–h Clips and coils. Various coils (**a–c**) and clips (**d–h**) of different configurations and from different companies.

a Tumark semicircular coil (SOMATEX Medical Technologies GmbH, Teltow, Germany).

b ClipLoc incompletely closed circular coil (Invivo Corp., Orlando, FL, USA).

c MMS Coil with spiral configuration (Cook Medical, Bloomington, IN, USA).

d Marker clip with barbs (Ethicon Endo-Surgery, Cincinnati, OH, USA).

e Ultra clip marker (Bard Biopsy Systems, Tempe, AZ, USA).

f Ultra clip marker with different configuration (Bard Biopsy Systems, Tempe, AZ, USA).

g Clip marker especially well-suited for marking tumor borders prior to neoadjuvant chemotherapy (Bard Biopsy Systems, Tempe, AZ, USA).

h Clip marker with ultrasound-visible sponge attachment (Bard Biopsy Systems, Tempe, AZ, USA).

Fig. 16.13a–d Clip marker with ultrasound-visible attachment.

a MammoMark sponges in unused condition (top) and in expanded condition after being soaked in fluid (bottom) (Ethicon Endo-Surgery, Cincinnati, OH, USA).

b MammoMark clip as seen on mammography.

c MammoMark expanded sponge as seen on ultrasound. Note the visible signal reflections caused by the metal clip in the center.

d Surgical specimen 12 days after vacuum-assisted biopsy and clip placement. Biopsy cavity (arrows). MammoMark sponge remnant (open arrows). Radiographically visible metal clip (arrowhead).

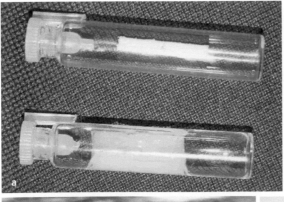
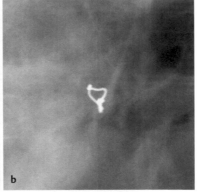
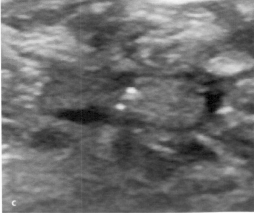
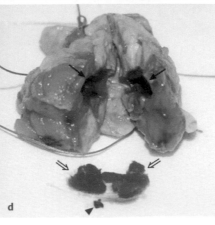

Procedure

MRI-Guided Preoperative Localization*

- Contrast enhanced breast MRI is performed with the localization equipment positioned on the affected side to reproduce the target lesion for the MRI-guided localization.
- If the target lesion is not or is only questionably reproduced, and the lesion is not histologically proven to be a carcinoma, the intervention should be discontinued and a short-term follow-up examination in 6 months recommended.
- If the target lesion is unequivocally identified, then the puncture coordinates (*x*-, *y*-, and *z*-axes) are calculated. The calculated puncture site (*x*- and *y*-axes) is marked with an external marker (e.g., oil-containing), and an MRI check is performed without additional contrast administration.
- If the marker position is incorrect, a new calculation is performed and the marker position corrected. If the marker position is correct, the skin is disinfected and local anesthesia may be administered. The puncture cannula is inserted 5–10 mm deeper than the calculated depth (*z*-axis).
- The position of the needle is checked by performing an MRI T1w series without contrast. If the position is incorrect, the needle is repositioned and rechecked. If the position is correct, the marker is advanced and released into the breast tissue (wire, coil/clip).
- Postlocalization MRI check (when indicated with contrast administration) as a final documentation of the correct wire or coil/clip marking. If the position is incorrect (> 10 mm from lesion), and the localization marker used is a repositionable wire, then the wire may be relocated. Alternatively, a second marker can be placed opposing the first, placing the localized lesion between the two markers. The position of coil/clip markers cannot usually be corrected.
- Conclusion of the localization procedure and taking of postlocalization mammograms in CC and ML projections for the surgeon.
- *Special case:* For nonmass lesions, a localization marker need not necessarily be placed within the finding. It is often better for the surgeon's orientation to place markers at relevant lesion borders (e.g., margins for segmental resection, **Fig. 16.15b,c**). In this situation, it is not necessary to correct the marker when it is more than 10 mm from the lesion.
- Before neoadjuvant chemotherapy, clip markers are placed at the original tumor borders.
- *Report:*
  - Was the target finding reproducible? (yes/no)
  - Position of the target finding (quadrant, clock time position, distance from the skin)
  - What marker was used? (single/double hook wire, J-wire, clip/coil)
  - Marker position relative to lesion (in cm)
  - Associated findings (e.g., hematoma after biopsy)
- *Specimen radiography:* Recommended, especially for confirmation and documentation of complete excision of the target lesion after coil or wire localization.
- *Documentation:*
  - MRI image of target finding (subtraction image, **Fig. 16.14a**)
  - MRI image documentation of the marker's position (T1w image, **Fig. 16.14b**)
  - Mammography in CC and ML projections
- *Quality assurance criteria:*
  - Distance of marker to lesion < 10 mm in 90% of cases†
  - Complete surgical excision in > 95% of cases‡
  - Correlation of histopathology with MRI findings‡

* Recommendations of the German Radiological Society Breast Diagnostics Working Group 2007.

† Not applicable for diffusely enhancing lesions with marking of surgically relevant borders.

‡ Final assessment made in an interdisciplinary conference.

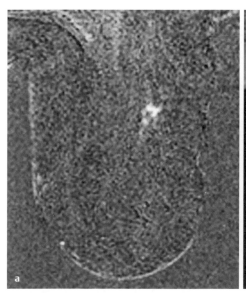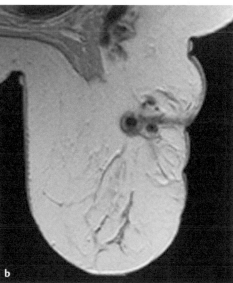

Fig. 16.14a, b MRI-guided tumor localization.

a Subtraction slice image: clear identification of focal hypervascularization in the left breast. Histologically verified breast carcinoma in the right breast.

b T1w postlocalization image: Localization wire in the correct position.

Histology: high grade DCIS.

Checklist

MRI-Guided Preoperative Localization

- Establish the indication.
- Confirm that there is no correlative finding on mammography and/or (second-look) ultrasonography.
- Obtain informed consent (in advance).
- Position the patient Properly and comfortably in an open breast surface coil with localization option.
- Choose the appropriate puncture equipment (grid, post-and-pillar).
- Position external markers at the estimated target position (arbitrary zero-point).
- Carry out dynamic MR mammography examination with image subtraction.
- Identify the target.
- Calculate appropriate x-, y-, and z-coordinates.
- Move external markers to the appropriate puncture site and perform an MRI check.
- Disinfect the breast skin and administer local anesthesia if necessary.

- Choose the localization material (wire, coil/clip).
- Introduce the localization needle.
- Perform an MRI check of the needle position in relation to the target lesion and correct the position if necessary.
- Release markers.
- Remove the localization needle.
- If necessary, repeat the procedures for placement of additional markers.
- Perform a final MRI check of marker position(s) in relation to target lesion (if necessary with additional contrast administration).
- Release the breast from the puncture device while applying compression to the puncture site. Move the patient to a reclining chair, apply compression, and cool.
- Obtain final mammograms in two orthogonal planes.
- Optional creation of photomontage showing individual lesions and marker positions (Fig. 16.15 d, e).

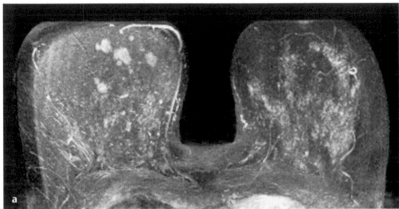
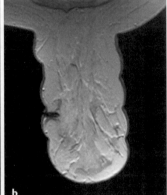
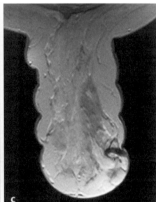

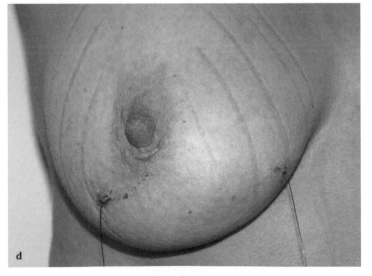
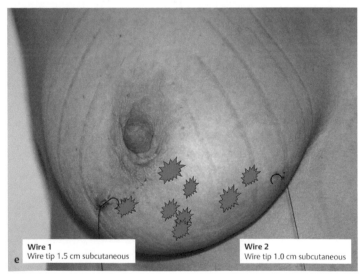
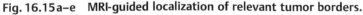

Fig. 16.15a–e   MRI-guided localization of relevant tumor borders.

a Diagnostic subtraction MIP: several tumor manifestations in both lower segments of the right breast.

b T1w postlocalization slice image: localization wire tip marking the medial border of the target volume.

c T1w postlocalization slice image: localization wire tip marking the lateral border of the target volume.

d Postinterventional photographic documentation showing both localization wires.

e Postinterventional photomontage showing the depth of wire tips and the location of tumor manifestations for the surgeon's orientation.

Histology: multifocal breast carcinoma. Quadrantectomy achieved R0 resection.

17 Indications for Breast MRI

The expedient use of breast MRI requires several aspects to be taken into consideration:

- Widely accepted indications for the performance of breast MRI include the **differentiation between scar tissue and local recurrence** in women after breast-conserving therapy, and the search for the primary tumor site in women with **cancer of unknown primary origin** (CUP).
- Recent studies have shown that it is expedient to perform breast MRI for **preoperative local staging** of patients with an invasive lobular carcinoma and for **early detection in women with a highly increased breast cancer risk profile**. Some national guidelines (e.g., German, American Cancer Society [ACS]) currently include specific recommendations for the use of breast MRI.
- Current study data have shown that breast MRI yields significant additional information when performed in the framework of **pretherapeutic breast cancer staging**, for **monitoring during neoadjuvant chemotherapy**, and in women with **breast implants**.
- The most common use of breast MRI in the diagnostic breast clinic is as a **problem solver** in cases where ambiguous findings are still present after the diagnostic work-up with clinical examination and/or mammography, and/or breast when ultrasound has been completed.
- The significant value of the information provided by breast MRI, especially in comparison with that provided by other breast imaging modalities, makes it an examination that should be considered in the framework of the **diagnostic work-up of an ambiguous breast finding** and **early breast cancer detection**. As a consequence, the application of modified examination protocols (e.g., **Göttingen Optipack**) and the primary use of breast MRI in early breast cancer detection (**MRI screening**) may provide an alternative to the diagnostic breast examination.

Differentiation between Scar and Local Recurrence after Breast-Conserving Therapy

Clinical examination, mammography, and breast ultrasonography cannot always reliably differentiate between a postoperative scar and breast cancer, or between a postoperative scar after breast-conserving therapy (BCT) and a local recurrence.

Vascularization. MRI makes possible the differentiation between nonvascularized scar tissue and a strongly vascularized malignancy, and is therefore the ideal examination technique for this indication. If breast MRI shows no enhancement in the scar tissue area after surgery, the presence of a carcinoma or recurrence can be reliably excluded (**Figs. 17.1, 17.2**). If localized enhancing areas are present in the scar area, then the presence of a malignancy must be considered (**Figs. 17.3, 17.4**). The dynamic signal characteristics are usually not relevant in this context as carcinoma tissue within a scar often displays an unspecific TIC. Apparently tumor angiogenesis of a carcinoma within fibrotic scar tissue is often increased to a lesser degree than that of carcinomas at other locations. It must be noted, however, that not all enhancing areas within a scar are necessarily an indication of malignancy or recurrence. Occasionally reactive hyperemia may be present.

> *!*
> The recommended interval between a diagnostic excision and a breast MRI examination is 6 months.
> The recommended interval between the end of radiation therapy after breast-conserving therapy and a breast MRI examination is 12 months.
> **Note:** there is great interindividual variability of tissue enhancement after radiation therapy.

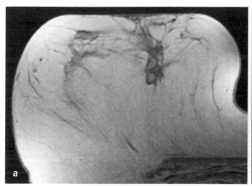 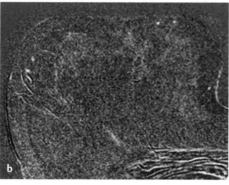

Fig. 17.1a, b   Postoperative scar after diagnostic excision.
  a T1w precontrast slice image: architectural distortion and several hyperintense fat necroses in the surgical region.
  b Subtraction slice image: no enhancement in the scar region. No pathological findings during the follow-up period.

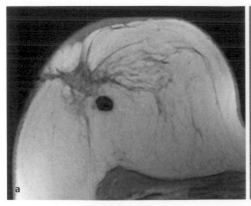
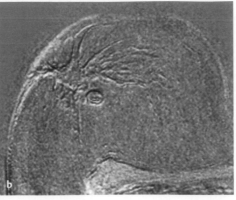

Fig. 17.2a, b Postoperative scar after breast-conserving surgery.

a T1w precontrast slice image: typical architectural distortion in the region of surgery. Susceptibility artifact due to clip marker.

b Subtraction slice image: no enhancement in the scar region rules out recurrence reliably. No pathological findings during the follow-up period.

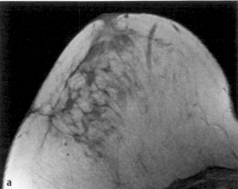
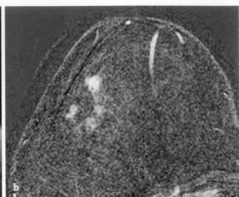

Fig. 17.3a, b Recurrence in the surgical region after breast-conserving surgery.

a T1w precontrast slice image: several, non-lipomatous, masslike lesions in the surgical region after breast-conserving therapy without radiation therapy (rejected by the patient).

b Subtraction slice image: nodular enhancement within these lesions with discrete enhancement of surrounding tissue areas.

Histology: bifocal invasive ductal breast carcinoma (= recurrence with surrounding EIC).

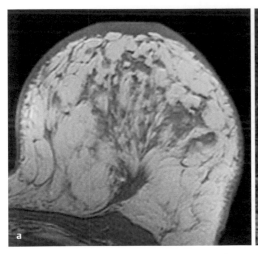
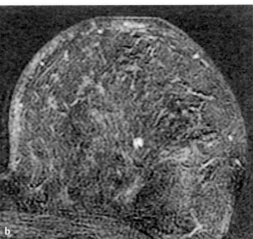
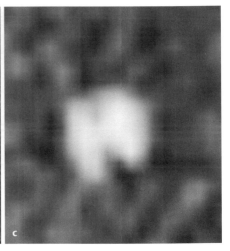

Fig. 17.4a–c Recurrence in the surgical region after breast-conserving surgery.

a T1w precontrast slice image: typical architectural distortion in the surgical region after breast-conserving therapy. Skin thickening due to radiation therapy.

b Subtraction slice image: focal enhancement in the ventral aspect of the scar area shows endotumoral dark septation, not typical of malignancy.

c Zoomed partial view of the hypervascularized lesion.

Histology: recurrence of invasive lobular breast carcinoma.

Detection of breast cancer recurrence in breast MRI. Several working groups have reported that breast MRI has a sensitivity of up to 100% for the detection of a recurrence of breast cancer after BCT. Most breast cancer recurrences develop in areas of preexisting extensive intraductal component that were not excised at the time of primary breast cancer surgery. Typically, these recurrences are detected 2–3 years after breast-conserving surgery (BCS) and have a diameter of 5–15 mm. Compared with other breast imaging modalities, breast MRI is significantly superior in detecting these recurrences. If a tumor recurrence has already been histologically verified, breast MRI allows the evaluation of breast areas near the chest wall and possible tumor infiltration of the pectoral muscle.

Importantly, breast MRI allows the reliable exclusion of breast cancer recurrence when there is no enhancement in the scar region. False-negative breast MRI findings are practically unknown.

Scheduling. There are no concrete recommendations for the scheduling of breast MRI examinations after BCT. From our experience, however, it seems expedient to routinely perform breast MRI one year after the end of adjuvant radiation therapy and at 2-year intervals thereafter.

New possible therapeutic strategies. Due to cumulative side-effects, it is not possible to perform a second course of radiotherapy in a woman who has had BCS with adjuvant radiation therapy. The detection of an ipsilateral breast cancer recurrence therefore generally results in mastectomy. However, the great reliability

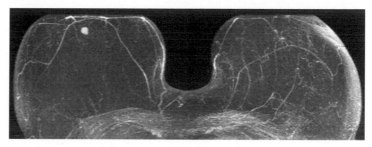

Fig. 17.5   A theoretical constellation of findings that could make possible a second BCS for breast cancer recurrence after BCS + radiation therapy. New hypervascularized mass lesion with a diameter of 6 mm in the scar area of the right breast, 8 years after BCS with radiation therapy. High transparency (MRI density I) without further suspicious findings.

Histology: IDC, pT1b.

of high-quality high-resolution (HR) breast MRI examinations in excluding breast cancer makes it conceivable that this strategy, which originated in the era of x-ray mammography and ultrasonography, might change in the future. It is imaginable, for example, that a second BCS could be performed when a metachronous, ipsilateral breast cancer recurrence has been detected in a woman who has already undergone earlier BCS with adjuvant radiation therapy. This could be the case when the recurrence is a solitary finding without signs of extensive intraductal component in a breast with high breast MRI transparency (MRI density I, **Fig. 17.5**). Such speculation has not yet been substantiated by scientifically acquired data.

Carcinoma of Unknown Primary

The term *CUP syndrome* is used to denote the presence of cancer cells, i.e., metastases, without knowledge of the primary tumor site from which these originate. A typical constellation leading to diagnostic breast examinations is the detection of an axillary lymph node metastasis (locoregional metastasis) without prior identification of the primary tumor site (e.g., in the breast, **Fig. 17.6**). In a broader context, it is sometimes reasonable to search for the primary tumor site in the breast when metastatic spread into other body regions (hematogenous metastasis) has occurred.

! The most common sites of metastatic spread from breast cancer are:
- Lymphogenous locoregional spread: primarily to the axillary, clavicular, and parasternal lymph nodes
- Hematogenous spread: to bone, lung, liver, and brain.

Diagnostic strategy. X-ray mammography is the diagnostic imaging method of choice in such a setting. Ultrasonography of the breast is a useful complementary method depending on parenchymal density. Dynamic MR mammography is indicated when both these diagnostic techniques have failed to identify an intramammary primary tumor (**Figs. 17.7, 17.8**).

! When searching for the primary tumor of a locoregional lymph node metastasis, *every* ipsilateral ambiguous breast MRI finding must be considered a potential primary lesion and be submitted to a diagnostic work-up.

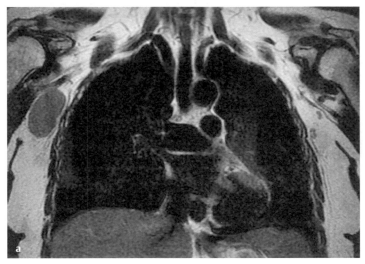 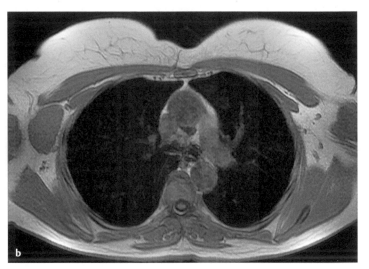

Fig. 17.6a, b   Carcinoma of unknown primary (CUP) with axillary lymph node metastasis. Enlarged right axillary lymph node with histologically verified adenocarcinoma cells (US-guided core biopsy). At this time there were no clinical or mammographic signs of breast cancer making this a CUP.
a T1w precontrast coronal slice image: upper thoracic aperture.   **b** T1w precontrast axial slice image.

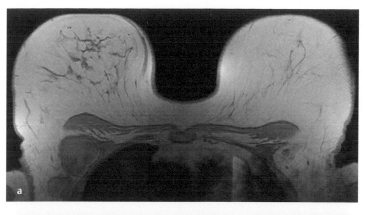

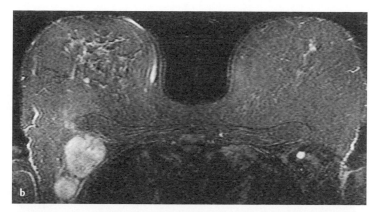

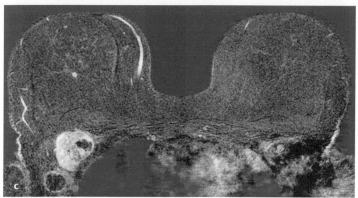

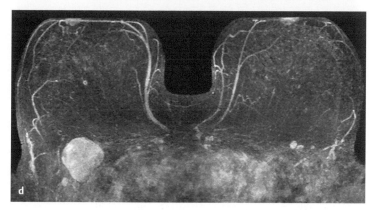

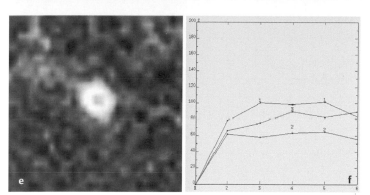

Fig. 17.7 a–f   CUP with primary tumor found on breast MRI. Enlarged right axillary lymph node as sole clinical symptom. Unremarkable mammogram and breast ultrasound examination.

a T1w precontrast slice image: several pathologically enlarged right axillary lymph nodes.
b IR T2w slice image.
c Corresponding subtraction slice image: hypervascularized focus with a diameter of 4 mm and little central perfusion (rim sign).
d Subtraction MIP.
e Zoomed subtraction slice image: better visualization of rim-enhancement and poorly defined borders.
f TIC: unspecific.

Histology: invasive ductal breast carcinoma (pT1a) as the primary tumor with extensive locoregional lymph node metastases.

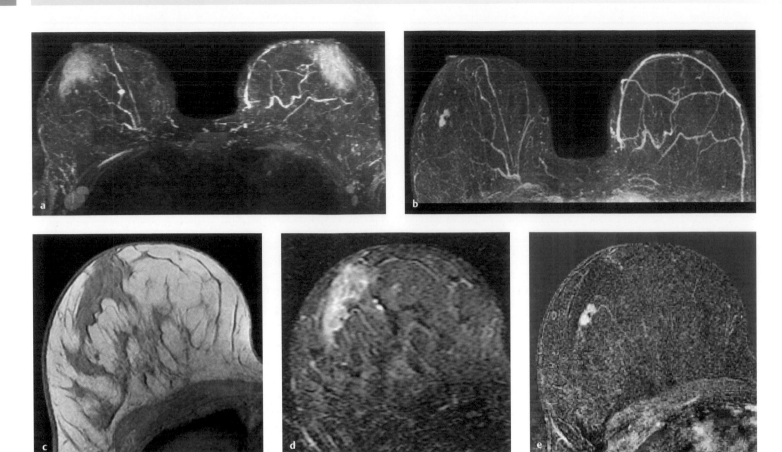

Fig. 17.8 a–e CUP with primary tumor found on breast MRI. Enlarged right axillary lymph node as sole clinical symptom. Unremarkable mammogram and breast ultrasound examination.

a T2w MIP: pathologically enlarged right axillary lymph node.
b Subtraction MIP: solitary barbell-shaped enhancement in the lateral aspect of the right breast.
c T1w precontrast slice image (right breast): unremarkable findings.
d IR T2w slice image (right breast): unremarkable findings.

e Corresponding subtraction slice image: good visualization of primary tumor.

Histology: bifocal invasive ductal breast carcinoma.

Preoperative Local Staging

One of the most important indications for use of breast MRI preoperatively. Of all breast imaging techniques, breast MRI has the greatest sensitivity for the detection of breast cancer. It is for this reason that MR mammography is especially suited to give additional preoperative information about the tumor extent, the presence of an extensive intraductal component (EIC), possible multifocality or multicentricity, and the presence of contralateral breast cancer. Numerous studies convincingly document the importance of preoperative MRI staging for the effective planning of the appropriate stage-dependent treatment strategy.

!
• The purpose of preoperative local MRI staging in breast cancer patients is assessment of:
  • Tumor size
  • EIC
  • Multifocality
  • Multicentricity
  • Contralateral tumor
  • Lymph node involvement

Tumor Size

Studies comparing the preoperative estimation of tumor size by breast imaging techniques (mammography, ultrasonography, MRI) with the histological tumor measurements show that MR mammography is superior to the other imaging modalities (**Fig. 17.9**). Current data show no significant difference in the size estimated by breast MRI and that measured in the histological specimen. In contrast, x-ray mammography and ultrasonography significantly underestimate the tumor size.

Extensive Intraductal Component

An extensive intraductal component (EIC) is present when the intraductal component surrounding an invasive ductal carcinoma constitutes 25% or more of the tumor. An EIC is the primary cause of breast cancer local recurrence in the scar area after BCT. Breast

MRI is superior to x-ray mammography and breast ultrasonography in the preoperative detection of EIC.

Criteria and procedures. The principal characteristic in breast MRI indicating the presence of an EIC is a contrast-enhancing area with linear (**Figs. 17.10, 17.11**), linear-branching (**Fig. 17.12**), or dendritic (**Fig. 17.13**) configuration adjacent to the primary tumor. The additional presence of small round or ovoid enhancing foci is often an indication of the presence of microinvasive tumor (**Fig. 17.14**). The signal analysis is usually not diagnostically helpful in such nonmasslike enhancing lesions. In the presence of the morphological changes described above, therefore, an unsuspicious time to signal intensity curve (TIC) cannot rule out an EIC.

An extensive intraductal tumor that contains areas indicative of invasive carcinoma should not be designated as an EIC, but rather as a ductal carcinoma in situ (DCIS) with signs of incipient localized invasion (**Fig. 17.15**). The percutaneous biopsy of such lesions should therefore preferably target areas most suspicious for invasive tumor so that, if it is confirmed, appropriate therapeutic procedures can be initiated (e.g., sentinel lymph node biopsy).

!
• **EIC:** Intraductal tumor in the periphery of an invasive breast carcinoma.

Infiltration of the Pectoral Muscle

Preoperative confirmation of breast cancer infiltration into the pectoral muscle is significant because it occasionally leads to a change in the indicated surgical procedure to include a fasciotomy or myotomy of the affected muscle areas. Here also, breast MRI is the favored imaging technique because it allows overlap-free visualization of the pectoral muscle in the entire retroparenchymal space.

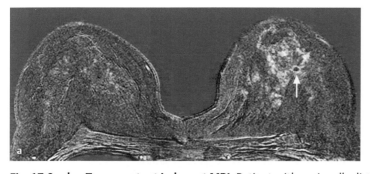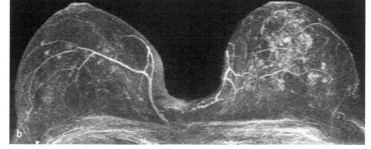

Fig. 17.9a, b   Tumor extent in breast MRI. Patient with regionally distributed, pleomorphic microcalcifications in the upper outer quadrant of the left breast. Histology revealed DCIS after stereotactic VAB.

a Subtraction slice image: linear/dendritic enhancement pattern in both upper breast quadrants of the left breast. Biopsy cavity (arrow).

b Subtraction MIP: improved visualization of tumor extent.

Procedure: percutaneous histological confirmation of DCIS in the left upper inner quadrant resulted in primary mastectomy of the left breast.

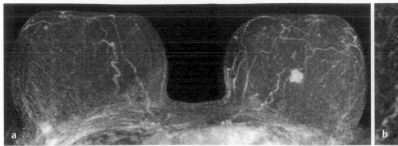
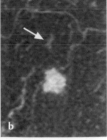

Fig. 17.10a, b   Intraductal component in breast MRI.
a Subtraction MIP: invasive ductal breast carcinoma in the central aspect of the left breast.
b Zoomed partial view of subtraction slice image: discrete linear enhancement (4 mm long) ventrally of the index tumor as the imaging correlate of an intraductal component.

Histological confirmation.

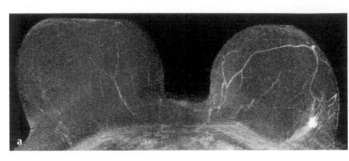
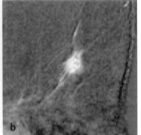

Fig. 17.11a, b   EIC in breast MRI.
a Subtraction MIP: invasive ductal breast carcinoma in the lateral aspect of the left breast.
b Zoomed partial view of subtraction slice image: linear enhancement ventrally and dorsally of the index tumor as the imaging correlate of EIC.

Histological confirmation.

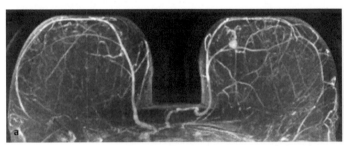
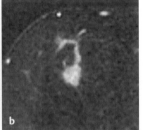

Fig. 17.12a, b   EIC in breast MRI.
a Subtraction MIP: invasive ductal breast carcinoma in the craniomedial aspect of the left breast.
b Zoomed partial view of the subtraction slice image: microlobulated index carcinoma with ventral linear-branching enhancement as the imaging correlate of EIC.

Histological confirmation.

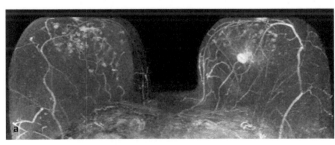
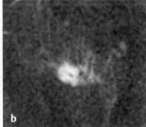

Fig. 17.13a, b   EIC in breast MRI.
a Subtraction MIP: invasive ductal breast carcinoma in the central aspect of the left breast.
b Zoomed partial view of the subtraction slice image: peritumoral dendritic enhancement of the index tumor as the imaging correlate of EIC.

Histological confirmation.

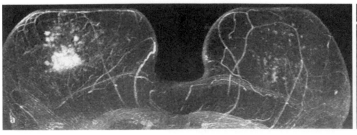
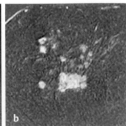

Fig. 17.14a, b   EIC in breast MRI.
a Subtraction MIP: large invasive ductal breast carcinoma in the central aspect of the right breast.
b Zoomed partial view of the subtraction slice image: multiple peritumoral hypervascularized foci as the imaging correlate of EIC with microinvasive tumor components at several locations.

Histological confirmation.

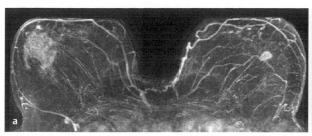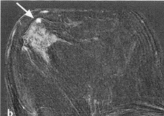

Fig. 17.15a, b   Bilateral breast cancer. DCIS with focal invasive tumor component in the right breast. Breast MRI performed in the preoperative setting for local staging of mammographically and sonographically detected breast carcinoma in the left breast.
a Subtraction MIP: regional enhancement in the upper outer quadrant of the right breast without correlative findings on mammography or breast ultrasound. Mass lesion correlating with mammographically and sonographically detected breast carcinoma in the left breast.
b Subtraction slice image (right breast): non-masslike enhancement with small, localized area of significantly stronger enhancement (arrow) as the correlate of area of invasive tumor.

Histology: extensive area of high-grade DCIS with small invasive component (IDC pT1b) in the right breast. IDC (pT1c) in the left breast.

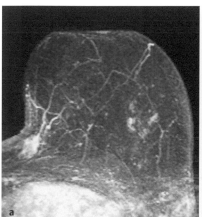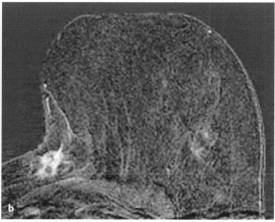

Fig. 17.16a, b   Breast carcinoma near the chest wall with enhancement of muscle fascia.
a Subtraction MIP (left breast): breast carcinoma in the far medial aspect of the left breast, very near the pectoral muscle.
b Subtraction slice image (left breast): enhancement of the index tumor and discrete enhancement of the adjacent pectoral fascia.

Histology: IDC (pT1c) without infiltration of the pectoral muscle.

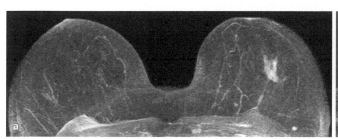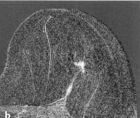

Fig. 17.17a, b   Breast carcinoma far from the chest wall with enhancement near the muscle fascia.
a Subtraction MIP: breast carcinoma in the central aspect of the left breast with long dorsal linear enhancement reaching the pectoral muscle.
b Subtraction slice image (left breast): better visualization of linear enhancement that reaches the ventral surface of the pectoral muscle.

Procedure: segment resection including the pectoral muscle fascia.
Histology: ILC (pT2) with CLIS extending to the pectoral muscle fascia.

Criteria and procedures. When a breast carcinoma is located near the chest wall (**Fig. 17.16**), more rarely further ventrally (**Fig. 17.17**), the finding of enhancing areas near the pectoral fascia should be communicated to the attending surgeon as a possible indication of muscle infiltration. In this context, imaging of an intact prepectoral fat lamella in the T1w precontrast image plays an important diagnostic role (**Fig. 17.18**). The diagnostic value of a breast MRI is limited, however, if motion artifacts are present near the chest wall. Motion artifacts can then result in the appearance of a nonexistent "pathological enhancement" near the chest wall in the subtraction images (**Fig. 17.19**). If this is suspected to be the case, MRI images should be reviewed in the so-called *cine mode* to more easily distinguish between artifact and true enhancement.

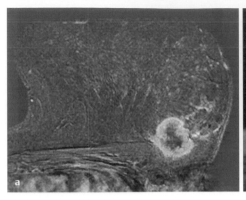 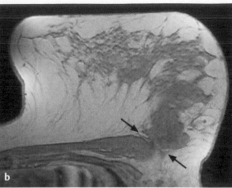

Fig. 17.18a, b Breast carcinoma with infiltration of the muscle fascia.
a Subtraction slice image (left breast): large breast carcinoma in the craniolateral aspect of the left breast immediately adjacent to the pectoral muscle, causing an indentation. No enhancement with muscle structures.
b T1w precontrast slice image: the fat lamella is not intact and does not separate the tumor from muscle tissue (arrows). Ventral surface of the pectoral muscle.

Histology: triple-negative breast carcinoma with beginning infiltration of the pectoral muscle fascia.

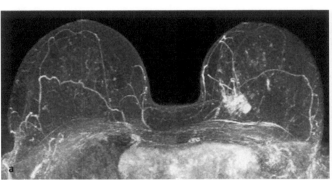 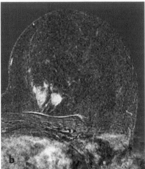

Fig. 17.19a, b Breast carcinoma with false appearance of muscle fascia infiltration.
a Subtraction MIP: large breast carcinoma with EIC in the caudomedial aspect of the left breast. Apparent enhancement of the ventral pectoral muscle surface.
b Subtraction slice image: findings compatible with motion artifact. Confirmation of motion artifact made by viewing examination in cine mode.

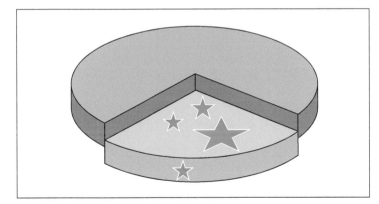

Fig. 17.20 Multifocality. Schematic diagram.

Multifocality

Many definitions of the term *multifocality* can be found in the medical literature. Most work groups base their accounts on the interpretation made by Lagios and colleagues, defining multifocality as two or more lesions within one quadrant of the breast. Other definitions are based on the maximum distance between the multiple breast cancer manifestations. Ultimately, the term multifocality is used to denote multiple tumor manifestations that can reasonably be excised by BCS completely and with adequate tumor-free margins (**Figs. 17.21, 17.22, 17.23**). Generally, one-quarter of the breast tissue is considered the maximum amount that can be removed during BCS (quadrantectomy) (**Fig. 17.20**). It should be noted, however, that a quadrantectomy is not restricted to the classic quadrants (upper outer, upper inner, lower outer, lower inner). Instead, the one-quarter of the breast

removed can be in any location (e.g., the 1-o'clock position to the 4-o'clock position).

> **! Multifocality:** Two or more carcinoma manifestations within one breast quadrant. Breast-conserving surgery can be performed as a segmental resection, up to a quadrantectomy.

Incidence. The reported incidence of multifocal breast cancer varies between 25% and 50%. The mammographic detection rate of multifocality is ~15%. In our own patient cohort, using a strict definition of multifocality, ~ 8% of breast carcinomas were shown to be multifocal. Over 70% of these were recognized as such solely in the preoperative breast MRI.

Multicentricity

There are also various definitions of *multicentricity*. Ultimately, the term multicentricity should be used to denote multiple tumor manifestations that cannot reasonably be excised by BCS due to their distant locations from each other in different breast quadrants (**Figs. 17.24, 17.25**). It should be understood, of course, that the complete removal of all breast tissue may not be performed on the basis of breast imaging alone. Histological verification of two tumor manifestations by percutaneous biopsy, confirming the presence of multicentricity, is a requirement before primary mastectomy may be performed (see **Fig. 17.27**).

> **! Multicentricity:** One or more carcinoma manifestations present in a breast quadrant other than the one harboring the primary lesion. No reasonable option for BCS

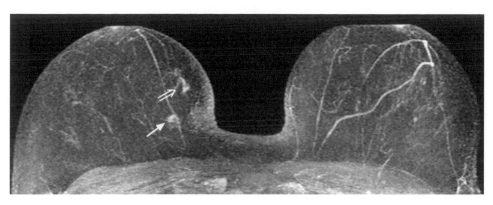

Fig. 17.21   Bifocal breast carcinoma (multifocality). Subtraction MIP shows small breast carcinoma as rim-enhancement in the lower inner quadrant of the right breast, primarily detected in mammography and breast ultrasound (solid arrow). Histological confirmation by US-guided core biopsy. Additional finding: linear-branching enhancement ventrally of the index tumor without correlative finding on mammography or second-look ultrasonography (open arrow).

Histology (in the resected breast segment): bifocal breast carcinoma with small IDC (solid arrow) and separate high-grade DCIS (double arrow).

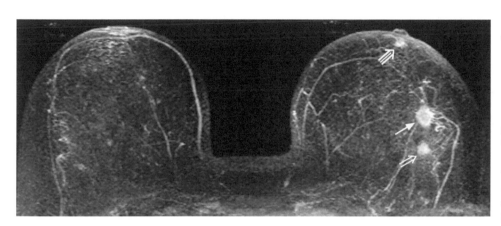

Fig. 17.22   Trifocal breast carcinoma (multifocality). Clinical examination showed slight retraction of the left nipple. Mammography revealed a mass lesion with typical signs of malignancy in the lateral aspect of the left breast. US-guided core biopsy confirmed an invasive ductal carcinoma. The subtraction MIP shows a mass lesion typical of malignancy in the lateral aspect of the left breast (solid arrow), corresponding to the histologically verified carcinoma. In addition, a small suspicious mass lesion 15 mm dorsally of the index lesion (open arrow) and a hypervascularized focus behind the mamilla (double open arrow, cause of clinical manifestation).

Histology (quadrantectomy with partial nipple resection): trifocal invasive breast carcinomas (IDC).

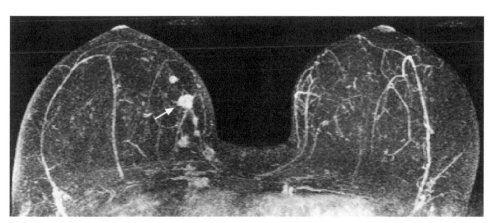

Fig. 17.23   Multifocal hypervascularized mass lesions. Suspicious mammographic and ultrasonographic lesion in the medial aspect of the right breast. US-guided core biopsy confirmed an invasive ductal carcinoma. The subtraction MIP shows a mass lesion typical of malignancy in the medial aspect of the right breast (arrow), corresponding to the histologically verified carcinoma. In addition, identification of several hypervascularized mass lesions and foci within the same quadrant as the primary tumor, some lying adjacent to the chest wall.

Histology (in the resected breast segment): ILC (pT1b). Additional verification of several hamartomas. No further malignancies.

Incidence. There is great discrepancy in the reported incidence of multicentric breast cancer, predominantly due to the use of different definitions. Histopathological studies have reported values between 40% and 60%. It must be mentioned, however, that some of the histologically proven intraductal lesions leading to the diagnosis of multicentricity will not progress to symptomatic invasive cancers and are therefore clinically insignificant. Realistic estimations of the incidence of multicentricity appear to be between 15% and 30%. Our own preoperative MRI studies have shown that multicentric tumors are found in ~12% of breast cancer patients. In half of these cases multicentricity was detected solely in MR mammography. Other working groups show an even greater proportion of the multicentric cases being detected solely in MR mammography.

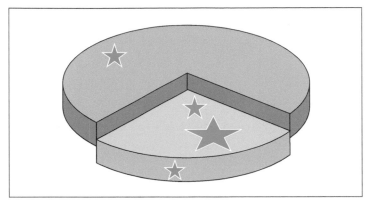

Fig. 17.24   Multicentricity. Schematic diagram.

Synchronous Bilateral Breast Cancer

When breast cancer is present in both breasts at the same time it is termed a synchronous, bilateral breast carcinoma (**Figs. 17.26, 17.27**).

Incidence. According to reports the synchronous presentation of bilateral breast cancer occurs in ~ 5% of all breast cancer patients. The incidence of bilateral invasive lobular carcinoma is reported to be significantly higher (up to 30%). In our own preoperative breast MRI studies, a contralateral carcinoma was detected in 5% of breast cancer patients. Approximately 75% of all synchronous contralateral carcinomas are detected by breast MRI.

N-Staging

MR mammography does not allow a reliable statement pertaining to metastatic axillary lymph node involvement. Unspecific lymph node enhancement (e.g., inflammatory lymph node reaction) may lead to false-positive findings. On the other hand, micrometastases do not necessarily result in pathological contrast enhancement (false-negative). The detection of a conspicuously enlarged lymph node, however, should raise suspicion of lymph node metastasis and lead to a targeted ultrasound examination and, if indicated, further cytological evaluation by FNAB or histological evaluation by percutaneous core biopsy. In addition, breast MRI images should be reviewed with special attention to the internal mammary lymph nodes in the retrosternal area as these may be enlarged when metastatically involved. Further information on the significance of MRI in the evaluation of axillary and mediastinal lymph nodes is found in Chapter 13.

Influence of Breast MRI on Therapeutic Strategy

The primary treatment of breast cancer is usually its surgical excision. Preoperative decisions must be made about whether breast-conserving therapy (lumpectomy, segment resection, quadrantectomy) is an option or not. Criteria making local excision less advisable or impossible are a large tumor size (usually over 2–3 cm, in case reports up to 5 cm), unfavorable tumor-to-breast size, and the presence of multicentric tumors. In addition, the informed patient's wishes must also be taken into consideration. Other primary forms of therapy include various combinations of chemotherapies and/or radiation therapy.

Therapy-relevant information yielded by breast MRI. Currently there is large collection of data regarding the additional relevant information that a local staging breast MRI examination yields in the preoperative setting, and the resulting modifications made in the primary treatment strategies. Studies performed with over 1500 patients showed that the preoperative breast MRI led to an appropriate alteration of the primary treatment strategy in 12%–32% of cases. The greatest proportion of these strategic corrections affected patients with invasive lobular breast carcinoma. Preoperative breast MRI information led to a change in therapy strategy in 24%–55% of these patients. This was less often the case

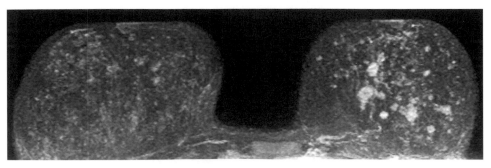

Fig. 17.25   Multicentric breast carcinoma. Bilateral stippled parenchymal enhancement pattern. Unremarkable findings in the right breast. Several hypervascularized foci and mass lesions in the medial, central, and lateral quadrants of the left breast (maximum diameter 8 mm). Percutaneous biopsy of two lesions in different breast quadrants confirmed malignancies and multicentricity.
　　Procedure: primary mastectomy. Verification of multiple carcinomas.

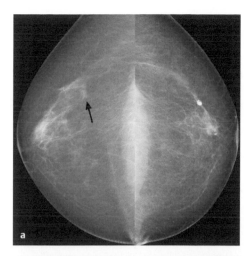

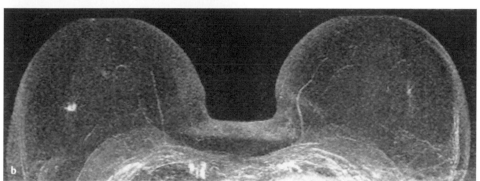

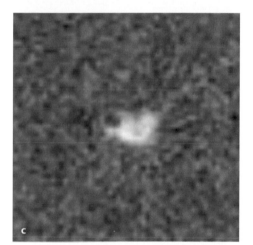
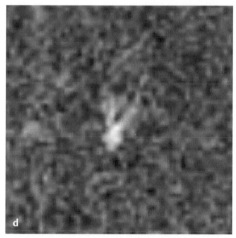

Fig. 17.26a–d Synchronous bilateral breast carcinomas.

a Mammography (CC projection): new suspicious mass lesion in the lateral aspect of the right breast.

b Subtraction MIP (preoperative staging): small hypervascularized mass lesion correlating with the mammographic finding in the right breast. Additional identification of linear-branching enhancement in the left breast.

c Zoomed partial view of the subtraction slice image (right lesion).

d Zoomed partial view of the subtraction slice image (left lesion).

Procedure: stereotactic VAB of the right lesion confirmed IDC. Preoperative wire-localization of the biopsy cavity in the right breast and MRI lesion in the left breast.

Histology: IDC (pT1b, pN0) in the right breast. High-grade DCIS (15 mm) in the left breast.

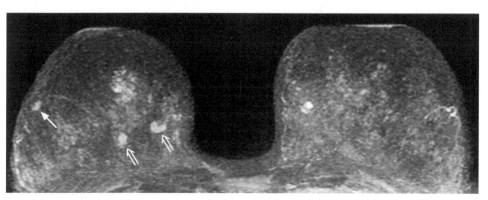

Fig. 17.27 Synchronous bilateral breast carcinomas. Unremarkable mammographic findings. Breast ultrasound revealed a suspicious lesion in the lateral aspect of the right breast. US-guided core biopsy confirmed an invasive ductal carcinoma. The subtraction MIP (preoperative local staging) shows a mass lesion in the lateral aspect of the right breast (solid arrow), corresponding to the histologically verified carcinoma. In addition, identification of two hypervascularized mass lesions in the upper inner and lower inner quadrants of the right breast (open arrows), and further suspicious mass lesion in the medial aspect of the left breast. Percutaneous VAB of lesions in the right upper inner quadrant and left breast confirmed invasive ductal carcinomas.

Procedure: primary mastectomy of the right breast and BCS of the left breast.

Histology: multicentric breast cancer in the right breast (IDC, pT1c, pN0). IDC in the left breast (pT1b, pN0).

for patients with an invasive ductal breast carcinoma. These study results are the major reason that current German national guidelines recommend the performance of a preoperative breast MRI in patients with a histologically verified ILC. In our patient cohort, additional diagnostic information provided by the preoperative breast MRI led to an appropriate modification of the surgical procedures performed in 14% of patients. This applied in particular to the widening of planned excision borders (e.g., quadrantectomy instead of lumpectomy), the performance of a mastectomy for verified multicentric tumors, and the performance of an additional contralateral lumpectomy for otherwise occult contralateral breast cancer.

False-positive findings. When appraising the value of the additional therapy-relevant information yielded by breast MRI examinations, one must also consider the possibility of false-positive findings that can influence the therapeutic strategy. Study data show that the quota of false-positive findings in breast MRI lies between 3% and 30%. In our breast cancer patient cohort this quota lies just under 10%. It is important to keep in mind that additional suspicious findings detected solely on breast MRI do not result in changes to therapeutic strategy without further diagnostic substantiation. Histological verification of additional findings by MRI-guided vacuum-assisted biopsy (VAB) is indicated to avoid unnecessary extension of the surgical procedures. This is especially true when considering primary mastectomy for multicentric MRI findings.

> **Good Practice Recommendations***
>
> Contrast-enhanced breast MRI should be recommended in the preoperative setting for the local staging of invasive lobular breast cancer and for patients with a relevantly increased breast cancer risk.
> * European S3 Guidelines: Early Breast Cancer Detection, Level of Evidence 3b, GCP (Grade of Recommendation B).
>
> **Good Practice Recommendations***
>
> Contrast-enhanced breast MRI should be coupled with provisions for the performance of MRI-guided interventions.
> * European S3 Guidelines: Early Breast Cancer Detection, GCP (Grade of Recommendation A).

Our strategies. In our women's health center, preoperative local staging breast MRI examinations are performed more often than the German national S3 guidelines recommend. Although the effectiveness of preoperative breast MRI for IDC is less than that for ILC, it is still very high, and we perform this examination preoperatively in almost all women with a histologically verified breast carcinoma.

Independently of this, it seems expedient to carry out breast MRI in women with a suspicious breast finding on clinical examination, mammography, and/or ultrasonography (BI-RADS 4 and 5) before the recommended percutaneous biopsy. Interfering enhancement patterns, sometimes resulting from prior large-core or vacuum-assisted biopsy, can thereby be avoided. And at least for mass lesions, absent enhancement on MRI allows reevaluation of the lesion and placement into the BI-RADS 3 category, avoiding the necessity for percutaneous biopsy. The prerequisite for this approach is, of course, a technically and methodically well-performed, high-resolution breast MRI examination.

Future prospects. The high sensitivity of breast MRI in the detection of breast carcinomas and the great reliability of high-quality HR breast MRI examinations in excluding breast cancer make it conceivable that current therapeutic strategies, which originated in the era of x-ray mammography and ultrasonography, may change in the future. It seems unreasonable, for example, that a patient with a bifocal breast cancer in multicentric locations (e.g., upper inner and lower outer breast quadrants) must obligatorily undergo mastectomy because of multicentricity. If the breast has high MRI transparency (e.g., MRI density I), only these two tumor manifestations and no signs of EIC, for example, then BCS seems a reasonable option. Such considerations have not yet, however, been substantiated by scientifically acquired data.

Increased Breast Cancer Risk

In industrialized countries, a normal woman's risk of being diagnosed with breast cancer during her lifetime is ~6%–8%. Women with a high risk profile have an increased lifetime risk of being diagnosed with breast cancer of over 30%. As a result, the average breast cancer risk is ~10%, that is, roughly every tenth woman in an industrialized country will develop breast cancer during her lifetime. Currently it is assumed that ~10% of all breast cancers are hereditary. Half of these (~5% of all breast cancers) are associated with mutations in the *BRCA1* or *BRCA2* genes. The other half are associated with mutations in other genes (e.g., *BRCA3* or *BRCA4*) for which no test is yet available. Women who have tested positive for a *BRCA1* or *BRCA2* gene mutation have a lifetime risk of developing breast cancer around 80% (**Fig. 17.28**), as well as a significantly increased risk of developing an ovarian carcinoma (*BRCA1*, ~50%; *BRCA2*, ~20%).

> ### Good Practice Recommendations*
>
> Breast MRI should be recommended as a supplementary diagnostic examination for women with an increased familial risk for breast cancer development (confirmed mutation in BRCA1 or BRCA2 genes, or having a heterozygote gene mutation risk of ≥20% or a lifetime risk of ≥30%).
> * European S3 Guidelines: Early Breast Cancer Detection, Level of Evidence 2a (Grade of Recommendation B).

In the current European S3 guidelines, an intensified early detection strategy is recommended for women with a confirmed mutation in the *BRCA1* or *BRCA2* genes, having a heterozygote gene mutation risk ≥20% or with a lifetime risk of ≥30%. The performance of a breast MRI examination is recommended for these women starting at age 25 years and continuing through to their 55th year of life, or until the mammographic density pattern shows involution breast parenchyma (ACR density I or II) (**Table 17.1**).

Significance of breast MRI. Studies to date regarding breast imaging diagnostics in women with a high risk profile have shown that breast MRI is significantly superior to x-ray mammography and/or breast ultrasound. In these studies, the sensitivity of breast MRI for the detection of breast cancer was ~95%, whereas mammography and ultrasonography each had a sensitivity of ~30%. The specificity was > 90% for all imaging modalities. In a prospective multicenter study including 687 asymptomatic women with an increased familial breast cancer risk (lifetime risk of ≥20%, EVA Study), breast MRI was vastly superior to all other breast imaging techniques (detection rate: US 6‰, Mx 5.4‰, Mx+US 7.7‰, breast MRI 14.9‰, breast MRI+US 14.9‰, breast MRI+Mx 16‰). It follows from these results that women with an increased familial breast cancer risk and unremarkable findings in a high-quality breast MRI examination can forgo the performance of x-ray mammography, especially when taking into consideration that these women have a higher vulnerability to the radiation exposure.

Specific characteristics. Hereditary breast cancer often has special characteristics that are less often found in breast carcinomas of women without a high-risk profile (**Table 17.2**). This results in the presence of special tumor features that are also relevant for the evaluation of breast MRI images: hereditary breast cancers tend to grow faster, are disproportionately often well-circumscribed, and are often associated with a rim-enhancement (**Fig. 17.29**).

Table 17.1 Intensified breast cancer early detection strategy for women with a high-risk profile[a]

Self-examination	At regular intervals	Beginning at 25 years of age[b]
Clinical examination	Every 6 months	Beginning at 25 years of age[b]
Breast US	Every 6 months	Beginning at 25 years of age[b]
Mammography	Yearly	Beginning at 25 years of age[b]
Breast MRI	Yearly	Beginning at 25 years of age[b]

[a] European S3-guidelines.
[b] Or at 5 years younger than the youngest affected family member.

Table 17.2 Specific characteristics of hereditary breast cancer

Young age at time of diagnosis (30–40 years)
More common incidence of multiple breast cancers (may be of differing histology)
More common development of aggressive tumor forms (high-grade, triple-negative)

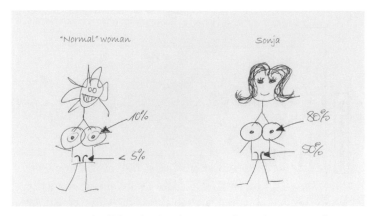

Fig. 17.28 Risk of developing breast and ovarian cancer for a woman with a *BRCA1* gene mutation. Scratch paper used to inform a patient (Sonja) with a positive *BRCA1* gene mutation test about her risk status.

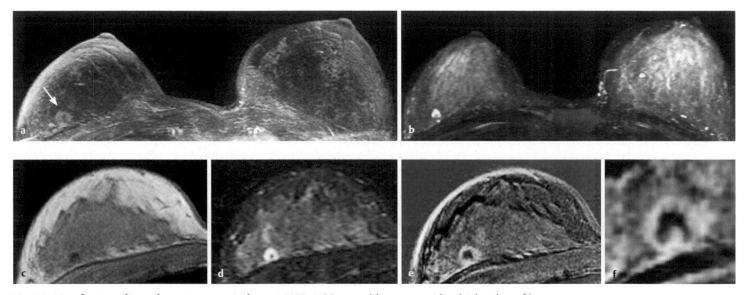

Fig. 17.29 a–f Hereditary breast cancer in breast MRI. A 28-year-old woman with a high risk profile.

a Subtraction MIP: hypervascularized mass lesion in the lateral aspect of the right breast (arrow).
b T2w MIP: high water content in the central portion of the mass lesion.
c T1w precontrast slice image (right breast): The tumor displays low signal intensity in its central portion.
d IR T2w slice image (right breast): The tumor displays high signal intensity (water content) in its central portion.

e Subtraction slice image (right breast): rim-enhancement.
f Zoomed partial view of the subtraction slice image (right breast): tumor proliferation within a central liquid (necrotic) portion of the tumor.

Histology: IDC, G3, triple-negative.

Monitoring during Neoadjuvant Chemotherapy

The expression *neoadjuvant chemotherapy* is used to denote the primary chemotherapy of breast cancer before surgical intervention. In the past, this therapeutic strategy was predominantly applied to inflammatory breast cancers because it is not usually possible to achieve tumor-free excision borders of such malignancies with primary surgery. Today, neoadjuvant chemotherapy is also being used for the therapy of locally advanced breast cancer, especially in younger women.

In the course of chemotherapy, clinical, ultrasonographic, and mammographic examinations are of limited use in providing information on the tumor response. As a slice imaging technique, breast MRI is especially suited to providing more accurate measurements for monitoring the tumor size and, importantly, also provides information pertaining to tumor vascularization.

Criteria and procedures. The key objective of image monitoring in this setting is to differentiate between "responders" (**Fig. 17.30**) and "nonresponders" (**Fig. 17.31**). Taking published evaluation criteria into account, the interpretation of MRI findings should not only consider metric tumor aspects (2-dimensional tumor diameters, 3-dimensional tumor volume) but should also include kinetic aspects (TICs) in making this differentiation. Breast MRI is normally performed after two and four cycles of neoadjuvant chemotherapy.

MRI criteria of tumor responsiveness to neoadjuvant chemotherapies (for so-called responders) are:
- Tumor size reduction > 25%
- Flattening of the initial signal increase in time–signal intensity curve
- Decrease of maximal contrast enhancement

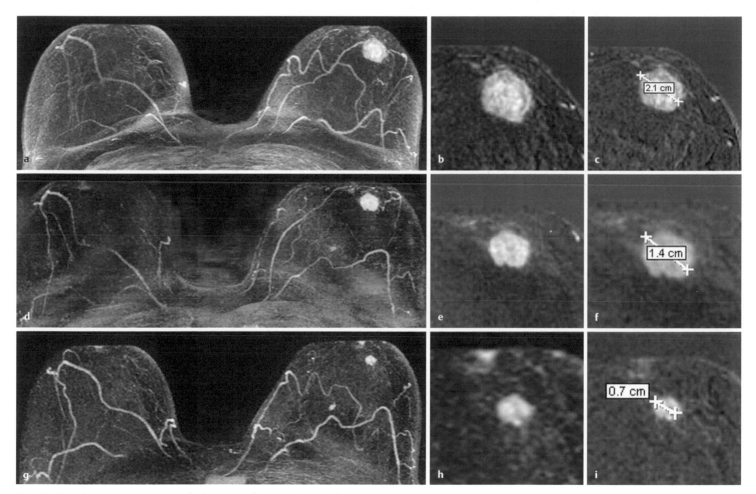

Fig. 17.30 a–i MRI monitoring during neoadjuvant chemotherapy.

a Subtraction MIP: primary findings before initiation of neoadjuvant chemotherapy.

b Zoomed partial view of the primary subtraction slice image (left breast).

c Zoomed partial view of the primary subtraction slice image (left breast): measurement for tumor metric comparisons (2-dimensional: 4.4 cm^2; 3-dimensional: 4.4 cm^3).

d Subtraction MIP after two cycles of neoadjuvant chemotherapy.

e Zoomed partial view of the subtraction slice image after two cycles of neoadjuvant chemotherapy (left breast).

f Zoomed partial view of the subtraction slice image after two cycles of neoadjuvant chemotherapy (left breast): measurement for tumor metric comparisons (2-dimensional: 1.96 cm^2; 3-dimensional 2.9 cm^3).

g Subtraction MIP after four cycles of neoadjuvant chemotherapy (preoperative images).

h Zoomed partial view of the subtraction slice image after four cycles of neoadjuvant chemotherapy (left breast).

i Zoomed partial view of the subtraction slice image after the last of four cycles of neoadjuvant chemotherapy (left breast): measurement for tumor metric comparisons (2-dimensional: 0.49 cm^2; 3-dimensional: 1.4 cm^3).

Interpretation: responder to neoadjuvant chemotherapy with tumor volume reduction of ~70%.

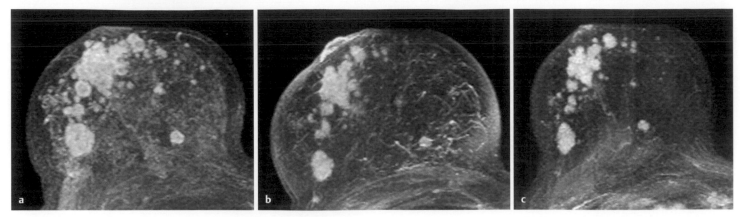

Fig. 17.31 a–c   MRI monitoring during neoadjuvant chemotherapy.

a Subtraction MIP (right breast): primary findings of multicentric breast cancer in the right breast before initiation of neoadjuvant chemotherapy.

b Subtraction MIP after two cycles of neoadjuvant chemotherapy (right breast): slight tumor volume reduction of < 25%.

c Subtraction MIP after four cycles of neoadjuvant chemotherapy (right breast): total tumor volume reduction of < 25%.

Interpretation: nonresponder to neoadjuvant chemotherapy.

Histology: IDC, ypT1c.

Follow-up after Breast Reconstruction with Prosthesis Implantation

The diagnostic value of conventional imaging techniques is very limited for patients with breast implants. This is true both for the evaluation with regard to complications of the prostheses and for the detection of periprosthetic and retroprosthetic carcinomas. Breast MRI examinations undertaken to answer the question of possible prosthesis complications employ specific sequence protocols. To rule out malignancy, contrast-enhanced dynamic breast MRI is performed in the usual way. Further details concerning the MRI examination of breast implants are found in Chapter 14.

The Problem Case in Mammography and/or Breast Ultrasound

The problem case in mammography and/or breast ultrasound is the most common indication for the performance of breast MRI in the everyday routine practice of a breast diagnostic clinic.

Breast MRI almost always allows a reliable assessment of an ambiguous mammographic and/or sonographic breast finding that is suspicious for an invasive breast tumor. If the ambiguous lesion shows no enhancement on breast MRI, then an invasive breast carcinoma can be ruled out with a high degree of reliability and percutaneous biopsy can be averted (**Figs. 17.32, 17.33**). If the corresponding MRI finding is also suspicious for malignancy or shows an unspecific enhancement, then histological verification is generally made by percutaneous biopsy (US-guided core biopsy or stereotactic VAB). Breast MRI is less reliable for the clarification of mammographic microcalcifications suspicious for DCIS.

! Breast MRI is superior to other breast imaging modalities in the diagnostic work-up of ambiguous findings.

Breast MRI often gives a patient with an ambiguous breast finding clear information about the nature and relevance of her lesion, and the consequences that may follow. When performed for the appropriate indications, breast MRI can genuinely solve a problem.

Current data show that an unremarkable breast MRI can almost certainly rule out an invasive breast carcinoma as the cause of an ambiguous mammographic finding (true-negative rate > 99%). In our experience, the rate of true-negative findings for DCIS is somewhat lower (90%–95%). The false-negative findings, however, are primarily prognostically favorable low-grade DCIS lesions.

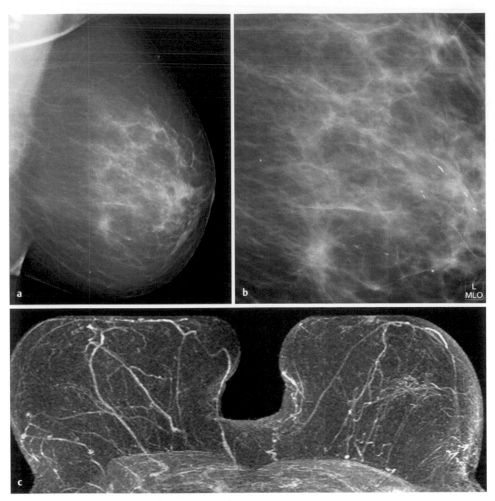

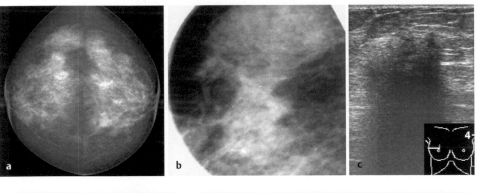

Fig. 17.32 a–c   Final resolution of a problem case with breast MRI. Unremarkable breast ultrasound findings.

a Mammography in MLO projection: Ambiguous spiculated density. No correlative finding in the CC projection.

b Spot compression: spiculated density appears unchanged. Incidental finding: calcifications indicating plasma cell mastitis.

c Subtraction MIP: MRI with high transparency. No hypervascularized findings correlating with spiculated mammographic density.

Procedure: no percutaneous biopsy. Follow-up over the following 3 years showed no carcinoma development.

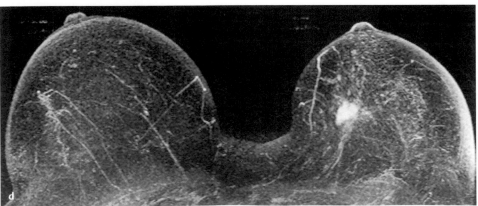

Fig. 17.33 a–d   Final resolution of a problem case with breast MRI.

a Mammography in CC projection: ambiguous density with retraction phenomenon (shrinking sign) in the lateral aspect of the right breast. No correlative finding in the MLO projection.

b Spot compression: better visualization of mammographic density.

c US: localized hypoechogenic area, possibly correlating with the mammographic density.

d Subtraction MIP: MRI with high transparency. The lack of any hypervascularized finding in correlation with the mammographic density in the right breast rules out malignancy here. Incidental detection of an otherwise occult breast carcinoma in the left breast.

Procedure: no percutaneous biopsy on the right breast. Follow-up over the following 2 years showed no carcinoma development here. Histological verification of an IDC (pT1c) in the left breast.

Early Breast Cancer Detection with Breast MRI

It is indisputable that a high-quality, high-resolution breast MRI examination is superior to all other breast imaging modalities in the detection of breast cancer. Thus it is logical to consider whether breast MRI examinations should be performed not only in women with a high-risk profile (e.g., women with a history of breast cancer or *BRCA* gene mutation), but also uniformly for early breast cancer detection in all women in the relevant age group. This diagnostic strategy is especially promising for those women with limited benefit from the currently implemented diagnostic imaging modalities (x-ray mammography, breast ultrasonography), that is, those with high parenchymal density (ACR density III and IV) and those with fibrocystic breast condition (inhomogeneous structures on breast ultrasound).

> ! The expression *early breast cancer detection* is used to denote breast cancer detected as a DCIS or, if invasive, with a diameter ≤10 mm. The presence of unremarkable clinical findings at the time of breast cancer detection does not necessarily signify early detection.

Göttingen Optipack. A diagnostic concept that has been employed for many years and includes a breast MRI examination is the *Göttingen Optipack*. The Göttingen Optipack combines digital x-ray mammography in one projection with high-resolution breast MRI. It allows the reliable detection of microcalcifications in mammography as a potential indication of an intraductal breast tumor, but with the breast MRI it also compensates for the limitations of x-ray mammography when parenchymal density is high. Our experience shows that the Göttingen Optipack is more reliable than other diagnostic concepts such as screening mammography and 2-view mammography + US. In addition, it is currently the technique with the least radiation exposure to the patient because the mammography is performed in only one projection.

The Göttingen Optipack is also the most cost-effective diagnostic concept in comparison with other early breast cancer detection strategies.

Further diagnostic work-up. If no conspicuous findings are present in an Optipack examination, an invasive breast carcinoma can be excluded with the greatest reliability presently possible (**Fig. 17.34**).

When an ambiguous finding is detected, further diagnostic work-up must follow. If ambiguous or suspicious microcalcifications have been detected (BI-RADS 3, 4, or 5), then further mammographic image(s) in the second projection and, if applicable, in magnification technique are performed. If an ambiguous finding is detected on breast MRI (BI-RADS 3, 4, or 5), then second-look ultrasonography with knowledge of the lesion location, size, and configuration is usually performed (**Fig. 17.35**). When a finding is finally categorized into the overall BI-RADS category 4 or 5 after taking all imaging results into consideration, then a percutaneous biopsy is performed to achieve a definitive histological diagnosis.

Examination intervals. Taking the average tumor doubling time of breast cancer (200–350 days) into consideration, the Göttingen Optipack concept allows systematic early breast cancer detection when performed at intervals of every 1 to 2 years. Breast MRI can reliably detect breast carcinomas as small as 3–4 mm in diameter. This implies that if smaller tumors are present at the time an unremarkable breast MRI has been performed, then the expected size that this tumor could grow to within the next 12 months would be 4 mm to maximally 7 mm in diameter. Within 24 months the expected tumor growth would result in a tumor with diameter of 8–20 mm (**Fig. 17.36**).

> ! Not taking the cost aspect into consideration, yearly performance of a Göttingen Optipack allows reliable early breast cancer detection of tumors under 1 cm in diameter.

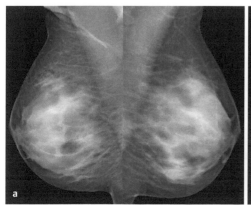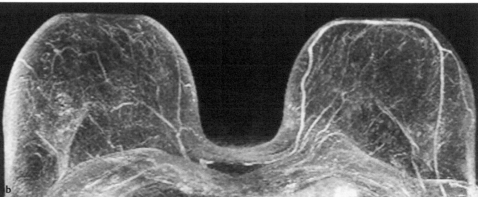

Fig. 17.34a, b Optipack implementation in early breast cancer detection: normal findings.
a Mammography in the MLO projection: unremarkable findings in breasts with high parenchymal density (ACR density IV).
b Subtraction MIP in HR-MRM: unremarkable findings (MRI BI-RADS right 1/left 1). No motion artifacts (MRM artifact level I). High transparency (MRI density I).

Interpretation: breast cancer can be ruled out reliably. Next examination at the normal interval for early breast cancer detection.

Study results. Results of our own studies on the significance of various breast imaging modalities in the examination of women without breast symptoms document the high value of the individualized and risk-adapted use of breast MRI in addition to the mammographic and breast ultrasound examinations in early breast cancer detection. Forty breast carcinomas were detected in a cohort of 3749 women with an average age of 53.7 years (10.67‰). Thirty of these carcinomas were detected by x-ray mammography (8.00‰). Three more carcinomas were detected by the adjunctive performance of breast ultrasonography (0.80‰). The adjunctive performance of breast MRI found 10 additional carcinomas (2.67‰). Of the radiographically occult carcinomas detected by breast MRI, 70% fulfilled the criteria of early breast cancer (two DCIS, two pT1a, three pT1b).

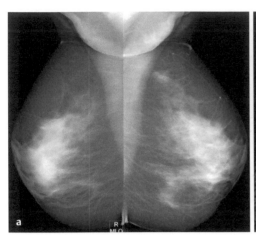
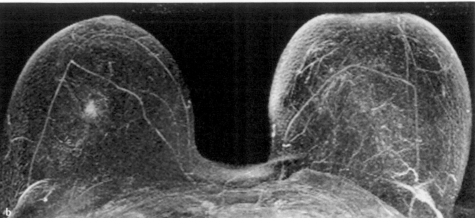

Fig. 17.35a, b Optipack implementation in early breast cancer detection: detection of mammographically occult breast carcinoma.

a Mammography in the MLO projection: harmless parenchymal asymmetry in the axillary tail of the left breast (unchanged over many years). High parenchymal density (ACR density IV).

b Subtraction MIP in HR-MRM: nonmasslike hypervascularized lesion in the right breast (MRI BI-RADS right 4c/left 1). No motion artifacts (MRM artifact level I). High transparency (MRI density I).

Procedure: second-look breast ultrasonography identified vague corresponding findings. US-guided core biopsy confirmed an invasive lobular carcinoma.

Histology (after BCS): ILC, pT1b, pN0.

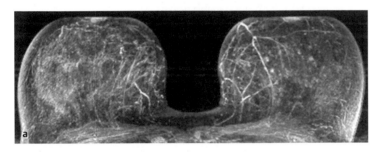
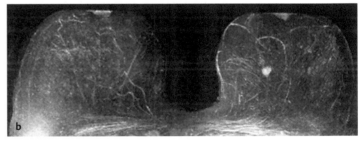
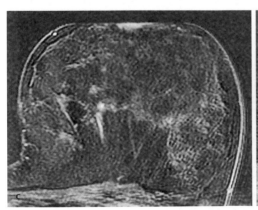
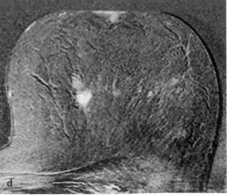

Fig. 17.36a–d Systematic implementation of the Optipack concept: detection of mammographically occult breast carcinoma.

a Subtraction MIP: unremarkable findings with several unsuspicious bilateral foci. Unremarkable mammography (not shown).

b Subtraction MIP 16 months later: hypervascularized mass lesion in the left breast.

c Subtraction slice image (first examination, left breast): subtle retrospective analysis shows a corresponding focus with a diameter of 2 mm.

d Subtraction slice image (second examination, left breast): tumor diameter of 11 mm at the time of diagnosis.

Procedure: no corresponding findings on mammography and second-look ultrasonography. MRI-guided VAB revealed an invasive ductal carcinoma.

Histology (after BCS): IDC, pT1c, pN0.

18 Differential Diagnosis and Strategy

Solitary Focus

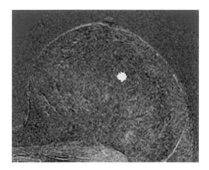

Common diagnoses. Focal adenosis, adenoma/fibroadenoma, papilloma.

Rare diagnoses. Lobulus, ductal carcinoma in situ (DCIS), invasive carcinoma, intramammary lymph node, phyllodes tumor.

Strategy. See **Table 18.1**.

! A solitary focus on breast MRI should preferably be followed up after 6 months. The risk of this lesion being malignant is somewhat higher than that of multiple foci. Should this focus be a malignant lesion, the expected lesion size after 6 months is maximally 5–6 mm. The initial performance of an MRI-guided vacuum-assisted biopsy (VAB) can and should be avoided.

Table 18.1 Diagnostic work-up strategy for solitary focus

Strategy: No correlative finding on mammography or breast ultrasound	
Mx/US BI-RADS 1	MRI follow-up[a] (**Figs. 18.1, 18.2, 18.3**).

Strategy: Correlative finding on mammography and/or breast ultrasound[b]	
Mx/US BI-RADS 2	Mx or US follow-up[a]
Mx/US BI-RADS 3	Mx or US follow-up[a]
Mx/US BI-RADS 4	Percutaneous biopsy (US-CB or Mx-VAB)
Mx/US BI-RADS 5	Percutaneous biopsy (US-CB or Mx-VAB)

[a] Follow-up interval usually 6 months.
[b] Small lesions often not found on second-look US.
Mx: x-ray mammography.
US: ultrasonography.
US-CB: US-guided core biopsy.
Mx-VAB: stereotactic vacuum-assisted biopsy.

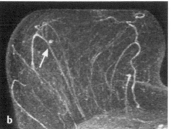
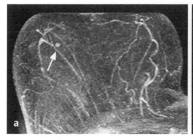

Fig. 18.1 a, b   Solitary focus. No change at follow-up breast MRI examination 6 months after detection.
a Subtraction slice image: initial detection of solitary focus in the right breast (arrow).
b Subtraction slice image (follow-up 6 months later): no progression (arrow).

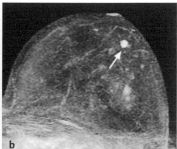
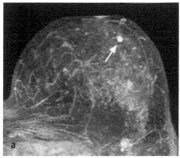

Fig. 18.2 a, b   Solitary focus. Size increase at follow-up breast MRI examination 6 months after detection.
a Subtraction slice image: initial detection of solitary focus in the left breast (arrow).
b Subtraction slice image (follow-up 6 months later): progression with focus size increase from 3 mm to 5 mm in diameter (arrow).
Histology: fibroadenoma (B2).

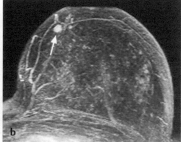
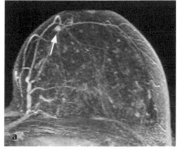

Fig. 18.3 a, b   Solitary focus. Size increase at follow-up breast MRI examination 6 months after detection.
a Subtraction slice image: initial detection of solitary focus in the left breast (arrow).
b Subtraction slice image (follow-up 6 months later): progression with focus size increase from 3 mm to 6 mm in diameter (arrow).
Histology: invasive ductal carcinoma (B5b).

Multiple Foci

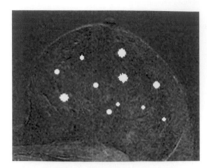

Common diagnoses. Lobuli (physiological enhancement), adenosis, adenomas/fibroadenomas.

Rare diagnoses. Papillomas, DCIS, invasive carcinoma (one of the multiple foci), multiple carcinomas, intramammary metastases.

Strategy. See **Table 18.2**.

> **!** Multiple foci on breast MRI should preferably be followed up in the normal early breast cancer detection interval of 1 year. Should one of these foci be a malignant lesion, the expected lesion size after 12 months is maximally 8–10 mm. The initial performance of an MRI-guided VAB is not expedient because "one will always biopsy the wrong focus."

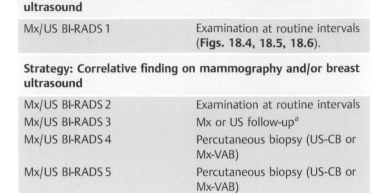

Table 18.2 Diagnostic work-up strategy for multiple foci

Strategy: No correlative finding on mammography or breast ultrasound	
Mx/US BI-RADS 1	Examination at routine intervals (**Figs. 18.4, 18.5, 18.6**).
Strategy: Correlative finding on mammography and/or breast ultrasound	
Mx/US BI-RADS 2	Examination at routine intervals
Mx/US BI-RADS 3	Mx or US follow-up[a]
Mx/US BI-RADS 4	Percutaneous biopsy (US-CB or Mx-VAB)
Mx/US BI-RADS 5	Percutaneous biopsy (US-CB or Mx-VAB)

[a] Follow-up interval usually 6 months.
Mx: x-ray mammography. US: ultrasonography. US-CB: US-guided core biopsy. Mx-VAB: stereotactic vacuum-assisted biopsy.

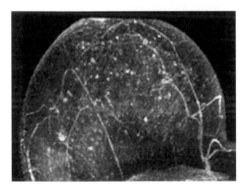

Fig. 18.4   Multiple foci. Subtraction MIP. The image is typical for physiological enhancement of lobuli.

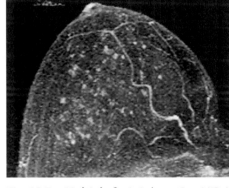

Fig. 18.5   Multiple foci. Subtraction MIP. Histologically confirmed adenosis (B2).

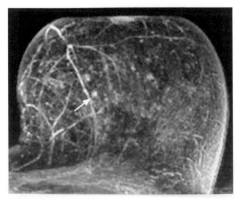

Fig. 18.6   Multiple foci. Subtraction MIP. In follow-up breast MRI 16 months later the most prominent focus (arrow) showed progression. Histology confirmed a DCIS (B5a).

Mass Lesion

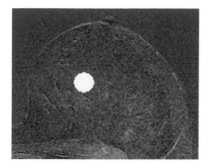

Common diagnoses. Adenoma/fibroadenoma, adenosis, tumor-forming adenosis, carcinoma, papilloma.

Rare diagnoses. Phyllodes tumor, hamartoma, granuloma, angiomatous hyperplasia, fibrosis, intramammary lymph node.

!
The Göttingen score is useful for the evaluation of a hypervascularized breast MRI lesion and allows its assignment to one of the five MRI BI-RADS categories (**Tables 18.3, 18.4**).

Table 18.3 Göttingen score

Criteria	0 points	1 point	2 points
Shape	Round, oval	Irregular	–
Margins	Well-circumscribed	Ill-circumscribed	–
Contrast pattern	Homogeneous	Inhomogeneous	Rim-enhancement
Initial signal increase	<50% (slow)	50%–100% (medium)	>100% (rapid)
Postinitial signal course	Continuous increase	Plateau	Washout

Strategy. See **Table 18.5**.

Table 18.4 Correlation between Göttingen score and MRI BI-RADS

	MRI BI-RADS 1	MRI BI-RADS 2	MRI BI-RADS 3	MRI BI-RADS 4	MRI BI-RADS 5
Göttingen score	1	2	3	4, 5	6–8

Table 18.5 Strategy for mass lesion work-up

	MRI BI-RADS 1	MRI BI-RADS 2	MRI BI-RADS 3	MRI BI-RADS 4	MRI BI-RADS 5
No correlative finding on mammography or breast ultrasound					
Mx/US BI-RADS 1	REI[a]	REI	MRI follow-up[b]	Percutaneous biopsy	Percutaneous biopsy
Correlative finding on mammography and/or breast ultrasound					
Mx/US BI-RADS 2	REI	REI	Follow-up	Percutaneous biopsy	Percutaneous biopsy
Mx/US BI-RADS 3	REI	REI	Follow-up	Percutaneous biopsy	Percutaneous biopsy
Mx/US BI-RADS 4	REI	Percutaneous biopsy	Percutaneous biopsy	Percutaneous biopsy	Percutaneous biopsy
Mx/US BI-RADS 5	REI	Percutaneous biopsy	Percutaneous biopsy	Percutaneous biopsy	Percutaneous biopsy

[a] REI: routine examination interval.
[b] Follow-up interval usually 6 months.

Mass Lesion—Differential Diagnosis

Rim-Enhancement (Figs. 18.7, 18.8, 18.9, 18.10)

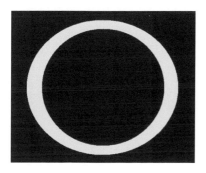

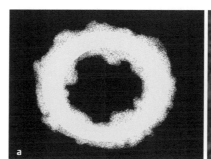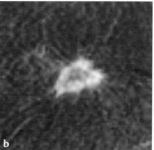

Fig. 18.7a, b Rim-enhancement. Ring-shaped enhancement of the tumor periphery with ill-defined internal and external margins. Diagnosis: carcinoma.

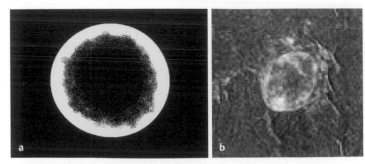

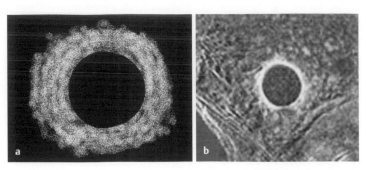

Fig. 18.8a, b   Rim-enhancement. Ring-shaped enhancement of the tumor periphery with ill-defined internal margins and well-circumscribed external margins. Diagnosis: fibroadenoma.

Fig. 18.9a, b   Rim-enhancement. Ring-shaped peripheral enhancement with well-circumscribed internal and ill-defined external margins. Diagnosis: inflamed cyst.

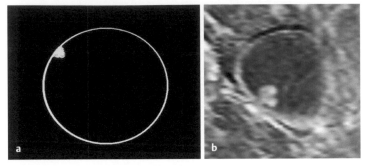

Fig. 18.10a, b   Rim-enhancement. Ring-shaped peripheral enhancement with a marginal area of localized enhancement (proliferation). Diagnosis: complicated cyst.

Endotumoral Changes (Figs. 18.11, 18.12, 18.13)

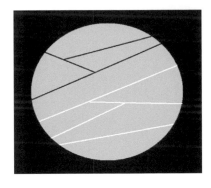

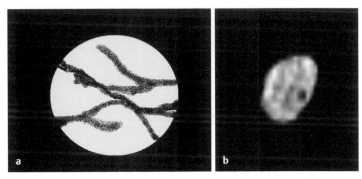

Fig. 18.11a, b   Endotumoral characteristics. Dark, nonenhancing septations within an enhancing matrix of mass lesion. Histological correlates are fibrotic strands with decreased circulation. Criterion indicative of benignity. Diagnosis: fibroadenoma.

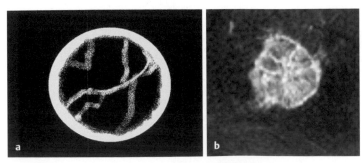

Fig. 18.12a, b   Endotumoral characteristics. Bright, enhancing septations within less enhancing matrix of mass lesion. Histological correlation with areas of increased cell proliferation and increased circulation. Criterion indicative of moderate to high-grade malignancy. Diagnosis: carcinoma.

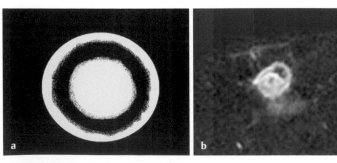

Fig. 18.13a, b   Endotumoral characteristics. Central area with bright, ring-shaped or round enhancement within a mass lesion also displaying rim-enhancement. Histological correlation with areas of increased cell proliferation and increased circulation. Criterion indicative of moderate to high-grade malignancy. Diagnosis: carcinoma.

Nonmasslike Lesion

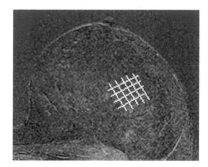

Common diagnoses.
- Parenchymal enhancement due to hormonal stimulation (physiological)
- Interstitial enhancement pattern: adenosis, ILC
- Ductal enhancement pattern: mastitis, papillomatosis, DCIS

Strategy. See **Table 18.6**.

! The evaluation of a nonmasslike lesion is based primarily upon morphological criteria. Because areas within nonmasslike lesions in which ROIs are placed typically include areas of nonenhancing lipomatous tissue in addition to the enhancing tumor tissue, TICs are rendered ineffective. Dynamic criteria of the Göttingen score system (Chapter 5) are therefore not applicable to these tumors.

As a rule, the interpretation of nonmasslike lesions should differentiate them into those with an **interstitial enhancement pattern** and those with a **ductal enhancement pattern**. Enhancement in the interstitium tends to be regional or diffuse (**Fig. 18.14**), whereas ductal enhancement shows an orientation along the milk duct system (**Fig. 18.15**). The enhancement pattern of a nonmasslike lesion is the basis for differential diagnostic considerations.

Table 18.6 Strategy for nonmasslike lesion work-up

Strategy: No correlative finding on mammography or breast ultrasound	
Mx/US BI-RADS 1	Percutaneous biopsy (MRI-VAB)

Strategy: Correlative finding on mammography and/or breast ultrasound	
Mx/US BI-RADS 2	Percutaneous biopsy (MRI-VAB)
Mx/US BI-RADS 3	Percutaneous biopsy (US-CB or Mx-VAB)
Mx/US BI-RADS 4	Percutaneous biopsy (US-CB or Mx-VAB)
Mx/US BI-RADS 5	Percutaneous biopsy (US-CB or Mx-VAB)

Mx: x-ray mammography. US: ultrasonography. MRI-VAB: MRI-guided vacuum-assisted biopsy. US-CB: US-guided core biopsy. Mx-VAB: stereotactic vacuum-assisted biopsy.

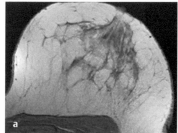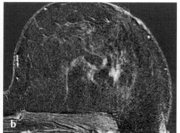

Fig. 18.14a, b Nonmasslike lesion with interstitial enhancement pattern. Enhancement distribution in the tissue spaces of the diffuse tumor area, leaving lipomatous structures intact. Diagnosis: ILC.

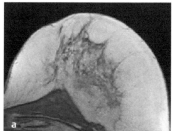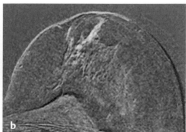

Fig. 18.15a, b Nonmasslike lesion with ductal enhancement pattern. Linear-branching enhancement distribution along a medially directed milk duct. Lipomatous structures are left intact. Diagnosis: DCIS.

Nonmasslike Lesion—Differential Diagnosis

Linear Enhancement (Figs. 18.16, 18.17, 18.18, 18.19)

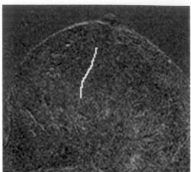

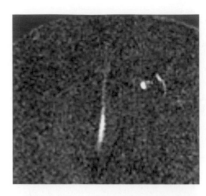

Fig. 18.16 Linear enhancement pattern. Linear enhancement in a single subtraction slice image, often subcutaneously located. In subtraction MIP typical vascular structures are recognizable. Diagnosis: vein.

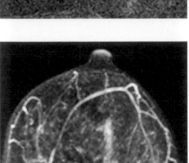

Fig. 18.17 Linear enhancement pattern. Linear ductal enhancement in MIP, often seen in the retromamillary area as double line (track phenomenon, enhancement of duct walls). Diagnosis: mastitis.

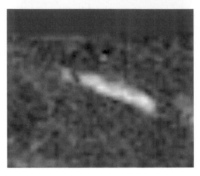

Fig. 18.18 Linear enhancement pattern. Linear intraductal enhancement in a single subtraction slice image. Occasionally seen as a pearl-necklace–like enhancement or interrupted linear enhancement. Diagnosis: papillomatosis.

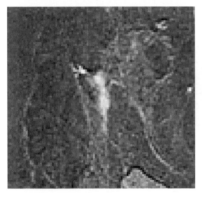

Fig. 18.19 Linear enhancement pattern. Linear ductal enhancement in a single subtraction slice image. Occasional presence of caliber fluctuations or inhomogeneous sections. Diagnosis: DCIS.

Linear-Branching Enhancement (Figs. 18.20, 18.21, 18.22)

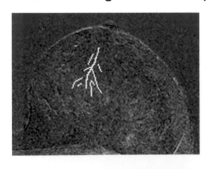

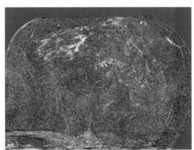

Fig. 18.20 Linear-branching enhancement pattern. Linear-branching ductal enhancement in a single subtraction slice image. Diagnosis: papillomatosis.

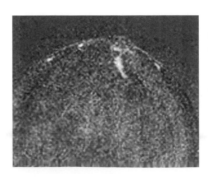

Fig. 18.21 Linear-branching enhancement pattern. Linear-branching intraductal enhancement in a single subtraction slice image. Diagnosis: DCIS.

Fig. 18.22 Linear-branching enhancement pattern. Linear-branching ductal enhancement in the retromamillary region (single subtraction slice image). Diagnosis: mastitis.

Segmental Enhancement (Figs. 18.23, 18.24, 18.25)

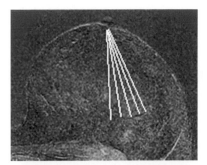

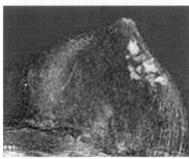

Fig. 18.23 Segmental enhancement pattern. A triangular area of enhancement with the base of the triangle near the chest wall (single subtraction slice image). Diagnosis: DCIS.

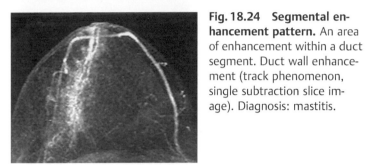

Fig. 18.24 Segmental enhancement pattern. An area of enhancement within a duct segment. Duct wall enhancement (track phenomenon, single subtraction slice image). Diagnosis: mastitis.

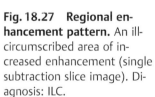

Fig. 18.25 Segmental enhancement pattern. A triangular area of blotchy enhancement within a duct segment (single subtraction slice image). Diagnosis: papillomatosis.

Regional Enhancement (Figs. 18.26, 18.27, 18.28)

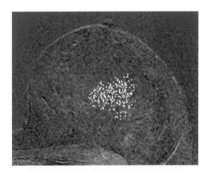

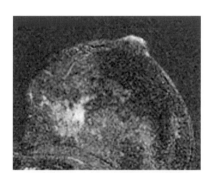

Fig. 18.26 Regional enhancement pattern. An ill-circumscribed area of increased enhancement (single subtraction slice image). Diagnosis: adenosis.

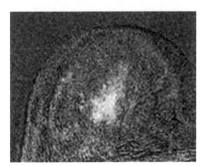

Fig. 18.27 Regional enhancement pattern. An ill-circumscribed area of increased enhancement (single subtraction slice image). Diagnosis: ILC.

Fig. 18.28 Regional enhancement pattern. An ill-circumscribed area of increased enhancement (single subtraction slice image). Diagnosis: nonpuerperal mastitis.

Unilateral Diffuse Enhancement (Figs. 18.29, 18.30, 18.31, 18.32, 18.33)

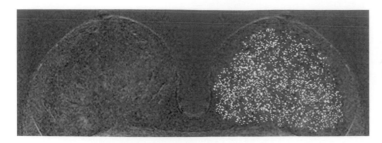

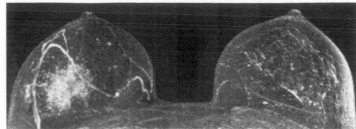

Fig. 18.29 Unilateral diffuse enhancement pattern. A large ill-circumscribed area of increased enhancement in the right breast (subtraction MIP). Diagnosis: adenosis.

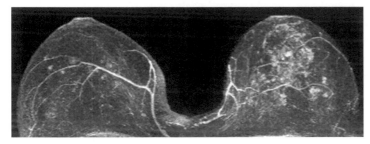

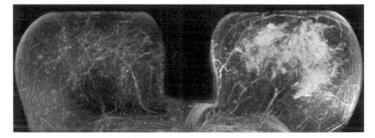

Fig. 18.30 Unilateral diffuse enhancement pattern. A diffuse increased enhancement of the entire left breast (subtraction MIP). Diagnosis: status after radiation therapy.

Fig. 18.31 Unilateral diffuse enhancement pattern. A diffuse increased enhancement of the entire left breast (subtraction MIP). Diagnosis: nonpuerperal mastitis.

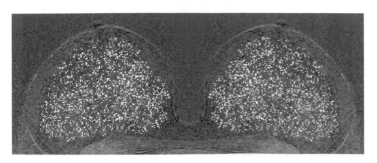

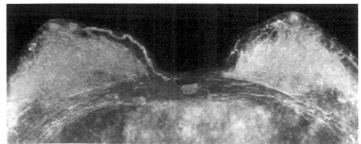

Fig. 18.32 Unilateral diffuse enhancement pattern. A diffuse spotty enhancement extending over a large area of the left breast (subtraction MIP). Diagnosis: DCIS.

Fig. 18.33 Unilateral diffuse enhancement pattern. A diffuse increased enhancement of the entire left breast (subtraction MIP). Diagnosis: ILC.

Bilateral Diffuse Enhancement (Fig. 18.34)

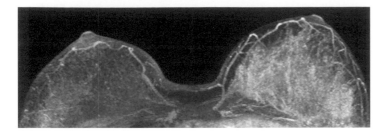

Fig. 18.34 Bilateral diffuse enhancement pattern. A diffuse increase of parenchymal enhancement in both breasts (subtraction MIP). Diagnosis: hormonal stimulation (MRI density IV).

Architectural Distortion

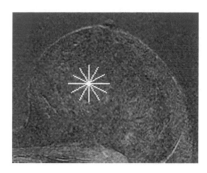

Common diagnoses. Postoperative scar, radial scar, carcinoma (especially of tubular histology) (**Figs. 18.35, 18.36, 18.37**)

Strategy. See **Table 18.7**.

! An architectural distortion is usually seen best in the T1w precontrast images. When there is no enhancement, malignancy can be ruled out with high reliability.

Table 18.7 Diagnostic work-up strategy for architectural distortion

Strategy: No correlative finding on mammography or breast ultrasound	
Mx/US BI-RADS 1	Open biopsy after preoperative MRI-guided wire localization

Strategy: Correlative finding on mammography and/or breast ultrasound	
Mx/US BI-RADS 2	Open biopsy after preoperative Mx- or US-guided wire localization
Mx/US BI-RADS 3	Open biopsy after preoperative Mx- or US-guided wire localization
Mx/US BI-RADS 4	Open biopsy after preoperative Mx- or US-guided wire localization
Mx/US BI-RADS 5	Open biopsy after preoperative Mx- or US-guided wire localization

Mx: x-ray mammography. US: ultrasonography.

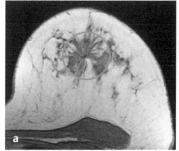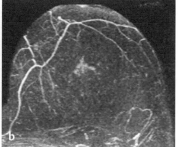

Fig. 18.35a, b   Architectural distortion.
a T1w precontrast slice image: initial detection of architectural distortion in the left breast (circle).
b Subtraction slice image: mild enhancement.

Histology: postoperative scar.

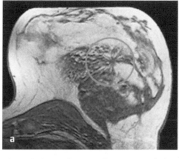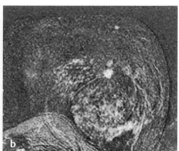

Fig. 18.36a, b   Architectural distortion.
a T1w precontrast slice image: architectural distortion in the left breast (circle).
b Subtraction slice image: focal enhancement in the center of the lesion.

Histology: radial scar with centrally located tubular breast carcinoma.

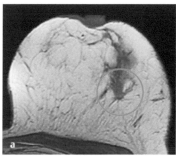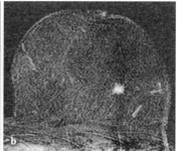

Fig. 18.37a, b   Architectural distortion.
a T1w precontrast slice image: a spiculated lesion in the left breast (circle).
b Subtraction slice image: the spiculated area of enhancement in the center of the lesion.

Histology: tubular breast carcinoma.

19 Quality Assurance

Minimum Requirements for Breast MRI Examinations

Recommendations for the performance of breast MRI examinations, based on a consensus of the members of the breast diagnostics working group of the German Association of Radiology in 2005, should be seen as the minimum requirements that need to be fulfilled to perform high-quality breast MRI examinations (**Table 19.1**).

Table 19.1 Minimum quality requirements for breast MRI[a]

Technique	Field strength	1–1.5 T
	Surface coil	Bilateral
	Breast fixation	Adequate compression (dedicated compression device, sports brassiere, cushions, or the like)
Methods	Time of examination	2nd (3rd) week of menstrual cycle (exception: preoperative staging)
	Hormonal influence	If disturbing enhancement is present: HRT should be discontinued for 4–6 weeks before repeat examination
	Influence of surgery	Time between surgery and MRI: >6 months Time between BCS and radiation therapy and MRI: >12 months
	Technique	2D or 3D
	Orientation	Axial or coronal
	Sequences	T1w GE, T2w (SE, TSE, IR)
	Dynamics	First measurement before CM administration; further measurements after CM administration over >6 minutes
	Paramagnetic contrast medium	0.1 mmol/kg BW for 2D examination 0.1–0.2 mmol/kg BW for 3D examination
	Contrast injection	Cubital vein, flow ~2–3 mL/s, followed by injection of at least 20 mL NaCl
	Spatial resolution	≤4 mm/slice
	Temporal resolution	<2.5 min/sequence
	Examination time	At least 6 minutes after CM administration
	FOV	300–350 mm
	Matrix	At least 256×256
	TR	Typical settings for 2D or 3D examination
	TE	Appropriate echo times for 1.0 and 1.5 T in-phase imaging
	Postprocessing	Subtraction (early–precontrast is obligatory)
	Examination evaluation	Morphological criteria, dynamic criteria, multimodal evaluation, T2w image information
	Documentation (obligatory)	T1w precontrast (complete) T1w early postcontrast (complete) Early subtraction (complete) TIC analysis + T2w (findings-oriented)
	Presentation	Hardcopy (film or paper)

[a]Mammadiagnostik der Deutschen Röntgengesellschaft AG. Empfehlungen zur MR-Mammographie. Rofo 2005;177:474

Quality Check in Breast MRI

After an examination has been performed, the following possible errors should be ruled out:

- Are both breasts completely imaged? (Possibilities of error on pp. 47 and 48).
- Did contrast material reach the breasts? (Reference points on p. 49).
- Are there motion artifacts? (Determine the MRI artifact level, see pp. 50–52.) If artifacts are pronounced (MRI artifact level III or IV), then examination should be repeated.

- How great is the parenchymal enhancement in the early subtraction images? (Determine MRI density, see p. 69). Should an earliest subtraction be performed? If parenchymal MRI density is high, then a repeat examination in an appropriate cycle phase or, if applicable, after discontinuing hormonal replacement therapy should be considered.
- Are the ROIs correctly placed? (Possibilities of error on p. 57.)

Written Report

The written breast MRI report should include a short reference to results of earlier examination results, any specific questions to be answered, and any relevant patient history information. This should be followed by information on the techniques used, sequences, and orientations, as well as the amount of contrast material administered.

The descriptive section should include details of apparent changes in the T1w precontrast and T2w images, and should especially provide information on signal changes after intravenous contrast administration. The evaluation of breast MRI findings into categories 1 to 5 should be performed for each side separately in accordance with the ACR BI-RADS Lexicon. Furthermore, correlation of the breast MRI findings with clinical, mammographic, and/or ultrasonographic findings (if possible) should be made, and recommendations for the further course of action expressed.

Written Report

Example of Written Report of Unremarkable Breast MRI Findings

Indication: Early breast cancer detection, reduced sensitivity of x-ray mammography and breast ultrasound. Mammography: ACR density IV, BI-RADS right 1/left 1. Breast US: Bilateral bland cysts, US BI-RADS right 2/left 2.

Risk profile: Increased familial risk (breast cancer detected in mother at age 67 years). Not considered high-risk.

MRI technique: Examination with HR technique (matrix 512×512) using a 1.5 T system and dedicated open breast surface coil. Acquisition of 46 IR T2w axial slice images. In identical slice position acquisition of 46 axial slice images once before and 5 times after IV administration of 0.1 mmol Gd-DTPA/kg BW. Image postprocessing for generation of subtraction slice images, TICs in appropriate regions, and presentation as MIP.

MRI findings: Unremarkable findings in the T1w precontrast images. No architectural distortions. In the IR T2w images depiction of multiple simple cysts up to 10 mm in diameter. After contrast administration, mild bilateral parenchymal enhancement (MRI density II) with the exception of the cystic spaces. No motion artifacts (MRI artifact level I). No areas of focal enhancement, no hypervascularized mass lesions, no nonmass-like areas of enhancement in either breast. MRI BI-RADS right 1/left 1.

Final evaluation: The present breast MRI examination shows no signs indicating the presence of a malignant breast tumor in either breast. Taking clinical, mammographic, and breast ultrasound findings into consideration results in the *cumulative BI-RADS* right 2 (cysts)/left 2 (cysts). The next examination for early breast cancer detection is recommended at a routine interval of 1 to 2 years.

Example of Written Report of Breast MRI Performed for Preoperative Local Staging

Indication: Preoperative local staging after histological verification of a breast carcinoma with a diameter of 1 cm in the upper outer quadrant of the left breast. *Mammography:* ACR density III, BI-RADS right 1/left 5. *US BI-RADS* right 1/left 5. *Cumulative BI-RADS* right 1/left 6.

Personal history: Diagnostic excision in the right breast 8 years ago (benign lesion).

Risk profile: No increased familial disposition.

MRI technique: Examination with HR technique (matrix 512×512) using a 1.5 T system and dedicated open breast surface coil. Acquisition of 46 IR T2w axial slice images. In identical slice position acquisition of 46 axial slice images once before and 5 times after IV administration of 0.1 mmol Gd-DTPA/kg BW. Image postprocessing for generation of subtraction slice images, TICs in appropriate regions, and presentation as MIP.

MRI findings: In the T1w precontrast images susceptibility artifacts are seen in the upper outer quadrant of the right breast after diagnostic excision. Unremarkable findings in the left breast. In the IR T2w images depiction of multiple simple cysts up to 3 mm in diameter. After contrast administration, no early enhancement in the right breast. In the upper outer quadrant of the left breast there is a hypervascularized, ill-circumscribed mass lesion with a diameter of 10 mm which displays an increased marginal enhancement (rim sign). TICs in appropriate ROIs show a rapid initial signal increase (>100%) and postinitial washout. MRI score: 7 points. Additional 15 mm linear enhancement originating from this index tumor and nearly reaching the nipple. High parenchymal transparency (MRI density I). No motion artifacts (MRI artifact level I). No pathologically enlarged axillary lymph nodes in the T1w and T2w images. MRI BI-RADS right 1/left 5.

Final evaluation: Confirmation of the histologically verified carcinoma in the upper outer quadrant of the left breast (diameter 1 cm). Additional findings indicative of an EIC between the primary tumor and the breast nipple. No indication of multifocality or multicentricity. No depiction of enlarged locoregional lymph nodes. On the basis of left breast image results we recommend segment resection and sentinel lymph node biopsy. The contralateral right breast is unremarkable. *Cumulative BI-RADS* right 1/left 6 (plus signs of EIC).

Quality Assurance in Special Cases

Quality Assurance: MRI BI-RADS 3 Findings

When a breast MRI finding is categorized as a MRI BI-RADS 3 lesion and has no correlating finding on mammography or breast ultrasound, then a follow-up MRI examination is typically recommended in 6 months. Results of such follow-up breast MRI examinations should be statistically analyzed and the rate of breast carcinomas detected at this time should be under 2%. It is also advisable to ensure that follow-up examinations are performed by sending a reminder or making a follow-up phone call to patients who do not show up on time (e.g., after 7 months).

Quality Assurance after MRI-Guided Vacuum-Assisted Biopsy

The histological evaluation of breast MRI findings in the MRI BI-RADS categories 4 or 5 that have no correlating finding on mammography or breast ultrasound is performed by MRI-guided vacuum-assisted biopsy, in accordance with recommendations. The results of histology are classified into histological B-categories, and must be checked for compatibility with image findings (**Table 19.2**).

Table 19.2   Consequences resulting from MRI-guided vacuum-assisted biopsy of MRI BI-RADS 4 or 5 findings depending on histological B-classification

Histological B-classification		Consequences
B1	No lesion	Incorrect biopsy probable: Follow-up? Repeat biopsy? Open biopsy?
B2	Benign lesion	Check for compatibility with imaging: If yes, follow-up in 6 months. If no, repeat biopsy?
B3	Borderline lesion	Interdisciplinary conference: Determination of further proceedings (open biopsy? follow-up? regular examinations?)
B4	Insufficient material	Repeat VAB? Open biopsy?
B5a	DCIS	Compatibility with imaging (possible underestimation)
B5b	Invasive carcinoma	Compatibility with imaging

Quality Assurance after MRI-Indicated Open Biopsy (Surgery)

It is recommended that breast MRI BI-RADS 4 and 5 findings and the corresponding histological results of open biopsy be statistically analyzed to document the rate, tumor type, and stage distribution of carcinomas in each BI-RADS category.

20 Current Standing, Problems, and Perspectives of Breast MRI

Current Standing

Value of Breast MRI

It is indisputable that due to the development of open surface coils with multiple channel systems and integrated compression devices, as well as the improvement of especially the spatial resolution in all three planes, HR breast MRI has become the most reliable imaging modality in breast diagnostics (**Fig. 20.1**). A technically and methodologically flawless breast MRI allows not only the detection of invasive breast carcinomas from a diameter of 3–4 mm (sensitivity 94%–98%) but also the detection of intraductal carcinomas with the highest accuracy (sensitivity 85%–90%). The technique thus demonstrates itself to be significantly superior to x-ray mammography and breast ultrasonography, especially in the early detection of breast cancer (pTis, pT1 a, pT1 b). The specificity of breast MRI, which has occasionally been criticized as being too low, is good when the examination is performed with appropriate quality and evaluated with high expertise. At 70%–80% it lies in the same range as that of other breast imaging techniques.

Indications for Breast MRI

Breast MRI examination is therefore generally to be recommended in those cases in which other breast imaging techniques (x-ray mammography, breast ultrasonography) have significant limitations. This is especially true for x-ray mammography when parenchymal density is high (ACR density III and IV) and the sensitivity is therefore reduced to as little as less than 50%. This limitation does not apply to breast MRI because the mammographic density of parenchyma does not correlate with parenchymal enhancement on MRI. Currently acknowledged indications for the performance of breast MRI particularly take into account women who have an increased risk of having or developing breast cancer. As a result, the following **indications for the performance of breast MRI** are generally accepted standards of good practice:

- Differentiation between a postoperative scar and breast cancer recurrence after breast-conserving surgery (BCS)
- Search for the primary tumor in the presence of a CUP syndrome
- Early breast cancer diagnostics in women with a high-risk profile
- Preoperative local staging in women with histologically verified breast cancer
- Response monitoring in women undergoing neoadjuvant chemotherapy

Apart from the indications listed above, breast MRI is often implemented as an efficacious "problem solver" when there are ambiguous findings in x-ray mammography and/or breast ultrasound. In such a situation, breast MRI often provides a definitive directive for or against performing a percutaneous biopsy.

Breast MRI is the method of choice for the evaluation of **prosthesis complications**. The use of special sequence protocols that allow selective imaging of the various prosthesis components, and the capability for slice imaging in multiple planes, make breast MRI superior to other imaging modalities for this indication (see chapter 14).

Göttingen Optipack

The combination of bilateral digital x-ray mammography in the MLO projection with HR breast MRI (known as the Göttingen Optipack) is presently the examination protocol with the most reliable detection of breast carcinomas and the least possible parenchymal radiation dose. This combination allows the detection of both invasive and intraductal carcinomas with very high sensitivity.

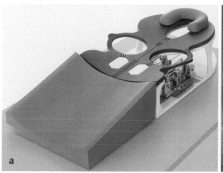 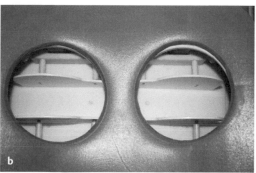

Fig. 20.1 a, b Open surface coil. Indispensable for high-quality breast MRI.
a Open surface coil.
b Breast compression device.

Problems and Solutions

Limitations of Breast MRI

Motion artifacts used to be a major limiting factor in the diagnostic value of breast MRI examinations. This methodological problem has been almost completely eliminated by the construction of open surface coils combined with a breast compression device.

A diagnostic limitation that remains is the occasional disturbing early enhancement of parenchyma due to **hormonal stimulation**, which can sometimes mask small tumor lesions. This "physiological problem" decreases breast MRI transparency and diagnostic reliability similarly to the way high parenchymal density does for mammography. Fortunately, in the relevant age group this phenomenon (early physiological enhancement) is only seen in fewer than 5% of all examined women. For comparison, mammographically dense breast tissue (ACR type III and IV) is found in at least 50% of these same women. Potential solutions to alleviate this problem in breast MRI are the generation of earliest subtraction slice images, and the discontinuation of stimulating hormone therapies, or even temporary antiestrogen therapy before performing the examination.

A further, solvable problem is the variable image quality seen area-wide. The main cause of suboptimal **image quality** is the use of substandard MRI equipment and methods. The excellent results for detection of DCIS in breast MRI, for example, can only be achieved when the examination is performed with a high matrix (512×512) and without motion artifacts.

Certification

The application of an adequate certification process which records and tests quality-relevant criteria for MRI equipment and examiner expertise can improve the current standards. Accordingly, the German working group for individualized breast diagnostics (AIM, a registered association) has prepared a conceptual plan for accreditation of physicians providing breast MRI examinations. This certification program provides for two expertise levels and is expressly individual-orientated and intended only for medical specialists (**Table 20.1**).

Table 20.1 Concept for breast MRI certification according to AIM[a]

		Level 01	Level 02
Technique	Field strength	≥1.5 T	≥1.5 T
	In-plane pixel size (bilateral acquisition, not interpolated)	≤1.0 mm × 1.2 mm	≤0.8 mm × 0.8 mm
	Spatial resolution	≤3 mm/slice	≤3 mm/slice
	Temporal resolution	≤2 minutes per dynamic sequence	≤2 minutes per dynamic sequence
	Surface coil	Open, bilateral	Open, bilateral, multiple channels
	Fixation device	Dedicated breast compression device	
	Postprocessing	Subtraction, MIP, findings-oriented TICs	
	Quality assurance	Classification of artifact level	
Interpretation		Mammograms are available for comparison	
		Mx and breast US findings are mentioned in breast MRI report (if applicable)	
		MRI assessment takes clinical, Mx and breast US findings into account	
		Categorization of findings according to BI-RADS	
Expertise of interpreting physician	No. of patients per interpreter per year	≥250	≥500
Interventions	Type of intervention	MRI-guided wire localization or cooperation with certified center	MRI-guided wire localization and MRI-guided VAB
	No. of interventions per examiner per year	>30 or cooperation with certified center	>30 MRI-guided wire localizations and >30 MRI-guided VABs
	Interventional equipment	MRI surface coil with specialized localization unit or cooperation with certified center	MRI surface coil with specialized localization unit for MRI-guided wire localization and MRI-guided VAB
	Assessment of intervention	Availability of further breast x-ray diagnostics (spot compression, magnification mammography, special views) Possibility of performing second-look breast US	
	Personal review of findings with the patient	Yes	Yes
Interdisciplinary aspects	Radiological–pathological correlation	Interdisciplinary consensus to correlate image findings with pathology for all BI-RADS 4 and 5 lesions. Documentation and archiving of histology results for quality assurance. Conference protocol.	
	Time from BI-RADS 6 diagnosis to preoperative MRI	<1 week	<3 working days
	Participation in AIM-certified advanced MRI-specific training	1 training unit/year	2 training units/year

[a] German working group for individualized breast diagnostics (www.aim-mamma.de).

Perspectives

Diagnostic and Therapeutic Strategies

Because breast parenchyma often shows high transparency on MRI, it can be expected that current diagnostic and therapeutic strategies, which are based predominantly on information gained by x-ray mammography and breast ultrasound examinations, will be modified in the future. Current recommendations—for example, that follow-up mammography of the ipsilateral breast after BCS be performed every 6 months—may be revised. Studies must be performed to evaluate whether or not yearly mammograms in this situation are sufficient when breast MRI is unremarkable. In addition, the recommendation that a multicentric breast carcinoma always be treated by mastectomy should also be reassessed. A bifocal lumpectomy followed by radiation therapy could be a good alternative to mastectomy when breast MRI shows high parenchymal transparency and both tumors in multicentric locations can be excised with BCS. Another strategy to be reevaluated is whether a late recurrence after BCS followed by radiation therapy must always be treated by mastectomy when the remaining breast tissues can be reliably followed up by breast MRI.

Early Breast Cancer Diagnostics

If one does not take the cost into consideration, breast MRI is the optimal diagnostic tool for early breast cancer detection in most women. Because breast MRI does not employ biologically hazardous ionizing radiation and has a very high sensitivity as well as good specificity for breast cancer detection, it seems rational to use it as the first-line diagnostic method in the future. Other, less reliable methods and/or methods using ionizing radiation can then be employed to supplement breast MRI when the situation requires it. In this context one should ask whether and what additional information can be obtained when a technically and methodologically well performed HR breast MRI (MRI artifact level I) shows high parenchymal transparency (MRI density I) and no or a definitely benign lesion (MRI BI-RADS 1 or 2) (**Fig. 20.2**). Can x-ray mammography yield any additional information at all when a breast MRI examination renders such results? If not, then we should not carry it out. Taking into consideration laws regulating the use of ionizing radiation for diagnostic purposes, one can also ask whether performance of x-ray mammography in such cases is even legally permissible.

Study results. In a retrospective study performed at our center of 2500 asymptomatic women who underwent a breast MRI examination for early breast cancer detection and had high mammographic parenchymal density (ACR density III or IV), 40% had the constellation of findings described above (MRI artifact level I, MRI density I, and MRI BI-RADS 1 or 2). In no cases did the additionally performed diagnostic examinations result in the detection of a breast carcinoma. Another 15% of these women had a parenchyma with MRI density II and no or a definitely benign lesion (MRI artifact level I, MRI-BI-RADS 1 or 2). Waiving further diagnostic examinations in these cases would have resulted in missing a carcinoma in 0.03% of the women having breast cancer.

Potential for cost reduction and modification of the breast MRI examination. The road to a pure breast MRI screening program is obstructed primarily by the costs it would incur. With the goal of reducing these costs, there needs to be consideration of modifications of technical and methodological aspects of MRI, as well as whether the cost of contrast material can be reduced. Other issues, such as the limited availability of breast MRI and insufficient examiner expertise are resolvable in the intermediate term.

Methods. The question arises whether, in the context of such a breast MRI screening program of asymptomatic women, with an average expected breast carcinoma detection rate of ~1%, all women need to undergo the entire examination with all measurement sequences. Pathological enhancement of a breast carcinoma statistically reaches its maximum ~3 minutes after intravenous contrast administration. If a breast MRI examination shows no pathological enhancement within the first 5 minutes after contrast administration (MRI BI-RADS 1) and an MRI density I or II, then breast cancer can be reliably ruled out. Additional time-consuming sequences, which serve to further characterize a detected lesion, are unnecessary in such a case. Thus the acquisition of later postcontrast images and water-sensitive T2w images is superfluous, as there is no lesion to further characterize (**Fig. 20.3**). As an alternative to prompt image evaluation by the examining physician, MRM-CAD systems could be helpful in determining the absence of enhancement in an ongoing examination (**Fig. 20.4**). Hence the time consumption of an unremarkable breast MRI could be shortened by eliminating the performance of superfluous sequences, resulting in a time saving of ~50%.

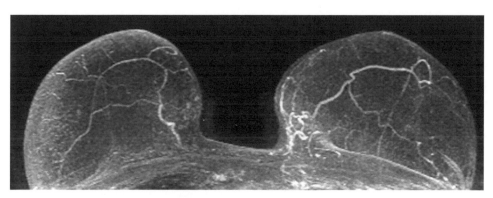

Fig. 20.2 Screening HR breast MRI—breast cancer is reliably ruled out. High-quality breast MRI (MRI-artifact level I) with high parenchymal transparency (MRI density I) and unremarkable findings (MRI BI-RADS 1). Asymptomatic woman with mammographic ACR density IV. Breast cancer is definitively ruled out.

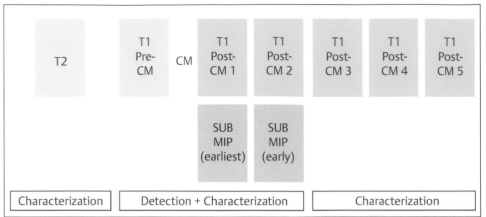

Fig. 20.3 Detection and characterization of findings in breast MRI. Relevant for the detection of pathological MRI findings are the T1w precontrast and the first two postcontrast measurements. The corresponding image subtractions facilitate detection and contribute to the morphological characterization. Later postcontrast measurements (third to fifth T1w postcontrast images) allow further characterization based upon dynamic criteria. The water-sensitive T2w images also contribute to the better characterization of MRI findings.

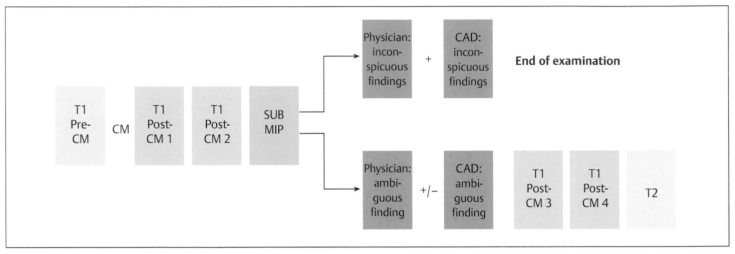

Fig. 20.4 A vision of one approach to breast MRI screening. The primary examination performed for the detection of pathological MRI findings includes the T1w precontrast, the first two postcontrast measurements, and the image subtraction. Prompt evaluation of subtraction images/MIP is done by the examining physician and the auxiliary MRM-CAD-system. If the examination is unremarkable, then the examination can be terminated (upper row). If a lesion is detected, then examination protocol is continued in the usual manner, performing the later T1w postcontrast measurements and the water-sensitive T2w measurements (lower row).

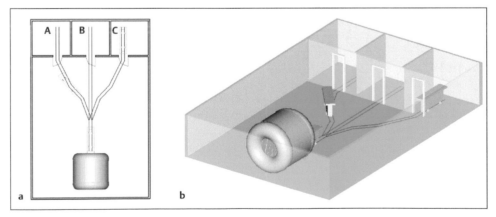

Fig. 20.5a, b Example of a breast MRI system with three examination tables.
a Floor plan of whole-body magnet with three separate examination tables (A–C).
b 3D illustration of back-to-back performance of breast MRI examinations without blocking the MRI system's capacity during patient preparation (Architekturbüro Weitemeier, Dransfeld, Germany).

Examination tables. Another possibility for lowering breast MRI costs further could lie in optimizing the operation of the practice by having 2–3 examination tables in separate cubicles for each MRI system. These could be installed so that they can be driven to the magnet bore on guiding tracks built into the examination room floor, either from one side (Fig. 20.5), or from opposing sides of the magnet. With this set-up it would be possible to start the breast MRI examination of woman B immediately after termination of woman A's examination. Patient positioning, arrangements for the examination (earplugs, music, mirror) and breast positioning and compression can be prepared in the calm atmosphere of the prep-cubicle without wasting MRI system capacity.

! Vision for 2020:
Breast MRI-screening—an early breast cancer detection program without X-rays.
"The better is the enemy of the good" (Voltaire)

Further Reading

Historical Review, Patient Preparation and Information, Breast MRI Technique and Methodology

Ballesio L, Savelli S, Angeletti M, et al. Breast MRI: are T2 IR sequences useful in the evaluation of breast lesions? Eur J Radiol 2009; 71(1):96–101

Baltzer PA, Freiberg C, Beger S, et al. Clinical MR-mammography: are computer-assisted methods superior to visual or manual measurements for curve type analysis? A systematic approach. Acad Radiol 2009;16(9):1070–1076

Baltzer PA, Renz DM, Kullnig PE, Gajda M, Camara O, Kaiser WA. Application of computer-aided diagnosis (CAD) in MR-mammography (MRM): do we really need whole lesion time curve distribution analysis? Acad Radiol 2009;16(4):435–442

Boetes CB, Barentsz JO, Mus RD, et al. MR characterization of suspicious breast lesions with a gadolinium-enhanced TurboFLASH subtraction technique. Radiology 1994;193(3):777–781

Buckley DL, Mussurakis S, Horsman A. Effect of temporal resolution on the diagnostic efficacy of contrast-enhanced MRI in the conservatively treated breast. J Comput Assist Tomogr 1998;22(1):47–51

Damadian R. Tumor detection by nuclear magnetic resonance. Science 1971;171(976):1151–1153

Demartini WB, Lehman CD, Peacock S, Russell MT. Computer-aided detection applied to breast MRI: assessment of CAD-generated enhancement and tumor sizes in breast cancers before and after neoadjuvant chemotherapy. Acad Radiol 2005;12(7):806–814

El Yousef SJ, Alfidi RJ, Duchesneau RH, et al. Initial experience with nuclear magnetic resonance (NMR) imaging of the human breast. J Comput Assist Tomogr 1983;7(2):215–218

Fischer U, von Heyden D, Vosshenrich R, Vieweg I, Grabbe E. [Signal characteristics of malignant and benign lesions in dynamic 2D-MRT of the breast]. [Article in German] Rofo 1993;158(4):287–292

Fischer U, Vosshenrich R, Kopka L, Kahlen O, Grabbe E. [Contrast medium assisted dynamic MR-mammography after diagnostic and therapeutic interventions on the breast]. [Article in German] Bildgebung 1996;63(2):94–100

Frahm J, Haase A, Matthaei D. Rapid three-dimensional MR imaging using the FLASH technique. J Comput Assist Tomogr 1986;10(2): 363–368

Haase A, Frahm J, Matthaei D, Hänike W, Merboldt KD. FLASH-Imaging: Rapid NMR imaging using low flip angle pulses. J Magn Reson 2011;213(2):533–541

Harms SE, Flamig DP, Hesley KL, et al. Fat-suppressed three-dimensional MR imaging of the breast. Radiographics 1993;13(2): 247–267

Harms SE, Flamig DP, Hesley KL, et al. MR imaging of the breast with rotating delivery of excitation off resonance: clinical experience with pathologic correlation. Radiology 1993;187(2):493–501

Heywang SH, Fenzl G, Beck R, et al. [Use of Gd-DTPA in the nuclear magnetic resonance study of the breast]. [Article in German] Rofo 1986;145(5):565–571

Heywang SH, Fenzl G, Edmaier M, Eiermann W, Bassermann R, Krischke I. [Nuclear spin tomography in breast diagnosis]. [Article in German] Rofo 1985;143(2):207–212

Heywang-Köbrunner SH, Beck R. Contrast-enhanced MRI of the breast. Berlin: Springer; 1995

Heywang-Köbrunner SH, Haustein J, Pohl C, et al. Contrast-enhanced MR imaging of the breast: comparison of two different doses of gadopentetate dimeglumine. Radiology 1994;191(3):639–646

Huang W, Fisher PR, Dulaimy K, Tudorica LA, O'Hea B, Button TM. Detection of breast malignancy: diagnostic MR protocol for improved specificity. Radiology 2004;232(2):585–591

Kaiser WA, Zeitler E. [Nuclear spin tomography of the breast—1st clinical results]. [Article in German] Rontgenpraxis 1985;38(7): 256–262

Kaiser WA. MR-mammography (MRM). Berlin: Springer; 1993

Kelcz F, Furman-Haran E, Grobgeld D, Degani H. Clinical testing of high-spatial-resolution parametric contrast-enhanced MR imaging of the breast. AJR Am J Roentgenol 2002;179(6):1485–1492

Kuhl CH, Bieling HB, Lutterberg G, et al. [Standardization and acceleration of quantitative analysis of dynamic MR mammographies via parametric images and automatized ROI definition]. [Article in German] RoFo 1996;164:475

Kuhl CK, Klaschik S, Mielcarek P, Gieseke J, Wardelmann E, Schild HH. Do T2-weighted pulse sequences help with the differential diagnosis of enhancing lesions in dynamic breast MRI? J Magn Reson Imaging 1999;9(2):187–196

Kuhl CK, Gieseke J, von Falkenhausen M, et al. Sensitivity encoding for diffusion-weighted MR imaging at 3.0 T: intraindividual comparative study. Radiology 2005;234(2):517–526

Kuhl CK, Jost P, Morakkabati N, Zivanovic O, Schild HH, Gieseke J. Contrast-enhanced MR imaging of the breast at 3.0 and 1.5 T in the same patients: initial experience. Radiology 2006;239(3): 666–676

Kuhl CK, Seibert C, Sommer T, Kreft B, Gieseke J, Schild HH. [Focal and diffuse lesions in dynamic MR-mammography of healthy probands]. [Article in German] Rofo 1995;163(3):219–224

Lauterbur PC. Image formation by induced local interactions: examples employing nuclear magnetic resonance. Nature 1973;242:190

Mansfield P, Morris PG, Ordidge R, Coupland RE, Bishop HM, Blamey RW. Carcinoma of the breast imaged by nuclear magnetic resonance (NMR). Br J Radiol 1979;52(615):242–243

Müller-Schimpfle M, Ohmenhäuser K, Claussen CD. Effect of age and menstrual cycle on mammography and MR mammography. [Article in German] Radiologe 1997;37(9):718–725

Müller-Schimpfle M, Rieber A, Kurz S, Stern W, Claussen CD. [Dynamic 3D MR mammography using a rapid gradient-echo sequence]. [Article in German] Rofo 1995;162(1):13–19

Nunes LW, Schnall MD, Siegelman ES, et al. Diagnostic performance characteristics of architectural features revealed by high spatial-resolution MR imaging of the breast. AJR Am J Roentgenol 1997;169(2):409–415

Perman WH, Heiberg EV, Herrmann VM. Half-Fourier, three-dimensional technique for dynamic contrast-enhanced MR imaging of both breasts and axillae: initial characterization of breast lesions. Radiology 1996;200(1):263–269

Schmitz AC, Peters NH, Veldhuis WB, et al. Contrast-enhanced 3.0-T breast MRI for characterization of breast lesions: increased specificity by using vascular maps. Eur Radiol 2008;18(2):355–364

Schorn C, Fischer U, Döler W, Funke M, Grabbe E. Compression device to reduce motion artifacts at contrast-enhanced MR imaging in the breast. Radiology 1998;206(1):279–282

Schorn C, Fischer U, Luftner-Nagel S, Grabbe E. Diagnostic potential of ultrafast contrast-enhanced MRI of the breast in hypervascularized lesions: are there advantages in comparison with standard dynamic MRI? J Comput Assist Tomogr 1999;23(1):118–122

Weinmann HJ, Laniado M, Mützel W. Pharmacokinetics of GdDTPA/ dimeglumine after intravenous injection into healthy volunteers. Physiol Chem Phys Med NMR 1984;16(2):167–172

Wong TZ, Lateiner JS, Mahon TG, Zuo CS, Buff BL. Stereoscopically guided characterization of three-dimensional dynamic MR images of the breast. Radiology 1996;198(1):288–291

Tumor Angiogenesis and Breast MRI

Aranda FI, Laforga JB. Microvessel quantitation in breast ductal invasive carcinoma. Correlation with proliferative activity, hormonal receptors and lymph node metastases. Pathol Res Pract 1996;192(2):124–129

Bicknell R, Harris AL. Mechanisms and therapeutic implications of angiogenesis. Curr Opin Oncol 1996;8(1):60–65

Brinck U, Fischer U, Korabiowska M, Jutrowski M, Schauer A, Grabbe E. The variability of fibroadenoma in contrast-enhanced dynamic MR mammography. AJR Am J Roentgenol 1997;168(5):1331–1334

Buadu LD, Murakami J, Murayama S, et al. Breast lesions: correlation of contrast medium enhancement patterns on MR images with histopathologic findings and tumor angiogenesis. Radiology 1996; 200(3):639–649

Buckley DL, Drew PJ, Mussurakis S, Monson JR, Horsman A. Microvessel density of invasive breast cancer assessed by dynamic Gd-DTPA enhanced MRI. J Magn Reson Imaging 1997;7(3):461–464

Engels K, Fox SB, Harris AL. Angiogenesis as a biologic and prognostic indicator in human breast carcinoma. EXS 1997;79:113–156

Fischer U. Aktuelle Aspekte der dynamischen MR-Mammographie. Habilitationsschrift Universität Göttingen; 1998

Folkman J, Klagsbrun M. Angiogenic factors. Science 1987;235(4787): 442–447

Folkman J. Seminars in Medicine of the Beth Israel Hospital, Boston. Clinical applications of research on angiogenesis. N Engl J Med 1995;333(26):1757–1763

Frouge C, Guinebretière JM, Contesso G, Di Paola R, Bléry M. Correlation between contrast enhancement in dynamic magnetic resonance imaging of the breast and tumor angiogenesis. Invest Radiol 1994;29(12):1043–1049

Furman-Haran E, Margalit R, Maretzek AF, Degani H. Angiogenic response of MCF7 human breast cancer to hormonal treatment: assessment by dynamic GdDTPA-enhanced MRI at high spatial resolution. J Magn Reson Imaging 1996;6(1):195–202

Hulka CA, Edmister WB, Smith BL, et al. Dynamic echo-planar imaging of the breast: experience in diagnosing breast carcinoma and correlation with tumor angiogenesis. Radiology 1997;205(3):837–842

Pluda JM. Tumor-associated angiogenesis: mechanisms, clinical implications, and therapeutic strategies. Semin Oncol 1997;24(2): 203–218

Sardanelli F, Iozzelli A, Fausto A, Carriero A, Kirchin MA. Gadobenate dimeglumine-enhanced MR imaging breast vascular maps: association between invasive cancer and ipsilateral increased vascularity. Radiology 2005;235(3):791–797

Siewert C, Oellinger H, Sherif HK, Blohmer JU, Hadijuana J, Felix R. Is there a correlation in breast carcinomas between tumor size and number of tumor vessels detected by gadolinium-enhanced magnetic resonance mammography? MAGMA 1997;5(1):29–31

Stomper PC, Herman S, Klippenstein DL, Winston JS, Budnick RM, Stewart CC. Invasive breast carcinoma: analysis of dynamic magnetic resonance imaging enhancement features and cell proliferative activity determined by DNA S-phase percentage. Cancer 1996;77(9):1844–1849

Szabó BK, Aspelin P, Kristoffersen Wiberg M, Tot T, Boné B. Invasive breast cancer: correlation of dynamic MR features with prognostic factors. Eur Radiol 2003;13(11):2425–2435

Teifke A, Behr O, Schmidt M, et al. Dynamic MR imaging of breast lesions: correlation with microvessel distribution pattern and histologic characteristics of prognosis. Radiology 2006;239(2): 351–360

Tuncbilek N, Unlu E, Karakas HM, Cakir B, Ozyilmaz F. Evaluation of tumor angiogenesis with contrast-enhanced dynamic magnetic resonance mammography. Breast J 2003;9(5):403–408

Weidner N, Folkman J, Pozza F, et al. Tumor angiogenesis: a new significant and independent prognostic indicator in early-stage breast carcinoma. J Natl Cancer Inst 1992;84(24):1875–1887

Weidner N, Semple JP, Welch WR, Folkman J. Tumor angiogenesis and metastasis—correlation in invasive breast carcinoma. N Engl J Med 1991;324(1):1–8

Diagnostic Criteria

Al-Khawari H, Athyal R, Kovacs A, Al-Saleh M, Madda JP. Accuracy of the Fischer scoring system and the Breast Imaging Reporting and Data System in identification of malignant breast lesions. Ann Saudi Med 2009;29(4):280–287

American College of Radiology. BI-RADS Breast Imaging Reporting and Data System. Breast Imaging Atlas: Mammography, Breast Ultrasound, Breast MR Imaging. Reston, VA: ACR; 2003

Baum F, Fischer U, Vosshenrich R, Grabbe E. Classification of hypervascularized lesions in CE MR imaging of the breast. Eur Radiol 2002;12(5):1087–1092

Buchbinder SS, Leichter IS, Lederman RB, et al. Computer-aided classification of BI-RADS category 3 breast lesions. Radiology 2004; 230(3):820–823

Buckley DL, Mussurakis S, Horsman A. Effect of temporal resolution on the diagnostic efficacy of contrast-enhanced MRI in the conservatively treated breast. J Comput Assist Tomogr 1998;22(1):47–51

Davis PL, McCarty KS Jr. Sensitivity of enhanced MRI for the detection of breast cancer: new, multicentric, residual, and recurrent. Eur Radiol 1997;7(Suppl 5):289–298

Fischer DR, Wurdinger S, Boettcher J, Malich A, Kaiser WA. Further signs in the evaluation of magnetic resonance mammography: a retrospective study. Invest Radiol 2005;40(7):430–435

Fischer U, von Heyden D, Vosshenrich R, Vieweg I, Grabbe E. [Signal characteristics of malignant and benign lesions in dynamic 2 D-MRT of the breast]. [Article in German] Rofo 1993;158(4):287–292

Goto M, Ito H, Akazawa K, et al. Diagnosis of breast tumors by contrast-enhanced MR imaging: comparison between the diagnostic performance of dynamic enhancement patterns and morphologic features. J Magn Reson Imaging 2007;25(1):104–112

Kaiser WA. Signs in MR-mammography. Berlin: Springer; 2008

Kim SJ, Morris EA, Liberman L, et al. Observer variability and applicability of BI-RADS terminology for breast MR imaging: invasive carcinomas as focal masses. AJR Am J Roentgenol 2001;177(3): 551–557

Kinkel K, Helbich TH, Esserman LJ, et al. Dynamic high-spatial-resolution MR imaging of suspicious breast lesions: diagnostic criteria and interobserver variability. AJR Am J Roentgenol 2000;175(1):35–43

Kuhl C. The current status of breast MR imaging. Part I. Choice of technique, image interpretation, diagnostic accuracy, and transfer to clinical practice. Radiology 2007;244(2):356–378

Kuhl CK, Bieling H, Gieseke J, et al. Breast neoplasms: T2* susceptibility-contrast, first-pass perfusion MR imaging. Radiology 1997; 202(1):87–95

Kuhl CK, Jost P, Morakkabati N, Zivanovic O, Schild HH, Gieseke J. Contrast-enhanced MR imaging of the breast at 3.0 and 1.5T in the same patients: initial experience. Radiology 2006;239(3): 666–676

Kuhl CK, Klaschik S, Mielcarek P, Gieseke J, Wardelmann E, Schild HH. Do T2-weighted pulse sequences help with the differential diagnosis of enhancing lesions in dynamic breast MRI? J Magn Reson Imaging 1999;9(2):187–196

Kuhl CK, Mielcareck P, Klaschik S, et al. Dynamic breast MR imaging: are signal intensity time course data useful for differential diagnosis of enhancing lesions? Radiology 1999;211(1):101–110

Kuhl CK, Schild HH, Morakkabati N. Dynamic bilateral contrast-enhanced MR imaging of the breast: trade-off between spatial and temporal resolution. Radiology 2005;236(3):789–800

Kvistad KA, Rydland J, Vainio J, et al. Breast lesions: evaluation with dynamic contrast-enhanced T1-weighted MR imaging and with T2*-weighted first-pass perfusion MR imaging. Radiology 2000; 216(2):545–553

Lazarus E, Mainiero MB, Schepps B, Koelliker SL, Livingston LS. BI-RADS lexicon for US and mammography: interobserver variability and positive predictive value. Radiology 2006;239(2): 385–391

Levman JE, Causer P, Warner E, Martel AL. Effect of the enhancement threshold on the computer-aided detection of breast cancer using MRI. Acad Radiol 2009;16(9):1064–1069

Liberman L, Abramson AF, Squires FB, Glassman JR, Morris EA, Dershaw DD. The breast imaging reporting and data system: positive predictive value of mammographic features and final assessment categories. AJR Am J Roentgenol 1998;171(1):35–40

Liberman L, Mason G, Morris EA, Dershaw DD. Does size matter? Positive predictive value of MRI-detected breast lesions as a function of lesion size. AJR Am J Roentgenol 2006;186(2):426–430

Liberman L, Morris EA, Dershaw DD, Abramson AF, Tan LK. Ductal enhancement on MR imaging of the breast. AJR Am J Roentgenol 2003;181(2):519–525

Liberman L, Morris EA, Lee MJ, et al. Breast lesions detected on MR imaging: features and positive predictive value. AJR Am J Roentgenol 2002;179(1):171–178

Marklund M, Torp-Pedersen S, Bentzon N, Thomsen C, Roslind A, Nolsøe CP. Contrast kinetics of the malignant breast tumour—border versus centre enhancement on dynamic midfield MRI. Eur J Radiol 2008;65(2):279–285

Matsubayashi R, Matsuo Y, Edakuni G, Satoh T, Tokunaga O, Kudo S. Breast masses with peripheral rim enhancement on dynamic contrast-enhanced MR images: correlation of MR findings with histologic features and expression of growth factors. Radiology 2000;217(3):841–848

Meeuwis C, van de Ven SM, Stapper G, et al. Computer-aided detection (CAD) for breast MRI: evaluation of efficacy at 3.0 T. Eur Radiol 2010;20(3):522–528

Morakkabati-Spitz N, Leutner C, Schild H, Traeber F, Kuhl C. Diagnostic usefulness of segmental and linear enhancement in dynamic breast MRI. Eur Radiol 2005;15(9):2010–2017

Mussurakis S, Gibbs P, Horsman A. Peripheral enhancement and spatial contrast uptake heterogeneity of primary breast tumours: quantitative assessment with dynamic MRI. J Comput Assist Tomogr 1998;22(1):35–46

Nunes LW, Schnall MD, Siegelman ES, et al. Diagnostic performance characteristics of architectural features revealed by high spatial resolution MR imaging of the breast. AJR Am J Roentgenol 1997; 169(2):409–415

Orel SG, Schnall MD, LiVolsi VA, Troupin RH. Suspicious breast lesions: MR imaging with radiologic-pathologic correlation. Radiology 1994;190(2):485–493

Penn A, Thompson S, Brem R, et al. Morphologic blooming in breast MRI as a characterization of margin for discriminating benign from malignant lesions. Acad Radiol 2006;13(11):1344–1354

Piccoli CW. Contrast-enhanced breast MRI: factors affecting sensitivity and specificity. Eur Radiol 1997;7(Suppl 5):281–288

Sakamoto N, Tozaki M, Higa K, et al. Categorization of non-mass-like breast lesions detected by MRI. Breast Cancer 2008;15(3):241–246

Schnall MD, Blume J, Bluemke DA, et al. Diagnostic architectural and dynamic features at breast MR imaging: multicenter study. Radiology 2006;238(1):42–53

Sherif H, Mahfouz AE, Oellinger H, et al. Peripheral washout sign on contrast-enhanced MR images of the breast. Radiology 1997; 205(1):209–213

Siegmann KC, Müller-Schimpfle M, Schick F, et al. MR imaging-detected breast lesions: histopathologic correlation of lesion characteristics and signal intensity data. AJR Am J Roentgenol 2002;178(6): 1403–1409

Thomassin-Naggara I, Salem C, Darai E, et al. [Non-masslike enhancement on breast MRI: interpretation pearls]. [Article in French] J Radiol 2009;90(3 Pt 1):269–275

Tokuda Y, Kuriyama K, Nakamoto A, et al. Evaluation of suspicious nipple discharge by magnetic resonance mammography based on breast imaging reporting and data system magnetic resonance imaging descriptors. J Comput Assist Tomogr 2009;33(1):58–62

Tozaki M, Fukuda K. High-spatial-resolution MRI of non-masslike breast lesions: interpretation model based on BI-RADS MRI descriptors. AJR Am J Roentgenol 2006;187(2):330–337

Tozaki M, Igarashi T, Fukuda K. Breast MRI using the VIBE sequence: clustered ring enhancement in the differential diagnosis of lesions showing non-masslike enhancement. AJR Am J Roentgenol 2006; 187(2):313–321

Tozaki M, Igarashi T, Matsushima S, Fukuda K. High-spatial-resolution MR imaging of focal breast masses: interpretation model based on kinetic and morphological parameters. Radiat Med 2005;23(1): 43–50

Van Goethem M, Schelfout K, Kersschot E, et al. Enhancing area surrounding breast carcinoma on MR mammography: comparison with pathological examination. Eur Radiol 2004;14(8):1363–1370

Warren RM, Thompson D, Pointon LJ, et al; Collaborators in the United Kingdom Medical Research Council Magnetic Resonance Imaging in Breast Screening (MARIBS) Study. Evaluation of a prospective scoring system designed for a multicenter breast MR imaging screening study. Radiology 2006;239(3):677–685

Wiener JI, Schilling KJ, Adami C, Obuchowski NA. Assessment of suspected breast cancer by MRI: a prospective clinical trial using a combined kinetic and morphologic analysis. AJR Am J Roentgenol 2005;184(3):878–886

Williams TC, DeMartini WB, Partridge SC, Peacock S, Lehman CD. Breast MR imaging: computer-aided evaluation program for discriminating benign from malignant lesions. Radiology 2007;244(1): 94–103

Normal Findings in Breast MRI

Da Costa D, Taddese A, Cure ML, Gerson D, Poppiti R Jr, Esserman LE. Common and unusual diseases of the nipple-areolar complex. Radiographics 2007;27(Suppl 1):S 65–S 77

Dean KI, Majurin ML, Komu M. Relaxation times of normal breast tissues. Changes with age and variations during the menstrual cycle. Acta Radiol 1994;35(3):258–261

Espinosa LA, Daniel BL, Vidarsson L, Zakhour M, Ikeda DM, Herfkens RJ. The lactating breast: contrast-enhanced MR imaging of normal tissue and cancer. Radiology 2005;237(2):429–436

Fowler PA, Casey CE, Cameron GG, Foster MA, Knight CH. Cyclic changes in composition and volume of the breast during the menstrual cycle, measured by magnetic resonance imaging. Br J Obstet Gynaecol 1990;97(7):595–602

Friedman EP, Hall-Craggs MA, Mumtaz H, Schneidau A. Breast MR and the appearance of the normal and abnormal nipple. Clin Radiol 1997;52(11):854–861

Graham SJ, Stanchev PL, Lloyd-Smith JOA, Bronskill MJ, Plewes DB. Changes in fibroglandular volume and water content of breast tissue during the menstrual cycle observed by MR imaging at 1.5 T. J Magn Reson Imaging 1995;5(6):695–701

Husstedt H, Prokop M, Becker H. Window width as a dosage-relevant factor in high-contrast structures in CT. [Article in German] Rofo 1998;168(2):139–143

Kaiser WA. [The lactating breast in the magnetic resonance tomogram. Spin-echo and fat-water images]. [Article in German] Rofo 1987;146(1):47–51

Kaiser WA, Mittelmeier O. [MR mammography in patients at risk]. [Article in German] Rofo 1992;156(6):576–581

Kuhl CK, Bieling HB, Gieseke J, et al. Healthy premenopausal breast parenchyma in dynamic contrast-enhanced MR imaging of the breast: normal contrast medium enhancement and cyclical-phase dependency. Radiology 1997;203(1):137–144

Kuhl CK, Seibert C, Sommer T, Kreft B, Gieseke J, Schild HH. [Focal and diffuse lesions in dynamic MR-mammography of healthy probands]. [Article in German] Rofo 1995;163(3):219–224

Lee NA, Rusinek H, Weinreb J, et al. Fatty and fibroglandular tissue volumes in the breasts of women 20-83 years old: comparison of X-ray mammography and computer-assisted MR imaging. AJR Am J Roentgenol 1997;168(2):501–506

Martin B, el Yousef SJ. Transverse relaxation time values in MR imaging of normal breast during menstrual cycle. J Comput Assist Tomogr 1986;10(6):924–927

Müller-Schimpfle M, Ohmenhäuser K, Claussen CD. [Effect of age and menstrual cycle on mammography and MR mammography]. [Article in German] Radiologe 1997;37(9):718–725

Müller-Schimpfle M, Ohmenhäuser K, Stoll P, Dietz K, Claussen CD. Menstrual cycle and age: influence on parenchymal contrast medium enhancement in MR imaging of the breast. Radiology 1997;203(1):145–149

Nelson TR, Pretorius DH, Schiffer LM. Menstrual variation of normal breast NMR relaxation parameters. J Comput Assist Tomogr 1985;9(5):875–879

Benign Findings

Farria DM, Gorczyca DP, Barsky SH, Sinha S, Bassett LW. Benign phyllodes tumor of the breast: MR imaging features. AJR Am J Roentgenol 1996;167(1):187–189

Fischer U, Kopka L, Brinck U, Korabiowska M, Schauer A, Grabbe E. Prognostic value of contrast-enhanced MR mammography in patients with breast cancer. Eur Radiol 1997;7(7):1002–1005

Fischer U, Vosshenrich R, von Heyden D, Knipper H, Oestmann JW, Grabbe E. [Inflammatory lesions of the breast: indication for MR-mammography?]. [Article in German] Rofo 1994;161(4):307–311

Friedrich M, Sickles EA. Radiological diagnosis of breast diseases. Berlin: Springer; 1997

Gallardo X, Sentís M, Castañer E, Andreu X, Darnell A, Canalías J. Enhancement of intramammary lymph nodes with lymphoid hyperplasia: a potential pitfall in breast MRI. Eur Radiol 1998;8(9):1662–1665

Gibbs P, Liney GP, Lowry M, Kneeshaw PJ, Turnbull LW. Differentiation of benign and malignant sub-1 cm breast lesions using dynamic contrast enhanced MRI. Breast 2004;13(2):115–121

Gilles R, Meunier M, Lucidarme O, et al. Clustered breast microcalcifications: evaluation by dynamic contrast-enhanced subtraction MRI. J Comput Assist Tomogr 1996;20(1):9–14

Harris JR, Lippman ME, Morrow M, Hellman P. Diseases of the breast. Philadelphia: Lippincott-Raven; 1996

Heywang-Köbrunner SH, Beck R. Contrast-enhanced MRI of the breast. Berlin: Springer; 1995

Hochman MG, Orel SG, Powell CM, Schnall MD, Reynolds CA, White LN. Fibroadenomas: MR imaging appearances with radiologic-histopathologic correlation. Radiology 1997;204(1):123–129

Jacobs MA, Barker PB, Bluemke DA, et al. Benign and malignant breast lesions: diagnosis with multiparametric MR imaging. Radiology 2003;229(1):225–232

Jansen SA, Fan X, Karczmar GS, Abe H, Schmidt RA, Newstead GM. Differentiation between benign and malignant breast lesions detected by bilateral dynamic contrast-enhanced MRI: a sensitivity and specificity study. Magn Reson Med 2008;59(4):747–754

Kaiser WA, Mittelmeier O. [MR mammography in patients at risk]. [Article in German] Rofo 1992;156(6):576–581

Kaiser WA. MR-mammography (MRM). Berlin: Springer; 1993

Kenzel PP, Hadijuana J, Hosten N, et al. Boeck sarcoidosis of the breast: mammographic, ultrasound, and MR findings. J Comput Assist Tomogr 1997;21(3):439–441

Kopans DB. Breast imaging. Philadelphia: Lippincott-Raven; 1997

Kuhl CK, Bieling HB, Gieseke J, et al. Healthy premenopausal breast parenchyma in dynamic contrast-enhanced MR imaging of the breast: normal contrast medium enhancement and cyclical-phase dependency. Radiology 1997;203(1):137–144

Kurtz B, Achten C, Audretsch W, Rezai M, Zocholl G. [MR mammography of fatty tissue necrosis]. [Article in German] Rofo 1996;165(4):359–363

Ogawa Y, Nishioka A, Tsuboi N, et al. Dynamic MR appearance of benign phyllodes tumor of the breast in a 20-year-old woman. Radiat Med 1997;15(4):247–250

Rovno HDS, Siegelman ES, Reynolds C, Orel SG, Schnall MD. Solitary intraductal papilloma: findings at MR imaging and MR galactography. AJR Am J Roentgenol 1999;172(1):151–155

Sittek H, Kessler M, Heuck AF, et al. [Dynamic MR mammography: is the course of signal intensification suitable for the differentiation of different forms of mastopathy?]. [Article in German] Rofo 1996;165(1):59–63

Solomon B, Orel S, Reynolds C, Schnall M. Delayed development of enhancement in fat necrosis after breast conservation therapy: a potential pitfall of MR imaging of the breast. AJR Am J Roentgenol 1998;170(4):966–968

Sydnor MK, Wilson JD, Hijaz TA, Massey HD, Shaw de Paredes ES. Underestimation of the presence of breast carcinoma in papillary lesions initially diagnosed at core-needle biopsy. Radiology 2007;242(1):58–62

Tomczak R, Rieber A, Zeitler H, Rilinger N, Kreienberg R, Brambs HJ. [The value of MR-mammography at 1.5 tesla in the differential diagnosis of non-puerperal mastitis and inflammatory breast carcinoma]. [Article in German] Rofo 1996;165(2):148–151

Unterweger M, Huch Böni RA, Caduff R, Hebisch G, Krestin GP. Inflammatory breast carcinoma versus puerperal mastitis. Difficulties in differentiation based on clinical, histological and MRI findings. [Article in German] Rofo 1997;166(6):558–560

van den Bosch MA, Daniel BL, Mariano MN, et al. Magnetic resonance imaging characteristics of fibrocystic change of the breast. Invest Radiol 2005;40(7):436–441

Weinstein D, Strano S, Cohen P, Fields S, Gomori JM, Degani H. Breast fibroadenoma: mapping of pathophysiologic features with three-time-point, contrast-enhanced MR imaging—pilot study. Radiology 1999;210(1):233–240

Westerhof JP, Fischer U, Moritz JD, Oestmann JW. MR imaging of mammographically detected clustered microcalcifications: is there any value? Radiology 1998;207(3):675–681

Yabuuchi H, Soeda H, Matsuo Y, et al. Phyllodes tumor of the breast: correlation between MR findings and histologic grade. Radiology 2006;241(3):702–709

Malignant Findings

Bartella L, Liberman L, Morris EA, Dershaw DD. Nonpalpable mammographically occult invasive breast cancers detected by MRI. AJR Am J Roentgenol 2006;186(3):865–870

Berg WA, Gutierrez L, NessAiver MS, et al. Diagnostic accuracy of mammography, clinical examination, US, and MR imaging in preoperative assessment of breast cancer. Radiology 2004;233(3):830–849

Bluemke DA, Gatsonis CA, Chen MH, et al. Magnetic resonance imaging of the breast prior to biopsy. JAMA 2004;292(22):2735–2742

Boetes C, Strijk SP, Holland R, Barentsz JO, Van Der Sluis RF, Ruijs JH. False-negative MR imaging of malignant breast tumors. Eur Radiol 1997;7(8):1231–1234

Boetes C, Veltman J, van Die L, Bult P, Wobbes T, Barentsz JO. The role of MRI in invasive lobular carcinoma. Breast Cancer Res Treat 2004;86(1):31–37

Boné B, Aspelin P, Bronge L, Isberg B, Perbeck L, Veress B. Sensitivity and specificity of MR mammography with histopathological correlation in 250 breasts. Acta Radiol 1996;37(2):208–213

Farria DM, Gorczyca DP, Barsky SH, Sinha S, Bassett LW. Benign phyllodes tumor of the breast: MR imaging features. AJR Am J Roentgenol 1996;167(1):187–189

Fischer U, Kopka L, Brinck U, Korabiowska M, Schauer A, Grabbe E. Prognostic value of contrast-enhanced MR mammography in patients with breast cancer. Eur Radiol 1997;7(7):1002–1005

Fischer U, Kopka L, Grabbe E. Invasive mucinous carcinoma of the breast missed by contrast-enhancing MR imaging of the breast. Eur Radiol 1996;6(6):929–931

Fischer U, Kopka L, Grabbe E. Breast carcinoma: effect of preoperative contrast-enhanced MR imaging on the therapeutic approach. Radiology 1999;213(3):881–888

Fischer U, Westerhof JP, Brinck U, Korabiowska M, Schauer A, Grabbe E. [Ductal carcinoma in situ in dynamic MR-mammography at 1.5 T]. [Article in German] Rofo 1996;164(4):290–294

Friedrich M, Sickles EA. Radiological diagnosis of breast diseases. Berlin: Springer; 1997

Gibbs P, Liney GP, Lowry M, Kneeshaw PJ, Turnbull LW. Differentiation of benign and malignant sub-1 cm breast lesions using dynamic contrast enhanced MRI. Breast 2004;13(2):115–121

Gilles R, Guinebretière JM, Lucidarme O, et al. Nonpalpable breast tumors: diagnosis with contrast-enhanced subtraction dynamic MR imaging. Radiology 1994;191(3):625–631

Gilles R, Zafrani B, Guinebretière JM, et al. Ductal carcinoma in situ: MR imaging-histopathologic correlation. Radiology 1995;196(2):415–419

Groves AM, Warren RM, Godward S, Rajan PS. Characterization of pure high-grade DCIS on magnetic resonance imaging using the evolving breast MR lexicon terminology: can it be differentiated from pure invasive disease? Magn Reson Imaging 2005;23(6):733–738

Harms SE, Flamig DP, Hesley KL, et al. MR imaging of the breast with rotating delivery of excitation off resonance: clinical experience with pathologic correlation. Radiology 1993;187(2):493–501

Hering M, Hagel E, Zwicker C, Krieger G. [Bilateral highly malignant centroblastic lymphoma of the breast]. [Article in German] Rofo 1996;165(2):198–200

Heywang-Köbrunner SH. Contrast-enhanced magnetic resonance imaging of the breast. Invest Radiol 1994;29(1):94–104

Jansen SA, Fan X, Karczmar GS, Abe H, Schmidt RA, Newstead GM. Differentiation between benign and malignant breast lesions detected by bilateral dynamic contrast-enhanced MRI: a sensitivity and specificity study. Magn Reson Med 2008;59(4):747–754

Jansen SA, Newstead GM, Abe H, Shimauchi A, Schmidt RA, Karczmar GS. Pure ductal carcinoma in situ: kinetic and morphologic MR characteristics compared with mammographic appearance and nuclear grade. Radiology 2007;245(3):684–691

Kaiser WA. [MR mammography]. [Article in German] Radiologe 1993;33(5):292–299

Kenzel PP, Hadijuana J, Hosten N, et al. Boeck sarcoidosis of the breast: mammographic, ultrasound, and MR findings. J Comput Assist Tomogr 1997;21(3):439–441

Ko ES, Lee BH, Kim HA, Noh WC, Kim MS, Lee SA. Triple-negative breast cancer: correlation between imaging and pathological findings. Eur Radiol 2010;20(5):1111–1117

Krämer S, Schulz-Wendtland R, Hagedorn K, Bautz W, Lang N. Magnetic resonance imaging and its role in the diagnosis of multicentric breast cancer. Anticancer Res 1998;18(3C):2163–2164

Kuhl CK, Schrading S, Bieling HB, et al. MRI for diagnosis of pure ductal carcinoma in situ: a prospective observational study. Lancet 2007;370(9586):485–492

Levrini G, Nicoli F, Borasi G, Mori CA, Zompatori M. MRI patterns of invasive lobular breast cancer. Eur J Radiol 2006;59(3):472

Lopez JK, Bassett LW. Invasive lobular carcinoma of the breast: spectrum of mammographic, US, and MR imaging findings. Radiographics 2009;29(1):165–176

Miller RW, Harms S, Alvarez A. Mucinous carcinoma of the breast: potential false-negative MR imaging interpretation. AJR Am J Roentgenol 1996;167(2):539–540

Mumtaz H, Hall-Craggs MA, Davidson T, et al. Staging of symptomatic primary breast cancer with MR imaging. AJR Am J Roentgenol 1997;169(2):417–424

Mussurakis S, Buckley DL, Horsman A. Dynamic MR imaging of invasive breast cancer: correlation with tumour grade and other histological factors. Br J Radiol 1997;70(833):446–451

Mussurakis S, Carleton PJ, Turnbull LW. MR imaging of primary non-Hodgkin's breast lymphoma. A case report. Acta Radiol 1997;38(1):104–107

Okafuji T, Yabuuchi H, Sakai S, et al. MR imaging features of pure mucinous carcinoma of the breast. Eur J Radiol 2006;60(3):405–413

Orel SG, Mendonca MH, Reynolds C, Schnall MD, Solin LJ, Sullivan DC. MR imaging of ductal carcinoma in situ. Radiology 1997;202(2):413–420

Orel SG, Schnall MD, Powell CM, et al. Staging of suspected breast cancer: effect of MR imaging and MR-guided biopsy. Radiology 1995;196(1):115–122

Qayyum A, Birdwell RL, Daniel BL, et al. MR imaging features of infiltrating lobular carcinoma of the breast: histopathologic correlation. AJR Am J Roentgenol 2002;178(5):1227–1232

Rieber A, Merkle E, Böhm W, Brambs HJ, Tomczak R. MRI of histologically confirmed mammary carcinoma: clinical relevance of diagnostic procedures for detection of multifocal or contralateral secondary carcinoma. J Comput Assist Tomogr 1997;21(5):773–779

Rieber A, Tomczak RJ, Mergo PJ, Wenzel V, Zeitler H, Brambs HJ. MRI of the breast in the differential diagnosis of mastitis versus inflammatory carcinoma and follow-up. J Comput Assist Tomogr 1997;21(1):128–132

Rodenko GN, Harms SE, Pruneda JM, et al. MR imaging in the management before surgery of lobular carcinoma of the breast: correlation with pathology. AJR Am J Roentgenol 1996;167(6):1415–1419

Rosen EL, Smith-Foley SA, DeMartini WB, Eby PR, Peacock S, Lehman CD. BI-RADS MRI enhancement characteristics of ductal carcinoma in situ. Breast J 2007;13(6):545–550

Sardanelli F, Bacigalupo L, Carbonaro L, et al. What is the sensitivity of mammography and dynamic MR imaging for DCIS if the whole-breast histopathology is used as a reference standard? Radiol Med (Torino) 2008;113(3):439–451

Schorn C, Fischer U, Luftner-Nagel S, Westerhof JP, Grabbe E. MRI of the breast in patients with metastatic disease of unknown primary. Eur Radiol 1999;9(3):470–473

Schouten van der Velden AP, Boetes C, Bult P, Wobbes T. The value of magnetic resonance imaging in diagnosis and size assessment of in situ and small invasive breast carcinoma. Am J Surg 2006;192(2):172–178

Seely JM, Nguyen ET, Jaffey J. Breast MRI in the evaluation of locally recurrent or new breast cancer in the postoperative patient: correlation of morphology and enhancement features with the BI-RADS category. Acta Radiol 2007;28:1–8

Sittek H, Perlet C, Untch M, Kessler M, Reiser M. [Dynamic MR-mammography in invasive lobular breast cancer]. [Article in German] Rontgenpraxis 1998;51(7):235–242

Stomper PC, Herman S, Klippenstein DL, et al. Suspect breast lesions: findings at dynamic gadolinium-enhanced MR imaging correlated with mammographic and pathologic features. Radiology 1995;197(2):387–395

Tesoro-Tess JD, Amoruso A, Rovini D, et al. Microcalcifications in clinically normal breast: the value of high field, surface coil, Gd-DTPA-enhanced MRI. Eur Radiol 1995;5:417–422

Tomczak R, Rieber A, Zeitler H, Rilinger N, Kreienberg R, Brambs HJ. [The value of MR-mammography at 1.5 tesla in the differential diagnosis of non-puerperal mastitis and inflammatory breast carcinoma]. [Article in German] Rofo 1996;165(2):148–151

Tominaga J, Hama H, Kimura N, Takahashi S. MR imaging of medullary carcinoma of the breast. Eur J Radiol 2009;70(3):525–529

Unterweger M, Huch Böni RA, Caduff R, Hebisch G, Krestin GP. [Inflammatory breast carcinoma versus puerperal mastitis. Difficulties in differentiation based on clinical, histological and MRI findings]. [Article in German] Rofo 1997;166(6):558–560

Weinstein SP, Orel SG, Heller R, et al. MR imaging of the breast in patients with invasive lobular carcinoma. AJR Am J Roentgenol 2001;176(2):399–406

Yeh ED, Slanetz PJ, Edmister WB, Talele A, Monticciolo D, Kopans DB. Invasive lobular carcinoma: spectrum of enhancement and morphology on magnetic resonance imaging. Breast J 2003;9(1):13–18

Autologous and Prosthetic Reconstruction

Ahn CY, Narayanan K, Gorczyca DP, DeBruhl ND, Shaw WW. Evaluation of autogenous tissue breast reconstruction using MRI. Plast Reconstr Surg 1995;95(1):70–76

Azavedo E, Boné B. Imaging breasts with silicone implants. Eur Radiol 1999;9(2):349–355

Baker JL Jr, Bartels RJ, Douglas WM. Closed compression technique for rupturing a contracted capsule around a breast implant. Plast Reconstr Surg 1976;58(2):137–141

Berg WA, Anderson ND, Zerhouni EA, Chang BW, Kuhlman JE. MR imaging of the breast in patients with silicone breast implants: normal postoperative variants and diagnostic pitfalls. AJR Am J Roentgenol 1994;163(3):575–578

Berg WA, Caskey CI, Hamper UM, et al. Diagnosing breast implant rupture with MR imaging, US, and mammography. Radiographics 1993;13(6):1323–1336

Berg WA, Caskey CI, Hamper UM, et al. Single- and double- lumen silicone breast implant integrity: prospective evaluation of MR and US criteria. Radiology 1995;197(1):45–52

DeAngelis GA, de Lange EE, Miller LR, Morgan RF. MR imaging of breast implants. Radiographics 1994;14(4):783–794

Everson LI, Parantainen H, Detlie T, et al. Diagnosis of breast implant rupture: imaging findings and relative efficacies of imaging techniques. AJR Am J Roentgenol 1994;163(1):57–60

Gorczyca DP. MR imaging of breast implants. Magn Reson Imaging Clin N Am 1994;2(4):659–672

Gorczyca DP, Brenner RJ. The augmented breast. Radiologic and clinical perspectives. Stuttgart: Thieme; 1997

Gorczyca DP, Sinha S, Ahn CY, et al. Silicone breast implants in vivo: MR imaging. Radiology 1992;185(2):407–410

Harms SE, Jensen RA, Meiches MD, Flamig DP, Evans WP. Silicone-suppressed 3 D MRI of the breast using rotating delivery of off-resonance excitation. J Comput Assist Tomogr 1995;19(3):394–399

Huch RA, Künzi W, Debatin JF, Wiesner W, Krestin GP. MR imaging of the augmented breast. Eur Radiol 1998;8(3):371–376

Kang BJ, Jung JI, Park C, et al. Breast MRI findings after modified radical mastectomy and transverse rectus abdominis myocutaneous flap in patients with breast cancer. J Magn Reson Imaging 2005;21(6):784–791

Kurtz B, Audretsch W, Rezai M, Achten C, Zocholl G. [Initial experiences with MR-mammography in after-care following surgical flap treatment of breast carcinoma]. [Article in German] Rofo 1996;164(4):295–300

Middleton MS, McNamara MP. Breast implant imaging. Philadelphia: Lippincott Williams & Wilkins; 2003

Monticciolo DL, Nelson RC, Dixon WT, Bostwick J III, Mukundan S, Hester TR. MR detection of leakage from silicone breast implants: value of a silicone-selective pulse sequence. AJR Am J Roentgenol 1994;163(1):51–56

Morgan DE, Kenney PJ, Meeks MC, Pile NS. MR imaging of breast implants and their complications. AJR Am J Roentgenol 1996;167(5):1271–1275

Mund DF, Farria DM, Gorczyca DP, et al. MR imaging of the breast in patients with silicone-gel implants: spectrum of findings. AJR Am J Roentgenol 1993;161(4):773–778

Piccoli CW, Greer JG, Mitchell DG. Breast MR imaging for cancer detection and implant evaluation: potential pitfalls. Radiographics 1996;16(1):63–75

Soo MS, Kornguth PJ, Walsh R, Elenberger CD, Georgiade GS. Complex radial folds versus subtle signs of intracapsular rupture of breast implants: MR findings with surgical correlation. AJR Am J Roentgenol 1996;166(6):1421–1427

Stroman PW, Rolland C, Dufour M, Grondin P, Guidoin RG. Appearance of low signal intensity lines in MRI of silicone breast implants. Biomaterials 1996;17(10):983–988

Youk JH, Son EJ, Kim EK, et al. Diagnosis of breast cancer at dynamic MRI in patients with breast augmentation by paraffin or silicone injection. Clin Radiol 2009;64(12):1175–1180

MRI of the Male Breast

Kaiser WA. Breast diseases in males. In: Kaiser WA, ed. MR-Mammography (MRM). Berlin: Springer; 1993: 80

Morakkabati-Spitz N, Schild HH, Leutner CC, von Falkenhausen M, Lutterbey G, Kuhl CK. Dynamic contrast-enhanced breast MR imaging in men: preliminary results. Radiology 2006;238(2):438–445

MRI-Guided Interventions

AG-Mammadiagnostik der DRG. Empfehlungen zur MR-gesteuerten Interventionen. Rofo 2007; 179:429

Chen X, Lehman CD, Dee KE. MRI-guided breast biopsy: clinical experience with 14-gauge stainless steel core biopsy needle. AJR Am J Roentgenol 2004;182(4):1075–1080

Daniel BL, Birdwell RL, Ikeda DM, et al. Breast lesion localization: a freehand, interactive MR imaging-guided technique. Radiology 1998;207(2):455–463

Döler W, Fischer U, Metzger I, Harder D, Grabbe E. Stereotaxic add-on device for MR-guided biopsy of breast lesions. Radiology 1996; 200(3):863–864

Fischer U, Baum F. Diagnostische Interventionen der Mamma. Stuttgart: Thieme; 2008

Fischer U, Kopka L, Grabbe E. Magnetic resonance guided localization and biopsy of suspicious breast lesions. Top Magn Reson Imaging 1998;9(1):44–59

Fischer U, Rodenwaldt J, Hundertmark C, Döler W, Grabbe E. MRI-assisted biopsy and localization of the breast. [Article in German] Radiologe 1997;37(9):692–701

Fischer U, Schwethelm L, Baum FT, Luftner-Nagel S, Teubner J. Effort, accuracy and histology of MR-guided vacuum biopsy of suspicious breast lesions—retrospective evaluation after 389 interventions. [Article in German] Rofo 2009;181(8):774–781

Fischer U, Vosshenrich R, Bruhn H, Keating D, Raab BW, Oestmann JW. MR-guided localization of suspected breast lesions detected exclusively by postcontrast MRI. J Comput Assist Tomogr 1995;19(1):63–66

Fischer U, Vosshenrich R, Keating D, et al. MR-guided biopsy of suspect breast lesions with a simple stereotaxic add-on-device for surface coils. Radiology 1994;192(1):272–273

Han BK, Schnall MD, Orel SG, Rosen M. Outcome of MRI-guided breast biopsy. AJR Am J Roentgenol 2008;191(6):1798–1804

Hauth EA, Jaeger HJ, Lubnau J, et al. MR-guided vacuum-assisted breast biopsy with a handheld biopsy system: clinical experience and results in postinterventional MR mammography after 24h. Eur Radiol 2008;18(1):168–176

Hefler L, Casselman J, Amaya B, et al. Follow-up of breast lesions detected by MRI not biopsied due to absent enhancement of contrast medium. Eur Radiol 2003;13(2):344–346

Heinig A, Heywang-Köbrunner SH, Viehweg P, Schaumlöffel U, Heske N. [A new needle system for the MR-guided localization and transcutaneous biopsy of suspicious breast lesions. In vitro studies with 1.0 tesla]. [Article in German] Rofo 1997;166(4):342–345

Helbich TH. Localization and biopsy of breast lesions by magnetic resonance imaging guidance. J Magn Reson Imaging 2001;13(6):903–911

Heywang-Köbrunner SH, Heinig A, Schaumlöffel U, et al. MR-guided percutaneous excisional and incisional biopsy of breast lesions. Eur Radiol 1999;9(8):1656–1665

Heywang-Köbrunner SH, Huynh AT, Viehweg P, Hanke W, Requardt H, Paprosch I. Prototype breast coil for MR-guided needle localization. J Comput Assist Tomogr 1994;18(6):876–881

Heywang-Köbrunner SH. MR-guided localization procedure. In: Heywang-Köbrunner SH, Beck R, eds. Contrast-enhanced MRI of the breast. Berlin: Springer; 1996: 53

Huber S, Wagner M, Medl M, Czembirek H. Benign breast lesions: minimally invasive vacuum-assisted biopsy with 11-gauge needles patient acceptance and effect on follow-up imaging findings. Radiology 2003;226(3):783–790

Kuhl CK, Elevelt A, Leutner CC, Gieseke J, Pakos E, Schild HH. Interventional breast MR imaging: clinical use of a stereotactic localization and biopsy device. Radiology 1997;204(3):667–675

Kuhl CK, Morakkabati N, Leutner CC, Schmiedel A, Wardelmann E, Schild HH. MR imaging–guided large-core (14-gauge) needle biopsy of small lesions visible at breast MR imaging alone. Radiology 2001;220(1):31–39

Lee JM, Kaplan JB, Murray MP, et al. Underestimation of DCIS at MRI-guided vacuum-assisted breast biopsy. AJR Am J Roentgenol 2007;189(2):468–474

Lehman CD, Deperi ER, Peacock S, McDonough MD, Demartini WB, Shook J. Clinical experience with MRI-guided vacuum-assisted breast biopsy. AJR Am J Roentgenol 2005;184(6):1782–1787

Li J, Dershaw DD, Lee CH, Kaplan J, Morris EA. MRI follow-up after concordant, histologically benign diagnosis of breast lesions sampled by MRI-guided biopsy. AJR Am J Roentgenol 2009;193(3):850–855

Liberman L, Bracero N, Morris E, Thornton C, Dershaw DD. MRI-guided 9-gauge vacuum-assisted breast biopsy: initial clinical experience. AJR Am J Roentgenol 2005;185(1):183–193

Liberman L, Bracero N, Vuolo MA, et al. Percutaneous large-core biopsy of papillary breast lesions. AJR Am J Roentgenol 1999;172(2):331–337

Liberman L, Holland AE, Marjan D, et al. Underestimation of atypical ductal hyperplasia at MRI-guided 9-gauge vacuum-assisted breast biopsy. AJR Am J Roentgenol 2007;188(3):684–690

Liberman L, Vuolo M, Dershaw DD, et al. Epithelial displacement after stereotactic 11-gauge directional vacuum-assisted breast biopsy. AJR Am J Roentgenol 1999;172(3):677–681

Morris EA, Liberman L, Dershaw DD, et al. Preoperative MR imaging-guided needle localization of breast lesions. AJR Am J Roentgenol 2002;178(5):1211–1220

Orel SG, Schnall MD, Newman RW, Powell CM, Torosian MH, Rosato EF. MR imaging-guided localization and biopsy of breast lesions: initial experience. Radiology 1994;193(1):97–102

Orel SG, Rosen M, Mies C, Schnall MD. MR imaging-guided 9-gauge vacuum-assisted core-needle breast biopsy: initial experience. Radiology 2006;238(1):54–61

Perlet C, Heywang-Kobrunner SH, Heinig A, et al. Magnetic resonance-guided, vacuum-assisted breast biopsy: results from a European multicenter study of 538 lesions. Cancer 2006;106(5):982–990

Perlet C, Schneider P, Amaya B, et al. MR-guided vacuum biopsy of 206 contrast-enhancing breast lesions. Rofo 2002;174(1):88–95

Rosen EL, Bentley RC, Baker JA, Soo MS. Imaging-guided core needle biopsy of papillary lesions of the breast. AJR Am J Roentgenol 2002;179(5):1185–1192

Schrading S, Simon B, Wardelmann E, et al. MR gesteuerte Vakuumbiopsie der Mamma. Rofo 2007;179:155

Schulz KD, Albert US. Stufe-3-Leitlinie Brustkrebs-Früherkennung in Deutschland. Munich: Zuckschwerdt; 2003

Siegmann KC, Wersebe A, Fischmann A, et al. [Stereotactic vacuum-assisted breast biopsy—success, histologic accuracy, patient acceptance and optimizing the BI-RADSTM-correlated indication]. [Article in German] Rofo 2003;175(1):99–104

Sittek H, Kessler M, Müller-Lisse U, Untch M, Bohmert H, Reiser M. [Technics for the preoperative marking of nonpalpable breast lesions in MRT]. [Article in German] Rofo 1996;165(1):84–87

Tozaki M, Yamashiro N, Suzuki T, et al. MR-guided vacuum-assisted breast biopsy: is it an essential technique? Breast Cancer 2009;16(2):121–125

van den Bosch MA, Daniel BL, Pal S, et al. MRI-guided needle localization of suspicious breast lesions: results of a freehand technique. Eur Radiol 2006;16(8):1811–1817

Viehweg P, Bernerth T, Kiechle M, et al. MR-guided intervention in women with a family history of breast cancer. Eur J Radiol 2006;57(1):81–89

Zuiani C, Mazzarella F, Londero V, Linda A, Puglisi F, Bazzocchi M. Stereotactic vacuum-assisted breast biopsy: results, follow-up and correlation with radiological suspicion. Radiol Med (Torino) 2007;112(2):304–317

Indications for Breast MRI

Abraham DC, Jones RC, Jones SE, et al. Evaluation of neoadjuvant chemotherapeutic response of locally advanced breast cancer by magnetic resonance imaging. Cancer 1996;78(1):91–100

Akazawa K, Tamaki Y, Taguchi T, et al. Preoperative evaluation of residual tumor extent by three-dimensional magnetic resonance imaging in breast cancer patients treated with neoadjuvant chemotherapy. Breast J 2006;12(2):130–137

Bagley FH. The role of magnetic resonance imaging mammography in the surgical management of the index breast cancer. Arch Surg 2004;139(4):380–383, discussion 383

Ballesio L, Maggi C, Savelli S, et al. Role of breast magnetic resonance imaging (MRI) in patients with unilateral nipple discharge: preliminary study. Radiol Med (Torino) 2008;113(2):249–264

Blair S, McElroy M, Middleton MS, et al. The efficacy of breast MRI in predicting breast conservation therapy. J Surg Oncol 2006;94(3):220–225

Bluemke DA, Gatsonis CA, Chen MH, et al. Magnetic resonance imaging of the breast prior to biopsy. JAMA 2004;292(22):2735–2742

Boetes C, Mus RDM, Holland R, et al. Breast tumors: comparative accuracy of MR imaging relative to mammography and US for demonstrating extent. Radiology 1995;197(3):743–747

Boné B, Aspelin P, Isberg B, Perbeck L, Veress B. Contrast-enhanced MR imaging of the breast in patients with breast implants after cancer surgery. Acta Radiol 1995;36(2):111–116

Braun M, Pölcher M, Schrading S, et al. Influence of preoperative MRI on the surgical management of patients with operable breast cancer. Breast Cancer Res Treat 2008;111(1):179–187

Brenner RJ, Rothman BJ. Detection of primary breast cancer in women with known adenocarcinoma metastatic to the axilla: use of MRI after negative clinical and mammographic examination. J Magn Reson Imaging 1997;7(6):1153–1158

Brown J, Buckley D, Coulthard A, et al; UK MRI Breast Screening Study Advisory Group. Magnetic resonance imaging screening in women at genetic risk of breast cancer: imaging and analysis protocol for the UK multicentre study. Magn Reson Imaging 2000;18(7):765–776

Buchberger W, DeKoekkoek-Doll P, Obrist P, Dünser M. [Value of MR tomography in inconclusive mammography findings]. [Article in German] Radiologe 1997;37(9):702–709

Causer PA, Jong RA, Warner E, et al. Breast cancers detected with imaging screening in the BRCA population: emphasis on MR imaging with histopathologic correlation. Radiographics 2007; 27(Suppl 1):S 165–S 182

Chen JH, Feig BA, Hsiang DJ, et al. Impact of MRI-evaluated neoadjuvant chemotherapy response on change of surgical recommendation in breast cancer. Ann Surg 2009;249(3):448–454

Chung A, Saouaf R, Scharre K, Phillips E. The impact of MRI on the treatment of DCIS. Am Surg 2005;71(9):705–710

Cilotti A, Iacconi C, Marini C, et al. Contrast-enhanced MR imaging in patients with BI-RADS 3–5 microcalcifications. Radiol Med (Torino) 2007;112(2):272–286

Crowe JP, Patrick RJ, Rim A. The importance of preoperative breast MRI for patients newly diagnosed with breast cancer. Breast J 2009;15(1):52–60

Dao TH, Rahmouni A, Campana F, Laurent M, Asselain B, Fourquet A. Tumor recurrence versus fibrosis in the irradiated breast: differentiation with dynamic gadolinium-enhanced MR imaging. Radiology 1993;187(3):751–755

Del Frate C, Borghese L, Cedolini C, et al. Role of pre-surgical breast MRI in the management of invasive breast carcinoma. Breast 2007;16(5):469–481

Demartini WB, Lehman CD, Peacock S, Russell MT. Computer-aided detection applied to breast MRI: assessment of CAD-generated enhancement and tumor sizes in breast cancers before and after neoadjuvant chemotherapy. Acad Radiol 2005;12(7):806–814

Diekmann F, Diekmann S, Beljavskaja M, et al. [Preoperative MRT of the breast in invasive lobular carcinoma in comparison with invasive ductal carcinoma]. [Article in German] Rofo 2004;176(4):544–549

Fischer U, Baum F. Trainer Mammadiagnostik. Stuttgart: Thieme; 2005

Fischer U, Kopka L, Grabbe E. Breast carcinoma: effect of preoperative contrast-enhanced MR imaging on the therapeutic approach. Radiology 1999;213(3):881–888

Fischer U, Vosshenrich R, Kopka L, Kahlen O, Grabbe E. [Contrast medium assisted dynamic MR-mammography after diagnostic and therapeutic interventions on the breast]. [Article in German] Bildgebung 1996;63(2):94–100

Fischer U, Vosshenrich R, Probst A, Burchhardt H, Grabbe E. [Preoperative MR-mammography in diagnosed breast carcinoma. Useful information or useless extravagance?]. [Article in German] Rofo 1994;161(4):300–306

Fischer U, Vosshenrich R, von Heyden D, Knipper H, Oestmann JW, Grabbe E. [Inflammatory lesions of the breast: indication for MR-mammography?]. [Article in German] Rofo 1994;161(4):307–311

Fischer U, Westerhof JP, Brinck U, Korabiowska M, Schauer A, Grabbe E. [Ductal carcinoma in situ in dynamic MR-mammography at 1.5 T]. [Article in German] Rofo 1996;164(4):290–294

Fischer U, Zachariae O, Baum F, von Heyden D, Funke M, Liersch T. The influence of preoperative MRI of the breasts on recurrence rate in patients with breast cancer. Eur Radiol 2004;14(10):1725–1731

Gilles R, Guinebretière JM, Lucidarme O, et al. Nonpalpable breast tumors: diagnosis with contrast-enhanced subtraction dynamic MR imaging. Radiology 1994;191(3):625–631

Gilles R, Guinebretière JM, Shapeero LG, et al. Assessment of breast cancer recurrence with contrast-enhanced subtraction MR imaging: preliminary results in 26 patients. Radiology 1993;188(2):473–478

Gilles R, Guinebretière JM, Toussaint C, et al. Locally advanced breast cancer: contrast-enhanced subtraction MR imaging of response to preoperative chemotherapy. Radiology 1994;191(3):633–638

Griebsch I, Brown J, Boggis C, et al; UK Magnetic Resonance Imaging in Breast Screening (MARIBS) Study Group. Cost-effectiveness of screening with contrast enhanced magnetic resonance imaging vs X-ray mammography of women at a high familial risk of breast cancer. Br J Cancer 2006;95(7):801–810

Hamilton LJ, Evans AJ, Wilson AR, et al. Breast imaging findings in women with BRCA1- and BRCA2-associated breast carcinoma. Clin Radiol 2004;59(10):895–902

Hata T, Takahashi H, Watanabe K, et al. Magnetic resonance imaging for preoperative evaluation of breast cancer: a comparative study with mammography and ultrasonography. J Am Coll Surg 2004;198(2):190–197

Heinig A, Heywang-Köbrunner SH, Viehweg P, Lampe D, Buchmann J, Spielmann RP. [Value of contrast medium magnetic resonance tomography of the breast in breast reconstruction with implant]. [Article in German] Radiologe 1997;37(9):710–717

Heywang SH, Hilbertz T, Beck R, Bauer WM, Eiermann W, Permanetter W. Gd-DTPA enhanced MR imaging of the breast in patients with postoperative scarring and silicon implants. J Comput Assist Tomogr 1990;14(3):348–356

Hlawatsch A, Teifke A, Schmidt M, Thelen M. Preoperative assessment of breast cancer: sonography versus MR imaging. AJR Am J Roentgenol 2002;179(6):1493–1501

Knopp MV, Brix G, Junkermann HJ, Sinn HP. MR mammography with pharmacokinetic mapping for monitoring of breast cancer treatment during neoadjuvant therapy. Magn Reson Imaging Clin N Am 1994;2(4):633–658

Krämer S, Schulz-Wendtland R, Hagedorn K, Bautz W, Lang N. Magnetic resonance imaging and its role in the diagnosis of multicentric breast cancer. Anticancer Res 1998;18(3C):2163–2164

Kriege M, Brekelmans CT, Boetes C, et al. MRI screening for breast cancer in women with familial or genetic predisposition: design of the Dutch National Study (MRISC). Fam Cancer 2001;1(3-4):163–168

Kriege M, Brekelmans CT, Boetes C, et al; Magnetic Resonance Imaging Screening Study Group. Efficacy of MRI and mammography for breast-cancer screening in women with a familial or genetic predisposition. N Engl J Med 2004;351(5):427–437

Kriege M, Brekelmans CT, Boetes C, et al; Dutch MRI Screening (MRISC) Study Group. Differences between first and subsequent rounds of the MRISC breast cancer screening program for women with a familial or genetic predisposition. Cancer 2006;106(11):2318–2326

Kronsbein H, Bässler R. Pathomorphologie und Diagnostik sogenannter Hamartome der Mamma. Pathologe 1982;3:310–318

Kuhl CK. High-risk screening: multi-modality surveillance of women at high risk for breast cancer (proven or suspected carriers of a breast cancer susceptibility gene). J Exp Clin Cancer Res 2002; 21(3, Suppl)103–106

Kuhl CK. [Familial breast cancer: what the radiologist needs to know]. [Article in German] Rofo 2006;178(7):680–687

Kuhl CK. Clinical Applications. Current status of breast MR imaging. Part 2. Clinical applications. Radiology 2007;244(3):672–691

Kuhl CK, Braun M. [Magnetic resonance imaging in preoperative staging for breast cancer: pros and contras]. [Article in German] Radiologe 2008;48(4):358–366

Kuhl CK, Kuhn W, Braun M, Schild H. Pre-operative staging of breast cancer with breast MRI: one step forward, two steps back? Breast 2007;16(Suppl 2):S 34–S 44

Kuhl CK, Schmutzler RK, Leutner CC, et al. Breast MR imaging screening in 192 women proved or suspected to be carriers of a breast cancer susceptibility gene: preliminary results. Radiology 2000;215(1):267–279

Kuhl CK, Schrading S, Leutner CC, et al. Mammography, breast ultrasound, and magnetic resonance imaging for surveillance of women at high familial risk for breast cancer. J Clin Oncol 2005;23(33):8469–8476

Kuhl CK, Schrading S, Weigel S, et al. [The "EVA" Trial: Evaluation of the Efficacy of Diagnostic Methods (Mammography, Ultrasound, MRI) in the secondary and tertiary prevention of familial breast cancer. Preliminary results after the first half of the study period]. [Article in German] Rofo 2005;177(6):818–827

Kurtz B, Achten C, Audretsch W, Rezai M, Urban P, Zocholl G. [MR-mammography assessment of tumor response after neoadjuvant radiochemotherapy of locally advanced breast carcinoma]. [Article in German] Rofo 1996;164(6):469–474

Kwong MS, Chung GG, Horvath LJ, et al. Postchemotherapy MRI over-estimates residual disease compared with histopathology in responders to neoadjuvant therapy for locally advanced breast cancer. Cancer J 2006;12(3):212–221

Leach MO, Boggis CR, Dixon AK, et al; MARIBS study group. Screening with magnetic resonance imaging and mammography of a UK population at high familial risk of breast cancer: a prospective multicentre cohort study (MARIBS). Lancet 2005;365(9473): 1769–1778

Lee CH, Smith RC, Levine JA, Troiano RN, Tocino I. Clinical usefulness of MR imaging of the breast in the evaluation of the problematic mammogram. AJR Am J Roentgenol 1999;173(5):1323–1329

Lee JM, Kopans DB, McMahon PM, et al. Breast cancer screening in BRCA1 mutation carriers: effectiveness of MR imaging—Markov Monte Carlo decision analysis. Radiology 2008;246(3):763–771

Lee SG, Orel SG, Woo IJ, et al. MR imaging screening of the contralateral breast in patients with newly diagnosed breast cancer: preliminary results. Radiology 2003;226(3):773–778

Lehman CD, Blume JD, Weatherall P, et al; International Breast MRI Consortium Working Group. Screening women at high risk for breast cancer with mammography and magnetic resonance imaging. Cancer 2005;103(9):1898–1905

Lehman CD, Gatsonis C, Kuhl CK, et al. MRI evaluation of the contralateral breast in women with recently diagnosed breast cancer. N Engl J Med 2007;356(13):1295–1303

Lehman CD, Isaacs C, Schnall MD, et al. Cancer yield of mammography, MR, and US in high-risk women: prospective multi-institution breast cancer screening study. Radiology 2007;244(2):381–388

Liberman L, Morris EA, Benton CL, Abramson AF, Dershaw DD. Probably benign lesions at breast magnetic resonance imaging: preliminary experience in high-risk women. Cancer 2003;98(2): 377–388

Liberman L, Morris EA, Dershaw DD, Abramson AF, Tan LK. MR imaging of the ipsilateral breast in women with percutaneously proven breast cancer. AJR Am J Roentgenol 2003;180(4):901–910

Liberman L, Morris EA, Kim CM, et al. MR imaging findings in the contralateral breast of women with recently diagnosed breast cancer. AJR Am J Roentgenol 2003;180(2):333–341

Lieberman S, Sella T, Maly B, Sosna J, Uziely B, Sklair-Levy M. Breast magnetic resonance imaging characteristics in women with occult primary breast carcinoma. Isr Med Assoc J 2008;10(6):448–452

Mameri CS, Kemp C, Goldman SM, Sobral LA, Ajzen S. Impact of breast MRI on surgical treatment, axillary approach, and systemic therapy for breast cancer. Breast J 2008;14(3):236–244

Moon WK, Noh DY, Im JG. Multifocal, multicentric, and contralateral breast cancers: bilateral whole-breast US in the preoperative evaluation of patients. Radiology 2002;224(2):569–576

Morris EA, Liberman L, Ballon DJ, et al. MRI of occult breast carcinoma in a high-risk population. AJR Am J Roentgenol 2003;181(3): 619–626

Morris EA. Diagnostic breast MR imaging: current status and future directions. Radiol Clin North Am 2007;45(5):863–880, vii

Morris EA, Schwartz LH, Dershaw DD, van Zee KJ, Abramson AF, Liberman L. MR imaging of the breast in patients with occult primary breast carcinoma. Radiology 1997;205(2):437–440

Morrogh M, Morris EA, Liberman L, Van Zee K, Cody HS III, King TA. MRI identifies otherwise occult disease in select patients with Paget disease of the nipple. J Am Coll Surg 2008;206(2):316–321

Müller RD, Barkhausen J, Sauerwein W, Langer R. Assessment of local recurrence after breast-conserving therapy with MRI. J Comput Assist Tomogr 1998;22(3):408–412

Mumtaz H, Davidson T, Hall-Craggs MA, et al. Comparison of magnetic resonance imaging and conventional triple assessment in locally recurrent breast cancer. Br J Surg 1997;84(8):1147–1151

Mumtaz H, Hall-Craggs MA, Davidson T, et al. Staging of symptomatic primary breast cancer with MR imaging. AJR Am J Roentgenol 1997; 169(2):417–424

Obdeijn IM, Kuijpers TJ, van Dijk P, Wiggers T, Oudkerk M. MR lesion detection in a breast cancer population. J Magn Reson Imaging 1996;6(6):849–854

Offodile RS, Daniel BL, Jeffrey SS, Wapnir I, Dirbas FM, Ikeda DM. Magnetic resonance imaging of suspicious breast masses seen on one mammographic view. Breast J 2004;10(5):416–422

Olivas-Maguregui S, Villaseñor-Navarro Y, Ferrari-Carballo T, et al. Importance of the preoperative evaluation of multifocal and multicentric breast cancer with magnetic resonance imaging in women with dense parenchyma. Rev Invest Clin 2008;60(5):382–389

Olson JA Jr, Morris EA, Van Zee KJ, Linehan DC, Borgen PI. Magnetic resonance imaging facilitates breast conservation for occult breast cancer. Ann Surg Oncol 2000;7(6):411–415

Orel SG, Reynolds C, Schnall MD, Solin LJ, Fraker DL, Sullivan DC. Breast carcinoma: MR imaging before re-excisional biopsy. Radiology 1997;205(2):429–436

Orel SG, Schnall MD, Powell CM, et al. Staging of suspected breast cancer: effect of MR imaging and MR-guided biopsy. Radiology 1995;196(1):115–122

Ozaki S, Tozaki M, Fukuma E, et al. Bilateral breast MR imaging: is it superior to conventional methods for the detection of contralateral breast cancer? Breast Cancer 2008;15(2):169–174

Pediconi F, Catalano C, Padula S, et al. Contrast-enhanced magnetic resonance mammography: does it affect surgical decision-making in patients with breast cancer? Breast Cancer Res Treat 2007; 106(1):65–74

Pediconi F, Catalano C, Roselli A, et al. Contrast-enhanced MR mammography for evaluation of the contralateral breast in patients with diagnosed unilateral breast cancer or high-risk lesions. Radiology 2007;243(3):670–680

Pediconi F, Venditti F, Padula S, et al. CE-Magnetic Resonance Mammography for the evaluation of the contralateral breast in patients with diagnosed breast cancer. Radiol Med (Torino) 2005;110(1–2): 61–68

Podo F, Sardanelli F, Canese R, et al. The Italian multi-centre project on evaluation of MRI and other imaging modalities in early detection of breast cancer in subjects at high genetic risk. J Exp Clin Cancer Res 2002; 21(3, Suppl)115–124

Porter BA, Smith JP, Borrow JW. MR-depiction of occult breast cancer in patients with malignant axillary adenopathy. Radiology 1995; 197:130

Prati R, Minami CA, Gornbein JA, Debruhl N, Chung D, Chang HR. Accuracy of clinical evaluation of locally advanced breast cancer in patients receiving neoadjuvant chemotherapy. Cancer 2009; 115(6):1194–1202

Price J, Chen SW. Screening for breast cancer with MRI: recent experience from the Australian Capital Territory. J Med Imaging Radiat Oncol 2009;53(1):69–80

Rieber A, Merkle E, Böhm W, Brambs HJ, Tomczak R. MRI of histologically confirmed mammary carcinoma: clinical relevance of diagnostic procedures for detection of multifocal or contralateral secondary carcinoma. J Comput Assist Tomogr 1997;21(5):773–779

Rieber A, Merkle E, Zeitler H, et al. [Doubtful mammographic findings: the value of negative MR mammography for tumor exclusion]. [Article in German] Rofo 1997;167(4):392–398

Rieber A, Merkle E, Zeitler H, et al. Value of MR mammography in the detection and exclusion of recurrent breast carcinoma. J Comput Assist Tomogr 1997;21(5):780–784

Rieber A, Zeitler H, Rosenthal H, et al. MRI of breast cancer: influence of chemotherapy on sensitivity. Br J Radiol 1997;70(833):452–458

Rodenko GN, Harms SE, Pruneda JM, et al. MR imaging in the management before surgery of lobular carcinoma of the breast: correlation with pathology. AJR Am J Roentgenol 1996;167(6): 1415–1419

Santamaría G, Velasco M, Farrús B, Zanón G, Fernández PL. Preoperative MRI of pure intraductal breast carcinoma—a valuable adjunct to mammography in assessing cancer extent. Breast 2008;17(2): 186–194

Sardanelli F, Giuseppetti GM, Panizza P, et al; Italian Trial for Breast MR in Multifocal/Multicentric Cancer. Sensitivity of MRI versus mammography for detecting foci of multifocal, multicentric breast cancer in fatty and dense breasts using the whole-breast pathologic examination as a gold standard. AJR Am J Roentgenol 2004;183(4): 1149–1157

Sardanelli F, Podo F, D'Agnolo G, et al; High Breast Cancer Risk Italian Trial. Multicenter comparative multimodality surveillance of women at genetic-familial high risk for breast cancer (HIBCRIT study): interim results. Radiology 2007;242(3):698–715

Schelfout K, Van Goethem M, Kersschot E, et al. Contrast-enhanced MR imaging of breast lesions and effect on treatment. Eur J Surg Oncol 2004;30(5):501–507

Schelfout K, Van Goethem M, Kersschot E, et al. Preoperative breast MRI in patients with invasive lobular breast cancer. Eur Radiol 2004;14(7):1209–1216

Schorn C, Fischer U, Luftner-Nagel S, Westerhof JP, Grabbe E. MRI of the breast in patients with metastatic disease of unknown primary. Eur Radiol 1999;9(3):470–473

Schott AF, Roubidoux MA, Helvie MA, et al. Clinical and radiologic assessments to predict breast cancer pathologic complete response to neoadjuvant chemotherapy. Breast Cancer Res Treat 2005; 92(3):231–238

Siegmann KC, Baur A, Vogel U, Kraemer B, Hahn M, Claussen CD. Risk-benefit analysis of preoperative breast MRI in patients with primary breast cancer. Clin Radiol 2009;64(4):403–413

Soderstrom CE, Harms SE, Farrell RS Jr, Pruneda JM, Flamig DP. Detection with MR imaging of residual tumor in the breast soon after surgery. AJR Am J Roentgenol 1997;168(2):485–488

Sperber F, Weinstein Y, Sarid D, Ben Yosef R, Shalmon A, Yaal-Hahoshen N. Preoperative clinical, mammographic and sonographic assessment of neoadjuvant chemotherapy response in breast cancer. Isr Med Assoc J 2006;8(5):342–346

Stoutjesdijk MJ, Boetes C, Jager GJ, et al. Magnetic resonance imaging and mammography in women with a hereditary risk of breast cancer. J Natl Cancer Inst 2001;93(14):1095–1102

Thibault F, Nos C, Meunier M, et al; Institut Curie Breast Cancer Group. MRI for surgical planning in patients with breast cancer who undergo preoperative chemotherapy. AJR Am J Roentgenol 2004; 183(4):1159–1168

Tilanus-Linthorst MM, Obdeijn AI, Bontenbal M, Oudkerk M. MRI in patients with axillary metastases of occult breast carcinoma. Breast Cancer Res Treat 1997;44(2):179–182

Tilanus-Linthorst MM, Obdeijn IM, Bartels KC, de Koning HJ, Oudkerk M. First experiences in screening women at high risk for breast cancer with MR imaging. Breast Cancer Res Treat 2000;63(1):53–60

Van Die LE, Boetes C, Barentsz JO, et al. Additional value of MR imaging of the breast in women with pathologic axillary lymph nodes and normal mammograms. Radiology 1996;201:214

Westerhof JP, Fischer U, Moritz JD, Oestmann JW. MR imaging of mammographically detected clustered microcalcifications: is there any value? Radiology 1998;207(3):675–681

Winnekendonk G, Krug B, Warm M, Göhring UJ, Mallmann P, Lackner K. [Diagnostic value of preoperative contrast-enhanced MR imaging of the breast]. [Article in German] Rofo 2004;176(5):688–693

Quality Control, Current Standing, Problems, and Perspectives of Breast MRI

AG-Mammadiagnostik der DRG. Empfehlungen zur MR-Mammographie. Rofo 2005;177:474–475

AG-Mammadiagnostik der DRG. Empfehlungen zur MR-gesteuerten Interventionen. Rofo 2007;179:429

Kreienberg R, Kopp I, Albert U, et al. Interdisziplinäre S 3-Leitlinie für die Diagnostik, Therapie und Nachsorge des Mammakarzinoms, 1. Aktualisierung 2008. Munich: W. Zuckschwerdt Verlag GmbH; 2008

Kreienberg R, Kopp I, Lorenz W et al. Diagnostik, Therapie und Nachsorge des Mammakarzinoms der Frau. Eine nationale S 3-Leitlinie. Deutsche Krebsgesellschaft e. V. 2008

Kuhl CK. The "coming of age" of nonmammographic screening for breast cancer. JAMA 2008;299(18):2203–2205

Kuhl CK, Weigel S, Schrading S, et al. Prospective multicenter cohort study to refine management recommendations for women at elevated familial risk of breast cancer: the EVA trial. J Clin Oncol 2010;28(9):1450–1457

Mann RM, Kuhl CK, Kinkel K, Boetes C. Breast MRI: guidelines from the European Society of Breast Imaging. Eur Radiol 2008;18(7): 1307–1318

Saslow D, Boetes C, Burke W, et al; American Cancer Society Breast Cancer Advisory Group. American Cancer Society guidelines for breast screening with MRI as an adjunct to mammography. CA Cancer J Clin 2007;57(2):75–89

Smith RA. The evolving role of MRI in the detection and evaluation of breast cancer. N Engl J Med 2007;356(13):1362–1364

Index

Note: page numbers in *italics* refer to figures and tables.

A

abscess 118
  nonpuerperal mastitis 115, *117*
accessory glandular tissue 66
adenoma 82–83, *84–86*
  etiology *82*
  internal septations 83
  lactating 82
  mammography findings *82*
  mass lesions 253
  multiple foci 252
  nipple 82, 86
  solitary focus 251
  T1-weighted sequences 83, *84–86*
  T2-weighted sequences 83, *84–86*
  tubular 82, *85*
  ultrasonography findings *82*
adenomyoepithelioma 102
adenosis 91, 92, *93–95*
  blunt duct 92, *94*
  etiology *92*
  focal 251
  mammography *92*
  mass lesions 253
  microcystic 92
  microglandular 92
  multiple foci 252
  nodular 92, *95*
  nonmasslike lesions 255, *257, 258*
  sclerosing 92, *93, 94*
  ultrasonography *92*
age, breast parenchyma 64
AIM working group *266*
alveolar hyperplasia 91
alveoli 63
American College of Radiology (ARC)
  BI-RADS lexicon 45–46
  see also BI-RADS assessment
androgens, decrease causing
  gynecomastia 213
angiogenesis 33
  in fibrotic scar tissue 229
angiogenetic growth factors 33
angioma, cutaneous *123*
angiomatous hyperplasia, mass
  lesions 253
angiosarcoma 189
apocrine metaplasia 145
architectural distortion, diagnosis 259
areola 63
areolar region, focal enhancement 67
arteriovenous shunts, carcinoma-
  associated 33

artifacts 47–56
  breast implants 55
  cardiac flow 55
  ghosting 61
  out-of-phase imaging 53
  surface coils 56
  susceptibility 54
    cauterization during surgery 130
    hemangioma 100
    scar tissue 130, *131*
  see also error sources; motion artifacts
atypical ductal hyperplasia (ADH) 151, *152*
  flat epithelial atypia *152*
  peripheral papillomatosis with *143, 144*
  radial scar coincidence 145
  risk for breast cancer 151
axial slice orientation 19

B

basic fibroblast growth factor (bFGF) 33
BI-RADS assessment 45–46
  MRI-guided biopsy 264
  quality assurance 263, *264*
biopsy
  MR mammography after 6
  open 6
  stereotactic vacuum-assisted 223, 247
  US-guided core 247
  see also MRI-guided biopsy
blood/bloody fluid, hemorrhagic cysts 108
blooming 42
body building, gynecomastia *215*
BRCA mutations 243, *244*
  male carriers 216
  risk 249
BRCA1 mutation 243, *244*
  triple-negative breast cancer 190
breast
  atypical location of tissues 66
  blood supply 63
  involution 64
  morphology 63
  normal findings 63–74
  size asymmetry 65
  stroma 63
breast augmentation 201
  silicone injection 211, *212*
breast compression 8
  motion artifact reduction 50
breast-conserving therapy
  local recurrence 231
    extensive intraductal component in
      scar tissue 235
  plus radiotherapy 231
  plus radiotherapy/mastectomy 133,
    134–135

R1 resection 136
  recurrence after 137, *138*
    local 231, 235
  second 231
breast implants *see* breast prostheses
breast parenchyma 63
  after mastectomy 133, *135*
  age 64
  alveoli 63
  asymmetry 65–66
    breast-conserving therapy 133, *134*
    enhancement 66
    focal 66
  cysts 103, *104*
  density patterns 69, *70*
  hemangioma 100, *101*
  hormone effects 71, 72
  hormone replacement therapy 72
  hyperemia 118
  interindividual variations 69, *70*
  intraindividual fluctuations 70–71
  lactation 73–74
  lobes 63
  lobules 63, 64
  menstrual cycle effects 70
  pregnancy 73
  residual after mastectomy 133, *135*
  signal intensity 17
  T1-weighted sequences 12
breast prostheses
  artifacts 55
  capsular contracture 206–207
  capsule 205
    fibrosis *207*
  capsulitis 206
  complications 265
    sagittal slice orientation with primary
      fat saturation sequences 19, *20*
  deformation 205, 207
  diagnostic MRI 203–211, *212*
    complications 206–211, *212*
    IR sequences 203–204
    normal findings 205–206
    orientation 203
    SE sequences 204
    swapped phase-encoding gradient *203*
  displacement 206
  double-lumen 205
  folds 206
  implant shell recession 207–208
  incomplete removal 211
  inverse type 205
  MRI follow-up after implantation 247
  periprosthetic capsule 207
  position 205
  prepectoral 205

radial folds 206, *210*
  silicone gel bleeding 207, *208*
reverse double-lumen 205
rupture
  complete 210, *211*
  extracapsular 209–210
  intracapsular 208–209, 210
shape 205, 207
shell 205
silicone gel bleeding 207, *208*
silicone leakage 209–210
single-lumen 205
subglandular 205
subpectoral 205
teardrop sign 207, *208*
breast reconstruction 201
  autologous, diagnostic MRI after 201,
    201–202
  flaps 201, *202*
  MRI follow-up 247
breast surgery
  abscess 118
  cauterization 130
  fat necrosis 125, *126–127*
  focal mastitis *116*
  R1 resection 136
  residual carcinoma 136
  scar tissue 130, *131–132*
  seroma 128

C

calcifications
  fat necrosis 125, *127*
  hemangioma 100, *101*
  medullary carcinoma 175
  periprosthetic with capsular contracture
    206, 207
  plasma cell mastitis 119
  see also microcalcifications
capsular contracture 206–207
  granulomatous inflammation 207
capsulitis, breast prostheses 206
carcinoma of unknown primary (CUP) 232,
  233–234
carcinomas
  adenosis differential diagnosis 92
  architectural distortion 259
  lymph node metastases *198*
  with lymphangioma *43*
  male 216
  mass lesions 253, *254*
  pseudoangiomatous stromal hyperplasia
    differential diagnosis 98
  radial scar 145
  residual after surgery 136
  signal intensity 17
  small 249, *250*
  subcutaneous *43*
  see also named types
cardiac flow artifacts 55
central tubular breast carcinoma, with
  radial scar *148*
certification of MRI 266

chemotherapy, neoadjuvant
  localization clips/coils 225
  MRI monitoring 245, *246*
chest wall, breast carcinoma
  location 237, *238*
chocolate cyst 108
choline peak 31
collagen, scar tissue 130
compression device
  coil-integrated mediolateral 8
  motion artifact reduction 50
computer-aided diagnosis/detection
  (CAD) 28, *29*
  MRM-CAD systems 267, *268*
contraindications to MR mammography 2
contrast-enhanced MRI 10
contrast medium (CM) 3, 5, 23
  improper administration 49
  materials 4
  motion artifacts 49
  paramagnetic 23–24, 33
  reference points 49
  T1-weighted precontrast examination
    34, *35*
  tolerance 23
  underdosage 49
  uptake
    fluctuations in breast parenchyma
      70–71
    by hypervascularized tumors 17
    by nipple 67
  washout phenomenon 17
Cooper's suspensory ligaments 63
coronal slice orientation 19, *20*
cutaneous changes 123, *124*
cystosarcoma phyllodes, malignant 188
cysts 91
  chocolate 108
  complicated 109, *110–111*, 254
    intracystic proliferation 109, *111*
    wall thickening 109, *110*
  hemorrhagic 108–109, *110–111*
  inflamed 105, *106–107*, 254
  intracystic proliferation 153, *154*
  oil 125, *127*
  simple 103, *104*

D

diagnosis/differential diagnosis 251–259
  architectural distortion 259
  foci
    multiple 252
    solitary 251
  mass lesions 253, *254*
  nonmasslike lesions 255, *256–258*
diagnostic criteria 34–46
diagnostic strategies 267
  early breast cancer detection 267–268
diagnostic work-up 249, *249–250*
diffusion-weighted MRI 32
duct ectasia, chronic nonpuerperal mastitis
  119, *120*
duct wall-enhancement, chronic nonpuerperal mastitis 119, *120*

ductal carcinoma in situ (DCIS) 155–163
  adenosis differential diagnosis 92
  classification 155–156, *157–162*
  comedo type 155
  cyst with intracystic proliferation *154*
  enhancement 41
  extensive intraductal component 156,
    162
  with focal invasive tumor component
    235, *237*
  high-grade *154*, 155, *159–161*
  intermediate type 155, *157–159*
  intracystic *154*
  intraductal papillary carcinoma 179
  linear-branching enhancement 156, *160*
  linear enhancement 156
  low-grade *154*, 155, *156, 157*
  masking by motion artifacts *51*, 52
  mass lesions 156, *157, 161*
  microcalcifications 247
  minimal invasion *162*
  MRI sensitivity 163
  multifocality *239*
  multiple foci 252
  non-comedo type 155
  nonmasslike lesions 255, *256, 257, 258*
  Paget disease of the nipple association
    186, *187*
  papilloma progression risk 139
  radial scar association *147, 148*
  solitary focus 251
  stromal fibrosis differential diagnosis 96
  synchronous bilateral *241*
  T1-weighted sequence
    contrast enhanced 155, *156, 157, 158,*
      159, 160, 161, 162
    precontrast 155, *156, 157, 158, 160, 161*
  T2-weighted sequence 155, *156, 157, 158*
  transformation from atypical ductal hy-
    perplasia 151
ductal dilatation, nonpuerperal mastitis
  115, *117*
ductal hyperplasia 91
  see also atypical ductal hyperplasia (ADH)
ductal intraepithelial neoplasia (DIN) 155
dynamic enhancement characteristics
  41–44
  initial signal increase 41–42

E

early breast cancer detection 249–250
  diagnostics 267–268
echo time (TE) 4, 14, *15*
  out-of-phase imaging 53
edema, peritumoral *43*
epitheliosis 91
error sources 47–48
  contrast medium improper administra-
    tion 49
  inadequate windowing 60
  incorrect pixel shifting 59
  incorrect positioning 47, *48*
  incorrect region of interest 58
  inhomogeneous fat suppression 62

inhomogeneous silicone suppression 62
insufficient spatial resolution 58, *59*
substandard process 59
see also artifacts
estrogens, gynecomastia 213
evaluation protocols 44–46
examination of patient 2
protocol 30
timing 5
unestablished techniques 31–32
examination tables 268
extensive intraductal component (EIC)
ductal carcinoma in situ 156, *162*
invasive ductal carcinoma 165, *168*
preoperative local staging 235, *236–237*

F

fast low-angle shot (FLASH) sequences 1
fat necrosis 125, *126–127*
fat saturation
T2-weighed sequences 16
see also primary fat saturation sequences
fat suppression
inhomogeneous 62
lipomas 90
primary 12, *13*
fibroadenolipoma 112
fibroadenoma 75–76, *77*, *78–79*, *80*, 81
etiology 75
fibrotic 75, 76, *78*, *79*, *80*
T1-weighted sequences 78–79, *80*
giant 79, 81
halo sign 76, *77*
intracanalicular 75
with invasive ductal carcinoma *168*
juvenile 79, 81
malignant phyllodes tumor differential
diagnosis 188
mammography findings *75*
mass lesions 253, *254*
multiple foci 252
pericanalicular 75
phyllodes 87, *88–89*
solitary focus 251
T1-weighted sequences 76, *77*, *78*, 79
T2-weighted sequences 76, *77*, *78*
ultrasonography findings *75*
see also myxoid fibroadenomas
fibroblast growth factor, basic (bFGF) 33
fibrocystic breast condition/change 91
fibrosis
breast prosthesis capsule *207*
mass lesions 253
nephrogenic systemic 24
stromal 91, 96, *97*
fibrous histiocytoma, malignant 189
field of view (FOV) 10, 18
coronal slice orientation 19, *20*
field strength 9
fine-needle aspiration
hematoma *129*
seroma *128*
fine-needle biopsy, MR mammography
after 6

flat epithelial atypia (FEA) *152*
flip angle 10
foci 37
adenomyoepithelioma 102
multiple 252
solitary 251
Fourier transform 11
frequency-encoding gradient 55

G

gadolinium-DTPA 23, 33
during lactation/pregnancy 24
renal insufficiency 24
underdosage 49
galactocele 74
galactography 6
galactophoritis 74, 119
gelatinous carcinoma *see* mucinous
carcinoma
ghosting 61
Göttingen Optipack 249, *250*, 265
Göttingen score 44, *45*, *46*
mass lesions 253
MRI BI-RADS comparison 46
nonmasslike lesions 255
gradient-echo (GE) sequences 3, 4, 14
granuloma, mass lesions 253
granulomatous mastitis
lobular 119
scar tissue *131*
growth factors, angiogenetic 33
gynecomastia 213, *214* 215
male breast cancer differential
diagnosis 216
pathological 213, *214–215*
physiological 213
T1-weighted sequence 213, *214–215*

H

halo sign 76, *77*
adenomas 83
hamartoma *112*
malignant phyllodes tumor 188
simple cysts 103, *104*
hamartoma 112, *113–114*
glandular component 112, *113*
lipomatous component 112, *114*
malignant phyllodes tumor differential
diagnosis 188
mass lesions 253
organoid internal structures 112, *113*,
114
pseudocapsular demarcation 112, *113*
hemangioma 100, *101*
hematogenous metastases 232
hematoma 129
hemorrhage, intramammary 129
hemosiderin precipitation, hematoma *129*
hereditary breast cancers 243, *244*
histiocytoma, fibrous malignant 189
hormonal stimulation
gynecomastia 213
limitations of MRI 266

nonmasslike lesions 255, *258*
hormone levels
breast parenchyma uptake of contrast
medium 71, 72
examination timing 5
fibrocystic breast conditions 91
lactation/pregnancy 192
hormone replacement therapy (HRT) 5
breast parenchyma 72

I

image
quality 266
reconstruction 11
volume 18
image-based reconstruction after Fourier
transform 11
image postprocessing 25, *26*, 27
automated 28, *29*
pixel shifting 59
image subtraction 25
T1-weighted sequences 12
implant shell recession 207–208
in-phase imaging 14, *15*
indications for breast MRI 229–250
carcinoma of unknown primary 232,
233–234
early detection 249–250
follow-up after breast reconstruction
with prosthesis implant 247
increased breast cancer risk 243, *244*
monitoring during neoadjuvant chemotherapy 245, *246*
preoperative local staging 235, *236*,
237–238, *239*, 240, *241*, *242*
problem cases 247, *248*
indurative mastopathy 145
infiltrating duct carcinoma, poorly
infiltrating 184
inflammation
capsulitis with breast prostheses 206
cysts 105, *106–107*
fat necrosis 125, *127*
granulomatous 130, *131–132*, 207
scar tissue 130, *131*, *132*
inflammatory breast cancer 184, *185*
information for patient 2
initial signal increase 41–42
intercostal artery 63
internal septations 39
adenomas 83
complicated cysts *109*
dark *39*, *77*, *78*, 79
enhancing *39*
hypervascularized 38–39
myxoid fibroadenomas 16, 36, 38–39
simple cysts 103
intracystic papillary carcinoma 179
intracystic papilloma *111*
intracystic septations, simple cysts 103
intraductal carcinoma *see* ductal carcinoma in situ (DCIS)
intraductal papillary carcinoma 179

intraductal tumors, adenosis differential diagnosis 92
invasive ductal carcinoma (IDC) 165, *166–169*
  contralateral to tubular carcinoma *183*
  definition 165
  extensive intraductal component 165, *168*
  with fibroadenoma *168*
  with high water content 165, *169*
  lymph node metastases *234*
    locoregional *233*
  male *216*
  mammographically occult *250*
  MRI influence on therapeutic strategy *242*
  MRI monitoring during neoadjuvant chemotherapy *246*
  MRI resolution of problem case *248*
  MRI sensitivity 194
  multicentricity *241*
  multiple foci *239*, 252
  pectoral muscle infiltration *237*
  peritumoral edema 165, *166, 167*
  recurrence *230*
  with rim-enhancement 165, *169*
  solitary focus *251*
  synchronous bilateral *241*
  T1-weighted sequence
    contrast enhanced 165, *166–169*
    precontrast 165, *166–167*
  T2-weighted sequence 165, *166–167, 169*
  time-signal intensity analysis 165, *167–168*
  triple-negative breast cancer *190, 191*
invasive lobular carcinoma (ILC) 170, *171–174*
  definition 170
  diffuse 170, *171–173*
  MRI influence on therapeutic strategy 240, 242
  MRI sensitivity 194
  multifocality *239*
  nodular 170, *173–174*
  nonmasslike lesions 255, *257, 258*
  papillomatosis with 144
  pectoral muscle infiltration *237*
  peritumoral edema 170, *173*
  recurrence *230*
  synchronous bilateral 240
  T1-weighted sequence
    contrast enhanced 170, *171–172, 174*
    precontrast 170, *171–172, 173–174*
  T2-weighted sequence 170, *173, 174*
  ultrasound 194
invasive papillary carcinoma 179, *180–181*
  differential diagnosis 179
  papilloma progression risk 139
  T1-weighted sequence 179, *180–181*
  T2-weighted sequence 179, *180–181*
invasive tubular carcinoma, MRI-guided vacuum-assisted biopsy *222*

inversion recovery (IR) sequence
  breast prosthesis diagnostic MRI 203–204
  silicone-sensitive/-suppressed 210
iris diaphragm phenomenon 42

K

k-space-based reconstruction before Fourier transform 11

L

lactation
  breast carcinoma 192, *192–193*
  breast parenchyma 73–74
  gadolinium-DTPA 24
  hormone levels 192
  mammary duct dilatation 74
  puerperal mastitis 115
lactiferous sinuses, subareolar 63
large-core biopsy, MR mammography after 6
Larmor frequency 3
latissimus dorsi myocutaneous flap technique 201
lesions
  detection time frame 17
  malignant and associated findings 43, *43–44*
  see also foci; masses/mass lesions; nonmasslike lesions
linguine sign 209, *210*
lipofibroadenoma 112
lipomas 90
lipomastia 213, *215*
lipomatous tissue
  scar tissue 130
  tumor recurrence 137, *138*
liponecrosis microcystica calcificata 125
lobular carcinoma in situ (LCIS) 149, *150*
  classification 149
  radial scar coincidence 145
lobular carcinoma, invasive 96
lobular hyperplasia 91
lobular intra-epithelial neoplasia (LIN) *222*
lobuli
  multiple foci 252
  solitary focus 251
local recurrence
  detection 231
  extensive intraductal component in scar tissue 235
  scar tissue
    differentiation 229, *230*, 231
    extensive intraductal component 235
localization clips/coils 225, *226*
localization wires 225
lumpectomy, MR mammography after 6
lymph nodes
  axillary *197, 198*
    metastases 232, *234*, 240
    diagnostics 195, *196–200*
    fatty hilus 195, *196, 198*
    inflammatory changes 195, *196, 198*

  intramammary *197, 199*
    mass lesions 253
    solitary focus 251
  locations 195, *196–197, 199*
  mass lesions 195, *196*, 253
  metastases 195, *198, 199, 200*
    carcinoma of unknown primary 232, *233, 234*
    with inflammatory breast cancer *185*
    staging 240
  morphology 195, *198, 200*
  normal *196, 199*
  parasternal 195, *199, 200*
  reactive hyperplasia *199*
  rim-enhancement *196*
  size 195, *198, 200*
  T1-weighted sequence
    contrast enhanced 195, *196–197*
    precontrast 195, *196*
  T2-weighted sequence 195, *196, 198*
lymphadenopathy *44*
lymphangioma *43*
lymphogenous spread 195
  breast carcinoma during pregnancy *192*

M

macrocalcifications *see* calcifications
magnetic resonance elastography (MRE) 31
magnetic resonance imaging (MRI)
  BI-RADS 3 lesions 263
  BI-RADS 4/5 lesions *264*
  certification 266
  cost reduction 267
  density patterns 69, *70*
  detection rate 250
  diagnostic
    after autologous breast reconstruction 201, *202*
    breast prostheses 203–211, *212*
  examination modification 267
  examination tables 268
  findings detection/characterization *268*
  historical aspects 1
  indications 265
  invasive ductal/lobular carcinoma sensitivity 194
  limitations 266
  malignant changes 194
  men 213, *214–215*, 216
  methods *261*, 267, *268*
  minimum requirements for examination 261
  principles 3–4
  quality check 262
  screening approach *268*
  specificity 265
  technique *261*, 265
  value 265
magnetic resonance spectroscopy (MRS) 31
magnetization transfer (MT) 12
male breast cancer 216

malignancy
  BI-RADS risk assessment 45, *46*
  characteristics of male breast cancer 216
  radial scar coincidence 145
  scar tissue differential diagnosis 130
  vascularized 229
malignant change 165–194
  breast carcinoma during pregnancy/
    lactation 192, *192–193*
  inflammatory breast cancer 184, *185*
  invasive ductal carcinoma 165, *166–169*
  invasive lobular carcinoma *144*, 170,
    171–174
  invasive papillary carcinoma 179,
    180–181
    papilloma progression risk 139
  medullary carcinoma 175, *176*
  MRI 194
  mucinous carcinoma 177, *178*
  phyllodes tumor 188
  sarcoma 189
  triple-negative breast cancer 190,
    190–191
  tubular carcinoma 182, *183*
  ultrasound 194
malignant fibrous histiocytoma 189
malignant lesions, associated findings 43,
  43–44
malignant phyllodes tumor 188
mammary ducts 64
  dilatation in lactation 74
mammary dysplasia 91
mammary papilla *see* nipple
mammographically occult tumors 250
masses/mass lesions 37–39
  adenomyoepithelioma 102
  diagnosis 253, *254*
  differential diagnosis *253–254*
  endotumoral changes *254*
  enhancement pattern 38–39
  Göttingen score *45, 46*, 253
  granuloma 253
  margins 38
  motion artifacts *50*
  pseudoangiomatous stromal hyperplasia
    98, *99*
  shape 38
  stromal fibrosis differential diagnosis
    96, *97*
masslike enhancement, breast parenchyma uptake of contrast medium 71
mastectomy
  breast parenchyma 133, *135*
  recurrence after 137, *138*
  residual parenchyma 133, *135*
mastitis
  acute 115
  granulomatous
    lobular 119
    scar tissue *131*
  inflamed cysts *107*
  lobular 119
  nonmasslike lesions 255, *256, 257, 258*
  nonpuerperal 115, *116–117*
    chronic 119, *120*
    diffuse *117*

inflammatory carcinoma differential
    diagnosis 184
  nonmasslike lesions *258*
  plasma cell 119
  puerperal 115
    abscess 118
matrix 18
maximum intensity projection (MIP)
  technique 19, *20*, 27
  motion artifact 51
medullary carcinoma 175, *176*
  atypical 175
  T1-weighted sequence
    contrast enhanced 175, *176*
    precontrast 175, *176*
  T2-weighted sequence 175, *176*
men
  breast MRI 213, *214–215*, 216
  male breast cancer 216
menstrual cycle
  breast parenchyma uptake of contrast
    medium 70
  examination timing 5
  fibrocystic breast conditions 91
metal clips, susceptibility artifacts 54
metastases
  breast skin 137
  carcinoma of unknown primary
    syndrome 232, *233–234*
  hematogenous 232
  intramammary 252
  locoregional 232
  lymph nodes 195, *198, 199, 200*
    carcinoma of unknown primary 232,
      233, 234
    with inflammatory breast cancer *185*
    staging 240
microcalcifications
  ambiguous 249
  atypical ductal hyperplasia *151*
  ductal carcinoma in situ 247
  lobular carcinoma in situ 149
  radial scar *145*
  suspicious 249
  tubular carcinoma 182
microcysts *104*
mixed tubular carcinoma 182
Mondor disease 121, *122*
Montgomery gland, inflamed 67
Morgagni's tubercles 63
motion artifacts 8, 49, 50–52
  classification 51–52
  corrective measures 52
  documentation 51–52
  false-positive/-negative 51, *52*
  ghosting *61*
  limitations of MRI 266
  pectoral muscle infiltration 237, *238*
  postprocessing 59
  subtraction images 51
MRI-guided biopsy 1, 217
  biopsy and localization grid 217, *218*
  classification of pathological
    findings *221*
  computer-aided calculation of puncture
    coordinates 217

equipment 217, *218*
  large-core 219, *220*
  open 264
  percutaneous *221*
  post-and-pillar targeting equipment
    217, *218*
  vacuum-assisted
    checklist *223*
    diagnostic 219, *220–221, 222–223*
    equipment 219, *220*
    follow-up examination 222
    good practice recommendations 219
    hematoma *129*
    histological verification of findings 242
    indications 219
    mass lesion *222*
    objectives 219
    postbiopsy check 222
    quality assurance 263, *264*
    scar tissue 130, *131, 132*
    study results 223
    therapeutic 224
MRI-guided interventions 217–228
  equipment 217
  localization 225, *226–228*
    checklist *228*
    direct 225
    equipment 225, *225–226*
    procedure *227, 228*
    target volume 225
  procedures 217
  surface coils 217, *218*
MRM-CAD systems 267, *268*
mucinous carcinoma 177, *178*
multicentricity 238, 240, *241*
multifactorial evaluation protocols 44
multiplanar reconstruction (MPR) 27
myxoid fibroadenomas 75
  benign phyllodes tumor differential
    diagnosis 87
  internal septations 16, 36, 38–39, 77,
    78, 79
  T1-weighted sequences 76, 77, 78
  T2-weighed sequences 16
  T2-weighted sequences 76, 77

N

N-staging 240
needles, broken parts 54
neonatal gynecomastia 213
nephrogenic systemic fibrosis 24
nevus, skin *124*
nipple
  adenoma 82, 86
  creviced unilateral/bilateral 68
  form variants 68
  incorrect positioning *48*
  inverted 68
  Paget disease 186, *187*
  papillary adenoma 139
  physiological enhancement 67
  retraction *43*
  thickening *43*
  unilateral enhancement 68

nonmasslike enhancement 40–41
  asymmetry 41
  distribution 40
  internal enhancement characteristics/
    pattern 41
  motion artifacts 51
  nonpuerperal mastitis 115, *116*
  pseudoangiomatous stromal hyperplasia
    98, *99*
  symmetry 41
  tumor recurrence *138*
nonmasslike lesions
  diagnosis 255, *256–258*
  differential diagnosis *256–257*
  diffuse unilateral/bilateral enhancement
    258
  ductal enhancement 255
  Göttingen score 255
  interstitial enhancement 255
  linear-branching enhancement *256*
  linear enhancement *256*
  regional enhancement *257*
  segmental enhancement *257*
nutritional supply to tumors 33

O

occult inflammatory breast cancer (OIBC)
  184, *185*
oil cysts 125, *127*
open breast coils *4*, 5, 217, *265*
out-of-phase imaging 14, *15*, 53
ovarian carcinoma risk 243, *244*

P

Paget cells 186
Paget disease of nipple 186, *187*
pain, breast 5
papillary adenoma of the nipple 139
papilloma 139, *140–144*
  benign 139
  classification 139
  etiology *140*
  galactography *140*
  intraductal
    large solitary 139, *141*
    peripheral 139, *142–144*
    small solitary 139, *140, 141*
  mammography *140*
  mass lesions 253
  MRI-guided vacuum-assisted therapeutic
    biopsy 224
  multiple foci 252
  solitary focus 251
  solitary intraductal 139
  solitary retromamillary *141*
  transformation risk 139, *140*
  ultrasonography *140*
papillomatosis 91, 139
  classification 139
  hypervascularization *144*
  with invasive lobular carcinoma *144*
  juvenile 139
  linear *142*

nonmasslike lesions 255, *256, 257*
  peripheral
    with ADH *143, 144*
    regional *143*
    segmental *142*
parallel imaging 11
paramagnetic substances 23–24, 33
patient(s)
  movements during examination 50
  preparation 2
patient positioning 7
  examination tables 268
  incorrect 47, *48*
  lateral displacement *47*
  supine *48*
pectoral fascia 63
pectoral muscle 63
  relaxation causing motion artifact *50*
  tumor infiltration *44*
pectoral muscle infiltration
  motion artifacts 237, *238*
  preoperative local staging 235, 237, *238*
perimamillary enhancement, atypical 67
phase-encoding gradient 21, *22*, 55
phyllodes tumor
  benign 87, *88–89*, 188
    bifocal *89*
  malignant 188
  mass lesions 253
  solitary focus 251
pixels, incorrect shifting/negative 59
port systems, susceptibility artifacts 54
portacaths, susceptibility artifacts 54
postinitial signal course 42
precessional frequency 3
pregnancy
  breast carcinoma 192
  breast parenchyma 73
  gadolinium-DTPA 24
  hormone levels 192
preoperative local staging 235, *236*,
  237–238, 239, 240, *241*, 242
  extensive intraductal component 235,
    236–237
  false-positive findings 242
  MRI influence on therapeutic strategy
    240, 242
  multicentricity 238, *240, 241*
  multifocality 238, *239*
  N-staging 240
  pectoral muscle infiltration 235, 237, *238*
  reliability 242
  strategies 242
  synchronous bilateral breast cancer
    240, *241*
  therapy-relevant information 240, 242
  tumor size 235
primary fat saturation sequences
  sagittal slice orientation 19, *20*
  T1-weighted sequences 12, *13*
prosthesis expanders, metal plates causing
  susceptibility artifacts 54
pseudoangiomatous stromal hyperplasia
  (PASH) 98, *99*
pseudogynecomastia 213, *215*

pseudopapillary lesions, papilloma
  differential diagnosis 139
pubertal gynecomastia 213
pulse sequences 3

Q

quality assurance 261–264
  minimum requirements for MRI
    examination 261
  MRI-guided vacuum-assisted biopsy
    263, *264*
  quality check 262
  special cases 263–264
  written reports 262, *263*

R

R1 resection 136
radial scar 92, 145, *146–148*
  architectural distortion 259
  classification 145
  DCIS association *147, 148*
  MRI-guided vacuum-assisted biopsy *222*
  tubular carcinoma 182
    central *148*
radial sclerosing lesion 145
radiofrequency (RF) excitation 3
radiofrequency (RF) pulse 4
radiotherapy
  adjuvant with breast cancer surgery 231
  breast-conserving therapy 133, *134–135*,
    231
  MR mammography after 6
  nonmasslike lesions *258*
  skin thickening 133, *134*
  vascularization of breast *134*
recanalization, Mondor disease 121, *122*
receiver coils, quality assurance test *56*
recurrence
  after breast-conserving therapy 137, *138*
  after mastectomy 137, *138*
  detection 231
  lipomatous tissue 137, *138*
  scar tissue differential diagnosis 130
  see also local recurrence
reduction mammoplasty 201
region of interest (ROI) 25, *26*
  automatically defined 28
  contrast-enhancing 41
  incorrect 57
relaxation time 3
renal insufficiency, gadolinium-DTPA 24
repetition time (TR) 10
resection, R1 136
retraction phenomenon *248*
rim enhancement 38, 39
  complicated cysts *109*
  fat necrosis *126, 127*
  inflamed cysts 105, *106*
  intraductal papilloma 139
risk, increased 243, *244*
RODEO (rotating delivery of excitation off-
  resonance) sequence 12

S

sagittal slice orientation 19, *20*
salad-oil sign 209
saline, inadequate flushing 49
sandwich protocol 21, *22*
sarcoma 189
scar tissue 130, *131–132*
  hyperemia 137
  local recurrence
    differentiation 229, *230,* 231
    extensive intraductal component 235
  postoperative 259
  tumor angiogenesis 229
  vascularization *132*
sclerosing adenosis 145
sclerosing papillary proliferation 145
screening approach *268*
sedimentation, hemorrhagic cysts 108
segmentectomy, recurrence after *138*
senescent gynecomastia 213
seroma 128
serratus muscle, anterior 63
shear stiffness of lesions 31
shrinking sign *248*
signal intensity
  breast parenchyma 17
  carcinomas 17
  homogeneity assessment 56
  initial increase 41–42
  kinetic pattern 42
  postinitial course 42
  sufficiency assessment 56
silicone
  bleeding of gel 207, *208*
  free 211, *212*
  inhomogeneous suppression 62
  injection into breast material 211, *212*
  leakage 209–210
  resonant frequency 203–204
siliconoma 211
skin, breast 63
  changes 123, *124*
  inflammatory carcinoma 184
  metastases 137
  Paget disease of the nipple 186
  retraction *43*
  thickening after radiotherapy 133, *134*
slice images, subtraction 36
slice orientation 19, *20*
slice thickness 18
snow-peak effect *51*
sources of error *see* error sources
spatial encoding 3
spatial resolution 1, 18
  insufficient 58, *59*
  surface coils 4
spin-echo (SE) sequences 3, 4
  breast prostheses diagnostic MRI 204
  T2-weighed 16
sponge attachment, ultrasound-visible for
  localization clips/coils 225, *226*
sternal wire cerclages, susceptibility
  artifacts 54
stromal fibrosis 91, 96, *97*

stromal hyperplasia, pseudoangiomatous
  98, *99*
subareolar lactiferous sinuses 63
subcutaneous lipoma 90
subscapular artery 63
subtraction images 25, *26,* 27
  inadequate technique *58*
  motion artifacts 51, 52
  substandard process 59
subtraction slice images 36
surface coils 4–5
  artifacts 56
  magnetic resonance elastography 31
  MRI-compatible 217, *218*
  open breast *4,* 5, 217, *265*
swapping of phase-encoding gradient
  21, *22*

T

T1 relaxation time 3, 4
T1-weighted sequences 12, *13*
  contrast-enhanced examination 36–46
  dynamic enhancement characteristics
    41–44
  juvenile fibroadenoma 81
  lesion types 37–41
  precontrast examination 34, *35*
T2 relaxation time 3, 4
T2-weighted sequences 16
  assessment 36
  before dynamic examination 47
  water-sensitive 16
teardrop sign 207, *208*
temporal resolution 17
therapeutic strategy 267
  MRI influence in preoperative local
    staging 240, 242
thoracic arteries, internal/lateral 63
thoracoacromial artery 63
thoracodorsal artery 63
thoracoepigastric flap technique 201
three-dimensional (3D) techniques 3, 10
thrombophlebitis 121
time-signal intensity curve (TIC) 21
  analysis of enhancing lesions 25, *26*
  computer-aided diagnosis 28
  contrast-enhancing ROI 41
track phenomenon 119, *120*
TRAM (transverse rectus abdominis myocutaneous) flap technique 201, *202*
transmitters, quality assurance test *56*
triple-negative breast cancer 190, *190–191*
  hereditary *244*
  pectoral muscle infiltration *238*
  rim-enhancement 190, *191*
tubular carcinoma 182, *183,* 259
  central with radial scar *148*
  invasive *222*
tubulosaccular secretory units 63
tumor angiogenesis 33
tumors
  contrast enhancement 33
  intraductal 92
  mammographically occult 250

MRI-guided localization 225, *226–228*
nutritional supply 33
perfusion increase 33
size and slice thickness 18
see also named types
turbo spin-echo (TSE) sequences,
  T2-weighted 16
two-dimensional (2D) techniques 3, 10

U

ultrasound (US)
  adenomas *82*
  adenosis *92*
  benign phyllodes tumor *87*
  detection rate 250
  fibroadenoma *75*
  invasive ductal carcinoma
    sensitivity 194
  invasive lobular carcinoma
    sensitivity 194
  malignant change 194
  papilloma *140*
  problem cases 247
  second-look 249, *250*
ultrasound-visible sponge attachment for
  localization clips/coils 225, *226*

V

vascular endothelial growth factor
  (VEGF) 33
vein ectasia, Mondor disease 121
viscoelastic property of tissue 31

W

wall enhancement 38
  ductal in chronic nonpuerperal mastitis
    119, *120*
washout phenomenon 17, *23*
  angiogenetic processes 33
water-sensitive T2w images 16
windowing, inadequate 60
wound healing, scar tissue 130, *131*
written reports 262, *263*

X

x-ray mammography
  detection rate 250
  malignant change sensitivity compared
    with MRI/US 194
  problem cases 247, *248*

Z

zebra protocol 21, *22*